ETHICAL AND LEGAL ISSUES
FOR DOCTORAL NURSING STUDENTS

HOW TO ORDER THIS BOOK

BY PHONE: 877-500-4337 or 717-290-1660, 9AM–5PM Eastern Time

BY FAX: 717-509-6100

BY MAIL: Order Department
DEStech Publications, Inc.
439 North Duke Street
Lancaster, PA 17602, U.S.A.

BY CREDIT CARD: American Express, VISA, MasterCard, Discover

BY WWW SITE: http://www.destechpub.com

SECOND EDITION

ETHICAL *and* LEGAL ISSUES *for* DOCTORAL NURSING STUDENTS

A Textbook for Students and Reference for Nurse Leaders

Edited by

Anne G. Peirce, RN, PhD
Professor (Retired)
Adelphi University College of Nursing and Public Health

Jennifer A. Smith, RN, MBA, MPH, DNP
Senior Associate Dean (Retired)
Columbia University School of Nursing

DES*tech* Publications, Inc.

Ethical and Legal Issues for Doctoral Nursing Students

DEStech Publications, Inc.
439 North Duke Street
Lancaster, Pennsylvania 17602 U.S.A.

Printed in the United States of America
10   9   8   7   6   5   4   3   2   1

Main entry under title:
   Ethical and Legal Issues for Doctoral Nursing Students: A Textbook for
   Students and Reference for Nurse Leaders, Second Edition

A DEStech Publications book
Bibliography: p.
Includes index p. 357

Library of Congress Catalog Card No. 2019953330
ISBN No. 978-1-60595-596-4

To our husbands,
Nathaniel W. Peirce, EdD
and
Daniel H. Smith, MD
for their constant support and encouragement.

Contents

Preface to the Second Edition

We are delighted to offer a second edition of Ethical and Legal Issues for Doctoral Nursing Students. Since we first wrote this book, health care has become even more complex; presenting nurses with never ending and never imagined ethical challenges. Some of the challenges come from the attempts to contain spiraling costs, often by reducing nursing staff. The public often forgets that hospitals only exist because of the need for 24-hour nursing care. All other functions can be done on outpatient status; from surgery to physical therapy. When hospitals attempt to place manufacturing cost-saving strategies on the care of patients, care suffers. There is no manufactured product in health care, no two patients are the same and if there is profit, it means that either patients are not receiving the care they need or there is overcharging and perhaps fraud.

Other ethical challenges are a result of the increasing use of technology to augment and sometimes to replace human activity. As I write this preface the news is reporting on how robotic remote telehealth technology was used to report a hospitalized patient's terminal status to the patient and his family. According to the hospital system spokesperson "technology is an appropriate enhancement to the care team…" (as reported by Samuel Braslow in LA Magazine, March 11, 2019). While later denials were issued and the circumstances clarified, the situation reported may herald the future unless nurses step in and object to the reduction of common decency and emphasize the role humanity plays in health care. This situation arose because of money-saving attempts. The hospital is located in a heavily populated area, close to major cities and health centers, but rather than have the appropriate staff available, in this case physicians, the system shares specialists remotely, leaving patients vulnerable, but saving dollars.

The biggest ethical challenges may still be ahead of us as artificial intelligence, Big Data, algorithms and supercomputing are fundamentally altering our world. All professions are struggling to keep up with what this new world order means for health care. It is undeniable that there are many benefits to these technologies, but there are also profound downsides which are not often considered. I recently attended a nursing conference where the director of the IT department in a large hospital system was reviewing their upcoming technology. He ended the presentation by describing the hospital system's desire to implant RFID/ geolocating chips in patients in order to monitor activities. I stood up to voice my concerns (re: horror) at what he was proposing, citing privacy, autonomy and other issues. He countered that he had considered all the HIPAA issues, completely failing in my mind to consider the underlying ethical issues. It was interesting to me that mine was the only voice registering concerns and in fact, rather than arguing that what I purported was wrong, I was told by more than one nurse to sit down and be quiet.

As a result of our seminal role in hospital and health care functions, it is critical that nurses not be complacent about our future role in ethical discussions. Our book has been updated to reflect the changes facing nurses since 2013. First, we have brought our references up to date, including the new 2015 ANA ethical standards. We have also added the 2018 changes to the Common Rule and how they influence nursing research. Each of the clinically focused chapters has been updated to reflect specialty specific changes as well. Finally both the business and legal chapters have been updated to reflect the changes since 2013.

We hope that this book inspires advanced practice and doctoraly prepared nurses to be the voice that patients so desperately need today. For if we don't speak for patients who will?

ANNE G. PEIRCE, RN, PhD
JENNIFER A. SMITH, RN, MBA, MPH, DNP

Preface to the First Edition

Advanced practice nurses and researchers prepared at the doctoral level must be equipped with specialized knowledge and skills in all aspects of medical, research, legal and business ethics relevant to evidence-based practice and research in underserved and other populations. The editors of this text realized the need for such content after completing an article together in 2008 for the *Journal of Professional Nursing,* "The ethics curriculum for doctor of nursing practice programs" (24(5): September–October, 270–274).

Traditional bioethics content often does not address these issues and therefore there is need for an expanded view of required ethics content in the curriculum of Doctor of Nursing Practice (DNP) and PhD programs nationwide. Thus, we have edited this new textbook, *Ethical and Legal Issues for Doctoral Nursing Students: A Textbook for Students and Reference for Nurse Leaders.* In today's healthcare workplace, whether in practice, academia or in research settings, doctoral nursing students and faculty may face the following ethical dilemmas:

- Determining that a bodega (Spanish market) owner was selling unprescribed antibiotics over the counter
- Voting, as part of a committee, on whether a noncompliant patient deserved a second liver transplant
- Being asked by a collaborating physician to collect clinical information before IRB and HIPAA forms were completed
- Having to care for a child who was declared dead but whose parents refused to allow the ventilator to be shut down
- Deciding how to handle a suspected case of billing irregularity

These examples demonstrate that the rapidly expanding scope of advanced practice requires doctorally prepared-advanced practice nurses and nurse researchers to make more complex ethical decisions, often without the necessary background to do so competently and comfortably. This curricular gap can have serious consequences in access, quality and patient safety and can also mean that nurses may not be able to fully contribute to the ethical decision-making process. DNP and PhD graduates must understand how the legal definition of death, assisted suicide and euthanasia may affect medication prescription and decisions about site of care. DNPs and PhDs must fully comply with HIPAA regulations and understand how the Stark Acts and the False Claims Act affect their practices. Medicare, Medicaid and private insurer reimbursement also requires a deep understanding of how coding irregularities might be considered fraud. As is true with clinical knowledge, traditional APN or undergraduate nursing ethics curricula do not reflect the expanded vision needed to practice in the twenty-first century. Nursing education at the doctoral level necessitates stronger ethical knowledge and application in clinical practice.

By the year 2015, nurse practitioner education will transition from the master's level to the doctorate. This represents a fundamental change that will require a curriculum that reflects the advanced level of a doctoral degree program. PhD nursing programs also require an advanced level of ethical education. This text will utilize a definition of nursing ethics which includes elements of medical, legal, research and business ethics. The expanded content is taught within one major core course and provides a foundation for all major courses.

The rationale for expanded expertise is based on five premises that directly influence health care quality:

- As the scope and independence of practice of DNPs have expanded, so too have ethical dilemmas that directly influence such practice. There are major, unaddressed ethical dilemmas that influence DNPs' ability to provide quality care to all. Consider that as part of a transplant team, DNP-prepared nurses may directly influence who is placed on organ transplant lists.
- Knowledge of bioethics, with its focus on patient care and research, is important but not sufficient for DNP practice. Nurses who practice at an advanced level must also understand other ethical frameworks, including legal and business arenas. Coding practices may influence reimbursement as well as patient costs. A nurse prepared at the DNP level must understand the ramifications of under- and over-coding.
- As health care becomes more interdisciplinary, DNPs must understand how different ethical frameworks impact the workplace. Having an expanded foundational base for ethical decision-making

will increase the DNP's ability to participate at the highest level with multiple professions.

• There are tremendous issues of access and disparity in care provided to the underserved. These problems are directly influenced by ethical reasoning and in turn lead to further ethical discourse. Knowledge of funding mechanisms and cultural differences are necessary but not sufficient to solve these problems. These issues will not be solved by health professionals who do not have a firm grounding in ethics.

We believe that *Ethical and Legal Issues for Doctoral Nursing Students: A Textbook for Students and Reference for Nurse Leaders* will help guide faculty and students in the complex healthcare arena faced by both.

Throughout this text, the LACE (Licensure, Accreditation, Certification and Education) 2008 APRN Consensus Model definition of advanced practice nursing is used. The model was developed by the APRN Consensus Work Group and the National Council of State Boards of Nursing APRN Advisory Committee with input from the stakeholder communities. There are four roles defined in this model: certified registered nurse anesthetist (CRNA), certified nurse-midwife (CNM), clinical nurse specialist (CNS) and certified nurse practitioner. When the title APRN is used in the text, it represents all four of these roles.

The contents of the book reflect current knowledge and legislation. We would like to thank all the authors for their thoughtful and wise contributions to this volume.

ANNE G. PEIRCE, RN, PhD
JENNIFER A. SMITH, RN, MBA, MPH, DNP

Contributors

PAMELA BJORKLUND, PhD, RN, CNS, PMHNP-BC
Professor, Department of Graduate Nursing
The College of St. Scholastica
Duluth, MN

CAROLINE M. HEWITT, DNS, RN, WHNP-BC, ANP-BC
Director, Advanced Practice
Atrius Health
Newton, MA

RITA MARIE JOHN, EdD, DNP, CPNP, PMHS, FAANP
Special Lecturer
School of Nursing
Columbia University

KIM A. O'HARA, JD, MS, RN, CNE
Doctoral Student
Adelphi University
Garden City, NY

NANCY KING REAME, MSN, PhD, FAAN
Mary Dickey Lindsay Professor of Health Promotion, Risk Reduction (Emerita)
School of Nursing
Columbia University

COURTNEY REINISCH, DNP, RN, FNP-BC
Associate Professor & Undergraduate Program Director
School of Nursing
Montclair State University

JOAN VALAS, PhD, RN, ACNP-BC
Professor and Graduate Program Director
School of Nursing
Montclair State University

CHAPTER 1

Ethics: What it is, What it is Not and What the Future May Bring

ANNE G. PEIRCE

1.1. OVERVIEW

It must be asked who in the health care system will protect the vulnerable and what knowledge and resources are needed for that protection?

The ethics of care has been a strong thread in the fabric of nursing beginning with Florence Nightingale (Peirce, 2017). We have advised patients, negotiated with families, argued for and against treatment all in the name of nursing care. These singular efforts have not been in vain but are not enough for the changing role of advanced practice nurses. Nurses at the forefront of advanced practice (APRNs) must have an in-depth knowledge of the foundations of ethics in order to understand the future of ethics and how to best apply current ethics knowledge in the health care arena. With in-depth knowledge of ethics comes the nursing voice to assist patients when needed and to speak for them when they cannot, as well as to ensure fiduciary and legal compliance (Peirce & Smith, 2008). APRNs today cannot, and should not act solely as employees who carry out bioethical decisions made by others. Doctorally prepared nurses and APRNS, either in practice or research, must be the leaders to their colleagues, students, and other members of the health-care team. The following chapter will discuss the earliest writings on ethics as well as the newest work on neuroethics, technology ethics and microethics. This background can then be used as foundation for the chapters to come where specific patient populations and situations are explored by experts in those areas.

Ethics, bioethics, morals, morality and even the law have overlapping definitions and in fact may sometimes be used interchangeably. The following are brief definitions of some of the major terms used in this chapter:

ETHICS: A theory or system surrounding moral practices and beliefs. Ethics is also called the philosophy of morality or moral philosophy.

MORALITY: A specific judgment about actions or character. It is sometimes used to define right and wrong actions.

MORALS: A standard of behavior used to define a good act or action.

BIOETHICS: Applied ethical inquiry and moral responses specific to health care

NORMATIVE ETHICS: The study of the norms that make an act right or wrong.

VIRTUE ETHICS: The aspects of the human character that makes actions right or wrong.

UTILITARIANISM: The doctrine that an act is right if it produces happiness or benefits. It describes ethical acts that produce the greatest good for the greatest number of people.

DEONTOLOGY: The ethical approach to do with adherence to rules and obligations regardless of consequences.

PRAGMATIC ETHICS: This approach is situation dependent. In pragmatic ethics, all ethical dilemmas and their solutions are modifiable if the situation warrants.

NEUROETHICS: "An interdisciplinary research area that focuses on ethical issues raised by our increased and constantly improving understanding of the brain and our ability to monitor and influence it, as well as on ethical issues that emerge from our concomitant deepening understanding of the biological bases of agency and ethical decision-making." (Roskies, 2016).

MICROETHICS: The new understanding that ethics is important to the small events in health care as well as the large. Every patient encounter involves small ethical decisions as does the allocation of health care resources (Truong et al, 2015).

ETHICS OF TECHNOLOGY: The ethical questions that arise from modern technology including control by machines, social media, robotics, artificial intelligence, algorithm development and super computers. Also there are biotech questions that arise from technology in health care. (Franssen, Lokhorst, & van de Poel, 2018).

1.2. HISTORICAL VIEW

1.2.1. Greeks

The earliest Greek philosophers, including Plato, Socrates and Aristotle explored the same questions that we ask today: what is a good life and what is needed to live such a life? A significant part of that early discussion focused on virtue. Aristotle (384-322 BC), in the Nicoma-chean Ethics, wrote that a good life is living a life of virtue (Aristotle, 1980). To Aristotle, the virtues of a life well lived were somewhat de-pendent upon role. Whereas a soldier might need the virtue of courage, a nurse might need the virtue of compassion. He did however acknowl-edge the importance of core virtues needed by all, such as justice and wisdom (Pellegrino & Thomasma, 1993). Today nurses continue to be influenced by Aristotle; just consider that undergraduate fundamentals and professionalism books often contain a list or description of the im-plied virtues of nursing including but not limited to caring, honesty, and integrity.

Aristotle distinguished between moral and intellectual virtues (Ar-istotle, 1980). The former is knowledge based and the latter character or habit based. To have a good life it is important to both know what is good and act in ways that affirm that good. But this thought of good-ness, or what Aristotle called eudaimonia, is a term that is not fully cap-tured in translation. In part, Artistotle referred to the need for balance, or the Doctrine of the Mean (Armstrong, 2007, Kuczewski & Polansky, 2000). The Doctrine of the Mean is evocative of the Eastern philoso-phies where balance, evidenced by the concepts of ying and yang, un-derlie health and wellness. Aristotle considered that there is a necessary balance, and someone who is too virtuous can be as problematic as someone who is not at all.

Aristotle believed that there is a difference between being virtuous and acting virtuously. If one's character is virtuous, then one's action will be the same; it is part of the whole. However a non-virtuous person can be taught to act in a virtuous way through education, and in time achieve the habits of virtue. To do what is right for the right reasons, to the right extent, to the right person and at the right time is goodness (Armstrong, 2007).

1.2.2. Romans

Roman Stoics also considered virtues to be critical to a well-lived life. They perceived virtues to be so embedded in human life that they form natural laws. The notion that there are laws of nature that provide a guiding force to life is something we consider today as well (Baltzly, 2018). The human abhorrence of murder could be considered a reflec-tion of natural law, as could the instinctive reaction to incest. These forms of natural law virtues are seen by biologists, most notably Wilson (Wilson, 2007), as critical to genetic survival. Sociobiologists contend that the virtues such as cooperation and altruism can increase fitness for survival. They point to the presence of cooperation and altruism in both animal and human behavior as evidence of its deep routed presence in nature (Houchmandzadeh & Vallade, 2012, Roughgarden, 2012).

At least two important ethical doctrines flow from natural law. One is the Doctrine of Double Effect which is credited to Thomas Aquinas (Murphy, 2018). This doctrine proposes that if an act has two expected results, then both should be considered in making the decision (McIntyre, 2019). The use of morphine to reduce pain (primary effect), with its known effect of respiratory suppression (secondary effect), is a classic example.

The second doctrine of natural law is the Principle of Totality (Moore, 2011) Stoics, and later religious philosophers believed we are whole and perfect as we are. Cicero wrote that "The primary duty is that the creature should maintain itself in its natural constitution; next, that it should cleave to all that is in harmony with nature and spurn all that is not..." (Cicero, 1914)

The *Principle of Totality* would indicate that health care should only occur in instances when bodily wholeness is threatened. For example, surgery for illness or trauma would be considered permissible under the Principle of Totality. Surgery to alter the body for cosmetic reasons would not meet the strictest standard of this natural law. The Principle of Totality may become even more important with the advent of genetic enhancement. The current debate as to whether genetic alteration is good for humankind echoes the early work of the Stoics.

1.2.3. Hippocrates, Galen and Maimonides: Physicians as Philosophers

"As to diseases, make a habit of two things—to help, or at least to do no harm. The art (sic of medicine) has three factors the disease, the patient, the physician. The physician is the servant of the art. The patient must co-operate with the physician in combating the disease." (Hippocrates quoted in Bartz, 2000, p14).

The time of *Hippocrates* (460-370 BC) was one of magic as well as medicine. Hippocrates sought to codify the acts of medicine in order to prevent harm by magic practicing charlatans. Early physicians were compelled to write about basic behaviors of physicians in order to create a moral or ethical bottom line. Many of these writings are attributed to Hippocrates, a contemporary of Socrates, who lived around 460 BC. His approach to medicine was one of vigilant watchfulness allowing healing to occur naturally, but if it did not, to wait to intervene until it was clear that healing would not occur without intervention (Bartz, 2000).

Galen (131-200 AD) is considered one of the greatest physicians of all time. His influence on medicine remained strong up to the time of the enlightenment. Of all his contributions his work on the circulatory system was the most important. In addition to his work as an anatomist, Galen was also a philosopher. In fact he wrote a treatise entitled *The Best Physician is Also a Philosopher* (Drizis, 2008). His ethical focus, derived from the works of Hippocrates, was on the duties of the physician and not the patient-physician relationship.

At a later time Maimonides (1138-1204) wrote similarly about the virtues of medicine (Nuland, 2008). A disciple of Galen and Hippocrates, he sought to reconcile his religious life with the practice of medicine (Collins 2007). The duty of medicine was important to Maimonides because a healthy body was important to God. He did not think that prayer alone was enough to restore health. He also wrote of the importance of knowledge to the patient. While knowledge is important to autonomy, Maimonides did not see patients as fully autonomous but rather as dependent upon the knowledge of the physician and the will of God (Collins, 2007, Gesundheit, 2011)

1.2.4. Western Philosophy and Ethics

To the early European philosophers, moral goodness was less about education and character and more about faith. Important contributions to the thinking about ethics reemerged in medieval times with the writings of St. Thomas Aquinas and St. Augustine. Aquinas sought to reconcile the virtue ethics of Aristotle with the theological virtues of the Christian church. To Augustine and Aquinas, the duty to God as manifested in faith, hope, charity and obedience, were more important than the reasoned life advocated by Aristotle (Pellegrino & Thomasma, 1993).

The 17th century was a time of great philosophical debate. Labeled the Enlightenment or the Age of Reason, it was dominated by European philosophers, many of whom were also scientists. This group, which included Spinoza, Locke, Newton, Rousseau and Voltaire, advocated the primacy of science in explaining the world around us. With this new world view the notion of Church-driven unreasoned action was questioned. If murder was a sin, why was the taking of life in war not the same? The dialogue between the obedience to God and the reasoned action according to conscience continues today as evidenced by the early discussions surrounding AIDS when it was seen by some as a punishment for sinful behavior.

1.2.5. The Reformation, Kant and Deontology

Immanuel Kant (1724-1804) is credited with the development of the major ethical schools of thought of *deontology*. (Kant, 1998). Writing after the time of the Reformation, he conceptualized Moral Law as not so much a replacement of Divine Law, but as an outgrowth. Kant was raised as a deeply religious conservative Protestant but began his career as a mathematical physicist. He later turned to the broader questions of philosophy. He strove to identify those actions or virtues that can be universally accepted. Kant wrote that there is a categorical imperative where there are certain acts that all agree are right. According to Kant, if one knows of these acts, then one should follow them. Kant's basic premise was that "A person ought to act in accordance with the rule that, if generally followed, would produce the greatest balance of good over evil, everyone considered." (Mappes & DeGrazia, 2001, p.13). He focused on adherence to the rules but not the consequences of such adherence. Kant argued instead for the respect of rules as guiding forces as long as they are universal in acceptance or can be universally accepted. Or in other words, one's actions should be such that they could serve as a model for universal law if everyone were to adopt them. A high standard indeed! There are many articles and videos on this topic, including an amusing but illustrative example from the BBC on *youtube* (https://www.youtube.com/watch?v=x_uUEaeqFog).

Kant's influence on ethics can be summarized as follows (Blackburn, 2001, Kant, 1998, Rohlf, 2018):

1. Ethics should not be concerned with consequences of the act but with duty to the act (rule adherence).
2. The right act is universally right. Others can and should act in the same way.
3. The right act treats humans as ends in themselves not as a means to an end.
4. The right act is a rational act, not a habit but rather one of free will.

1.2.6. Mill, Bentham and Utilitarianism

While Kant wrote that duty to laws and rules was more important than the outcome of that duty, not all philosophers concurred. There were many who felt that the consequences of actions do matter. To ignore the consequences seemed wrong sighted when such acts could result in harm. As a result, the consequentialist or utilitarian view evolved. The consequentialists said that the outcome was what was important; therefore the right actions that lead to the wrong outcome was the wrong thing to do. The two main proponents of this thinking were Jeremy Bentham (1748-1832) and John Stuart Mill (1806-1873).

Bentham's Utilitarianism was based on the notion of pleasure, or 'happiness', as the ultimate good (Bentham, 1861). To Bentham, acts that bring happiness are morally better than those that do not. In general, we now understand the Utilitarian view, not as Bentham did in terms of the individual but rather as the collective decisions whose actions bring the greatest good to the greatest number of people. The utility of the act is the happiness, pleasure, or goodness that it produces.

John Stuart Mill expanded upon the work of Bentham, considering not only the amount of pleasure but the quality of the pleasure (Mill, 1871). To Mill, some pleasures were worth more than others. The more a pleasure contributes to a human's growth; whether it be intellectually, spiritually or aesthetically, the better the quality of that pleasure. For example, the pleasure obtained from a successful work day as a nurse may be of better quality than a night spent in a bar even though both could bring pleasure. Mill argued that it is also the long term outcomes of such acts that are important. Thus moral guidelines developed should be devoted to maximization of pleasure and minimization of pain.

While Bentham and Mill focused on pleasure, in health care we use the notion of health utility to examine what health care actions produce the greatest good for the greatest number of people (Ahronheim, Moreno, & Zuckerman, 2000, Faden & Shebaya, 2016). For example, is it better to provide free immunizations for those who can't afford them or to rely on the herd response from those who can afford to be immunized? In the utilitarian view, costs, financial and otherwise would be considered in relation to the benefits derived.

Utilitarianism can be summarized as follows (Beauchamp & Childress, 2008, Bentham, 1861, Blackburn, 2001, Driver, 2014, Mill, 1871):

1. Consequences are of ultimate concern. Intentions are only as important as the consequences they produce.
2. The more people who benefit from the consequences the better.
3. The best consequences produce pleasure or what the person desires.
4. Each person's consequence is important but no more important than another's.

1.3. ETHICS IN HEALTHCARE

Ethical dilemmas in the health care system are different from those in other professions such as education and business. This has to do, in part, with the life and death results that may flow directly from any given decision and also from the sense that health care decisions should be made in such a way that reflects care for the group as well as the individual.

Many of the codes of ethics that guide health care share a history with research codes of ethics. The first general code of ethics grew out of the Nuremberg trials following World War II, when the world was first alerted to the human devastation wrought by Nazi doctors and nurses (Benedict & Kuhla, 1999, Mappes & DeGrazia, 2001). The trials uncovered evidence of the horrible experiments done on humans in the name of science. As a result, the following code, still used today, was developed. Its ten tenets (ORI, 2019) are:

1. The voluntary consent of the human subject is absolutely essential.
2. The experiment should be such as to yield fruitful results for the good of society.
3. The experiment should be so designed and based on the results of animal experimentation and knowledge of the natural history of the disease.
4. The experiment should be so conducted as to avoid all unnecessary physical and mental suffering and injury.
5. No experiment should be conducted where there is an a priori reason to believe that death or disabling injury will occur.
6. The degree of risk to be taken should never exceed that determined by the humanitarian importance of the problem to be solved by the experiment.
7. Proper preparations should be made and adequate facilities provided to protect the experimental subject against even remote possibilities of injury, disability, or death.
8. The experiment should be conducted only by scientifically qualified persons.
9. During the course of the experiment the human subject should be at liberty to bring the experiment to an end.
10. During the course of the experiment the scientist in charge must be prepared to terminate the experiment at any stage, if he has probable cause to believe, in the exercise of the good faith, superior skill and careful judgment required of him that a con

tinuation of the experiment is likely to result in injury, disability, or death to the experimental subject.

Following the Nuremberg Code, the Declaration of Helsinki sought to clarify and strengthen protection of humans. This document underscores the fundamental importance of human self-determination in participation in research but also influenced human rights in general. It also underscored the role the researcher in protecting the individual, as well as the care that must be given to vulnerable populations under study (Bulger, Heitman & Reiser, 2002). The Belmont Report, put forth by the National Commission for the Protection of Human Subjects of Biomedical and Behavioral Research in 1979, first identified three principles important with human research as being respect for persons, beneficence and justice (Bulger, Heitman & Reiser, 2002).

In addition to concerns with human research, the development of bioethics was driven by the technological advances of the 20th century. Antibiotics, the heart-lung machine, organ transplants, in vitro fertilization and other discoveries changed the health care landscape from one where nature had the last word to one where life could be prolonged and altered. It wasn't until 1968 that the Harvard Medical School, when organ transplants became possible, defined brain death. At that time brain death, labelled irreversible coma had three major criteria of unresponsiveness to painful stimuli, no movement and no reflexes (Ad Hoc Committee, Harvard, 1968). Since that time different definitions have evolved with each state having a defined definition. The 1980 Uniform Determination of Death was developed to give guidance to states (http://www.aopo.org/state-brain-death-laws/). Today both circulatory and neurological criteria are used to identify death, including an assessment of consciousness, brain-stem reflexes and the ability to breathe spontaneously. Recently there have been court challenges to how death is defined and who can decide when death has occurred (Grossman, 2014). For further information about the assessment of death by providers see the Brain Death Toolkit (https://www.neurocriticalcare.org/education/digital-education/brain-death-toolkit) and the Hastings Center Report (Truog, Berlinger, Zacharias, & Solomon, 2018) titled, "What does dead mean?" (https://www.thehastingscenter.org/publications-resources/special-reports-2/what-does-dead-mean/).

Nurses need to be cognizant of standing and changing rules about brain death, including legal challenges to who and how it is determined. In many state APRNs are able to pronounce death, in others they can also sign the death certificate. For example, in 2010 the New York State Senate passed legislation (S.2969) allowing certified nurse practitioners to sign death certificates ensuring the delivery of appropriate and medically-accurate postmortem care but not until 2012 did it go into effect as PBH 4141-A (https://www.nysenate.gov/legislation/laws/PBH/4141-A). APRNs should review their state rules and regulations pertaining to death pronouncement and signing of death certificates.

1.4. TECHNOLOGICAL ADVANCEMENTS

In the 21st century nurses face unprecedented ethical dilemmas from technology, particularly artificial intelligence. Artificial intelligence (AI) has begun to make health care decisions previously made only by doctors and nurses. Undoubtedly there are many potential benefits to AI, including fast sorting of signs and symptoms, ability to utilize large data sets, and expansive differential diagnoses. However, there are down sides as well including the consolidation of bias and amplification of risk (Char, Shah & Magnus, 2018). Other challenges come from the use of Big Data, algorithms, and technology in genomics.

1.4.1. Artificial Intelligence

Artificial intelligence is any computer based system that utilizes cues and data from the environment to solve problems, take actions and make decisions (Bringsjord & Govindarajula, 2018). The usage of AI is gaining momentum in many facets of life from self-driving cars, hiring systems, and even prediction of criminal recidivism. However, in these cases and others, problems of error and bias have been uncovered. To this point such error has been acknowledged after its appearance; an ethical problem. Health care AI faces the same benefits and risks as in other venues. Nurses need to ensure that ethics is part of all artificial intelligence discussions before, during, and after implementation.

1.4.2. Algorithms

Algorithms are a procedure or formula for solving a problem; based on a sequence of specified actions or calculations that translate input into output (Zsakó & Szlávi, 2012). Algorithms, as part of artificial intelligence and other computer based systems, drive much of computer based health care applications from electronic medical records to billing to assessment of vital signs. There is a misconception that mathematical analysis and algorithmic decisions are without error but nothing can be further from the truth. Algorithms have built in biases reflecting the biases of their creators. Recent discussions have pointed out that the creators of most algorithms are young men who may not see the same variables as important to decisions as other ages or genders (Simonite, 2015). It is critical that nurses question what data points are considered in clinical decision making algorithms. Unfortunately, there are barriers to such inquiry. Most decision focused algorithms are proprietary and as such the data used, and how it is weighted is unavailable. Nurses must be involved in purchasing to ensure that the products reflect the nursing ethos because once they are purchased and in place it may be too late to discern or fix any ethical decision making issues.

1.4.3. Big Data

Big Data is variously defined but recently definitions have focused both on the volume of data, variety of data, and the velocity with which it is analysed (Ienca, Vayena, & Blasimme, 2018). In many cases the information of Big Data is found data or what some call "digital exhaust" (McGowan, 2016). These data resources hold great promise, often allowing discovery of previously unknown connections. The NIH (2018) outlines its benefits in discovering new research possibilities. In addition they stress the importance of the FAIR principle of data; that is data should be Findable, Accessible, Interoperable, and Reusable.

The use of Big Data is also challenging traditional ethical norms. First access to Big Data is porous with no proven barriers. Without barriers such as that provided by HIPAA, it is possible to tie the individual to his or her digital exhaust. This means that shopping habits, driving data, use of over the counter medicines and other information assumed to be private is not. Anonymity as we have known it in the past is no longer possible. Without anonymity or in some cases even confidentiality there is a need to reconsider how to protect the individual. Several approaches have been put forth but to date there are no definitive guidelines.

The protection from harm is also critical. Big Data has until recently been presumed to be innocuous, with no threat of harm. But recently the invasion of privacy and loss of control over private information has come to be seen as a threat to contextual integrity and human dignity (Zimmer, 2018). Carpenter and Dittrich (2011) use "human harming" theory to explain how these threats are manifested. For further information see The Council for Big Data, Ethics and Society at https://bdes. datasociety.net/.

1.4.4. Genomics

Since the genome sequencing was finalized in the early 2000s, many research and commercial enterprises around genomics have sprung up using evolving technologies such as CRISPr. The rush to use genetic information is compelling. Take for example birth defects where there is irresistible urge to fix the genetic defect or to find a cure for cancer. While the upsides of genomics are without question, the downsides should not be ignored; such as the re-emergence of eugenics and the creation of a super class able to afford the cost of genetic alteration as well as the loss of insurability or employment opportunities. Today, as this chapter is written there is unverified news coming from China of fetal genetic alteration. While world scientists have condemned such research, its possibility in unregulated laboratories is a real threat.

1.4.5. Questions

In nursing we need to habituate ethical questioning of all these emerging technologies. While the ethical questions are also emergent, as creation has surged ahead of ethics, we offer the following as a place to begin:

1. How can we assure privacy with Big Data?
   a. What are the protections needed with the use of technological driven machines, such as IV pumps that collect and transmit data? Who receives the data and what privacy protections are in place with the end user?
   b. Are there surveillance and other recording devices in the institution? Where is the data store, with whom is it shared and how long is it kept? Are patient and health care worker data protected?
   c. What data elements are collected as part of Big Data and why?
      i. For example, does the data collected include pharmacy, grocery, fast food, and gasoline purchases as well as travel, education, zip code, census data, hospitalization, laboratory tests, provider encounters, and entertainment preferences? All of these examples (plus many others) together or separately, are possible data points used to determine health related care pathways. (Ask yourself if you want your health insurance rate determined by anyone of these elements, and if so why?)
   d. Does the institution or health care provider share information about individuals and if so why, are consents in place and what protections are offered?

2. What is the role of the institution and of providers in the protection of the individual when current anonymization strategies are ineffective?
3. Should there be soft, or hard censorship of health information found online?
   a. Do the internet based educational systems used by the institution have bias, such as funding by groups with commercial interest?
   b. Are patient educational systems kept current with the newest vetted information?
   c. What is the role/responsibility of the provider in directing patients to health information sources?
4. Are the algorithms used in any given program free from bias?
   a. Are certain diseases or conditions tagged, and if so how is the tag used?
   b. How are the financial algorithms developed and by whom; what is their goal and are there built in biases, such as gender, zip code, education level and so forth used in the formulation?
   c. What mechanisms are available to determine bias?
5. Are all consent forms transparent as to patient information and genetic material usage?
   a. Should third party usage of genetic material be consented with opt-in or opt out language?
   b. Should patients know specifically who will have access to their information, for example pharmaceutical companies, pharmacies, employers, insurers, researchers and so forth? This is particularly important when true anonymity is virtually impossible.
6. How is fairness determined in the artificial intelligence systems used by the institution or provider?
7. For proprietary AI and algorithms what information is available as to how decisions are made?
8. Is genetic information stored?
   a. Is genetic information shared and with whom?
   b. Who has access to the genetic information?
   c. What consent has been granted? And for how long?
   d. What privacy protections are in place?
   e. Are there secondary consents required for additional research?

While this list is incomplete, as the technology is evolving faster than questions can be raised, we hope that nurses will lend their voices to the ethical concerns raised in what many are calling the Fourth Industrial Revolution (Schwab, 2016). This discussion continues in Chapter 2 where research specific ethics is discussed, particularly in light of recent changes made to the Common Rule.

1.5. ETHICAL PRINCIPLES

Four major ethical principles have been identified as critical in health care by Beauchamp and Childress (2013). These so called major bioethical principles are autonomy, beneficence, nonmaleficence and justice. While these four principles are considered foundational, there are others that are also important. Ross (1930) speaks to prima facie duties that include fidelity, reparation, gratitude, and self- improvement. Other writers have added veracity and even care (Held, 2005). Privacy issues are also increasingly of concern.

1.5.1. Autonomy

Provision One of the ANA Code of Ethics for Nurses (Fowler, 2015) states that:

> *"The nurse practices with compassion and respect for the inherent dignity, worth, and unique attributes of every person"*

Autonomy is the notion that competent adults have the right of self-determination and this right should be respected by health care providers. Many ethicists consider autonomy to be the major overriding bio-ethical principle (Fry & Veatch, 2006). That is, adults have the right to decide what health care they want, as well as when, how and who will be involved in that care. It is taken for granted by most that no competent adult can be forced to have surgery or to undergo treatment if they do not want to do so. In fact, the ideal of autonomy posits that adults do not even have to seek care. In reality, the concept of autonomy is not so absolute. For example, tuberculosis patients can be forced into care if they are contagious, and soldiers can be forced to be immunized

In another deviation, children are not generally considered fully autonomous agents until they reach the age of 18. But even legal age is fungible and has changed over time. For example, an emancipated minor is in a different legal class than one who is not. A child undergoing surgery may not give consent but rather assent. The nuances of ethics and children's health care are more fully explored in Chapter 6.

Although autonomy is defined as self-determination or self-governance, there are qualifiers even for competent adults. To be autonomous an individual must have the will to act, the intention to act, the under-standing or knowledge needed, and freedom from extensive internal and external constraints. In other words, to qualify as an autonomous act it must be an intentional act, a knowledgeable act and the person must want to act in the way he or she did (Beauchamp & Childress, 2013). An accident is not an autonomous act. Nor is a person who agrees to experimental treatment without fully understanding the side effects acting autonomously, or thoughtfully. In the rush and confusion of hospitalization it is not unusual for accidental, or non-autonomous decisions to be made. Decisions may be made without complete infor-mation or real understanding of what the information means. Clinical research subjects may not truly understand what random assignment implies; that they may not receive the experimental treatment. Surgical patients may not comprehend the unintended consequences of surgery. In fact, it may not always be a singular decision made by an individual; sometimes decisions are shared by family and patient or by patient and provider. Understanding may be best thought of as a continuum, in which the goal is to achieve as complete an understanding as possible.

There are other barriers to autonomous actions. External barriers may also include judicial laws and physical restraints. Internal constraints may result from substance abuse, psychological disease or pain. Thus autonomy becomes the desired ideal, but not always the realized ideal.

Informed consent is representative of the principle of autonomy. When patients sign an informed consent document, it is assumed that they do so of their own free will, with an understanding of what is involved, and free from any constraints in coming to their decision. In reality, an individual may not fully understand what is involved and it also may not be pos-sible to explain every possible outcome. Patients may feel obligated to consent because of pressure from their physicians or family or they may be signing in times of pain or other physical constraints to autonomy. Ad-vanced practice nurses should be cognizant of these barriers and ensure that autonomy is actively promoted to the extent possible. Acceptance of the status quo, the expedient and the thoughtless approach to autonomy should never be tolerated by the nursing profession.

1.5.2. Beneficence

According to Beauchamp (2016) the word beneficence implies mer-cy, kindness and charity. While beneficence is the act, the moral virtue is benevolence. Many philosophers have explored what beneficence means in life. The philosopher David Hume (Morris & Brown, 2017) thought that beneficence was a central principle of human goodness, while Kant saw it as a duty (Kant, 1998). More recently, Beauchamp and Childress (2013) write of two aspects of this principle, positive beneficence and utility beneficence, both of which are important to bioethics.

Positive beneficence refers to the principle that individuals have positive obligations to others (Beauchamp &Childress, 2013). Beauchamp and Childress give examples of positive beneficence including rescuing people in danger, helping people with disabilities and so forth. They refer to these as moral rules of obligation.

There has been much recent discussion about moral obligations and how far they extend (Scheffler, 1997). In general terms, it appears that individuals feel more obligated to those with whom they are close in terms of friendship, kinship or proximity and less obligated to those further away (Murphy, 1993). Some modern philosophers see this as wrong and write that our concern should be for every human soul, not just the ones we may know (Singer, 1972, 1999). Peter Singer is a strong advocate for the general obligation of beneficence; to do what is good no matter our relationship. Other writers speak of situational or specific beneficence where one's obligation is only to those known (Murphy, 1993).

There are limits to our obligation to be beneficent. No one has the perfect gift of time, money, strength, compassion to meet all needs, yet that is what beneficence would ideally have us do. We all want health care providers to do good and contribute to the overall welfare of patients. Within the professional nursing role there is an obligation, a duty, to provide care. This also implies there is a duty to beneficence, although this is not directly stated in the ANA Code of Ethics. In part, the duty of beneficence is a reflection of reciprocity (Rawls, 1971). Nurses are paid to care, or at least to provide care, thus illustrating reciprocity. Within that arrangement, care is the unspoken obligation to work towards the welfare of the patient. The social contract between patient and nurse is one that is focused on what is best for the patient, both because it is a paid obligation but also because it is a professional and societal expectation.

The utility of beneficence is that the resultant good should outweigh the bad in all ethically-based decisions (Beauchamp & Childress, 2013). Many decisions in health care are firmly situated within utilitarianism, especially those of public health. For example, immunizations greatly benefit the whole population but still may entail harm to individuals. Every year a handful of people have bad outcomes, including death, from basic immunizations. These results are accepted, in the utilitarian sense, because the good so strongly outweighs the few bad outcomes. The utility approach is sometimes difficult, as the individual is not considered except as part of the whole.

Peirce and Ekhardt write of their ethical concerns (unpublished manuscript) with the wholesale acceptance of evidence-based practice, where the unusual or so called "Black Swan" events are overrode or ignored. Evidence-based practice is predicated on the view that one treatment, one medication and so forth is good for all, yet it may not be. Rather, evidence-based practice is good for the average and not for the outlier. Thus utilitarianism principles may override the rights of the individual in favor of the group. Because nursing's mandate has always been the care of the individual, there may be ethical issues for some compulsory aspects of evidence-based practice.

Paternalism may come into play with beneficence. Beneficence carries the "odor" of paternalism, in that health care providers sometimes use their own judgment to do what they believe is best for those who are ill or infirm, perhaps overriding the patients' preferences or failing to ascertain the preferences. There are no set rules for who decides what is good and what benchmarks are used for these decisions. There have been instances in the not too distant past in which women were sterilized without consent because the physician thought it wise (ACOG, 2017, Zumpano-Canto, 1996).

However, paternalism is not always problematic. Sometimes input cannot be obtained and then paternalism can make the difference between a good outcome and a bad. Paternalistic decisions are frequently made in emergency rooms and surgical suites as well as in times of natural and man-made disasters. At those times, it is desirable for a knowledgeable person to take charge and make decisions. While someone has to make decisions in times of crisis, it is hoped that the decision is in the best interest of those affected.

Beauchamp and Childress (2013) propose that paternalism is used to justify both beneficence and nonmaleficence. They list the four criteria that must be met before paternalism can be justified:

1. The patient is at risk for significant preventable harm
2. The paternalistic act will probably prevent the harm
3. The benefits of the act outweigh the risk to the patient
4. The least restrictive act is followed

1.5.3. Nonmaleficence

Nonmaleficence is distinguished by active, intentional actions that prevent the infliction of harm. To "not do harm" is viewed as separate from preventing harm or promoting good, both of which are generally labeled beneficence (Armstrong, 2007). Many ethicists write that the obligation to not cause or prevent harm is more important, "more stringent", to quote Beauchamp and Childress (2002) than the obligation to do good.

The distinction between these clearly overlapping concepts of preventing harm and promoting good are sometimes difficult to distinguish. Similar to Frankana's arguments (1988), it can be posited that there is a continuum over which these acts occur. At one end is the obvious intention to do harm solely for the sake of harm and on the other, the obvious intention to do good solely for the sake of good. In between there are acts, intentional or not, which promote the motion towards one end or another. Immunizing a child is done for good, both for the child and for the herd immunity it promotes. Yet this act also carries within it harm; at minimum it hurts and upsets the child, at maximum it leads to death. At the adult level, nurses who work in hospitals may be required to receive booster immunizations. This is done not on the volition of the individual, but as a mandate from the system. Is this a matter of nonmaleficence, of doing no harm, or of beneficence, the promotion of good and how does it relate to autonomy and justice? The answer varies as the viewpoint changes from person to system.

Nursing has always taken the threat of harm to patients seriously. The Nightingale Pledge and the Hippocratic Oath both echo one of the most common statements in health care; *above all do no harm* or in Latin: *primum non nocere*. In practice, nurses expend energy in preventing problems, whether it is falls, decubitus ulcers, or nosocomial infections. In fact the prevention of harm often serves as a nursing marker of quality. Organizations concerned with health care quality, including QSEN, IOM and JCAH, have all converged on preventable events as a marker of quality, but is this correct? Is the absence of harm or reduction in harm the same as quality? Is quality goodness, or is it the promotion of goodness? If so, shouldn't it be measured by activities that reflect beneficence and not just avoiding harm?

1.5.4. Justice

Justice has many definitions, but at its simplest, it is the act of being fair. Hume pointed out that it is only when there is a scarcity of resources that justice is questioned (Murphy & Brown, 2017). We all want what is fair, or our fair share of limited resources, whether it is food, fuel or health care. Justice is also defined as the punishment that is meted out when fairness is breached. Fair allocation of scarce resources appears to be a Natural Law; instinctive in humans and even some animals (Murphy, 2011). We instinctively respond to the idea that all are accorded what is due to them. However there are no simple answers to questions of justice. It is difficult to fairly allocate resources (distributive justice) and still reconcile the common and individual good (commutative justice).

The principle (and the virtue) of justice require health care decisions to be fair and equal (Fry & Veatch, 2006). Americans have come to expect that everyone has the same rights when it comes to access to, and provision of care. In addition there is a conception that health care is fairly distributed. All of this, of course, may not be true but rather the ideal. Allocation of limited resources poses many real as well as potential dilemmas in health care (Kahane, et al., 2018). Recently there have been debates as to how scarce influenza vaccine reserves might be allocated in a pandemic influenza outbreak. Various solutions have been discussed including vaccination of all first line providers, distribution based upon age, or even random distribution through a lottery. In each case, the choice to make the vaccine available to one group would mean that others would not have access to the resource. A system based upon immunizing the caregivers first might ensure better health care for the sick; a system based upon a national lottery would ensure fair distribution across all constituencies. Immunizing caregivers suggests utilitarianism as regulators look at the consequences of an act designed to care for as many of the sick as possible. The lottery system involves distributive justice, or the equitable allocation of resources among people. In either case, there will be devastating consequences for some but not for all.

Philosophers have begun to develop the concept of capability as a way of exploring social justice as well as beneficence. Capability theory proposes that the achievement of well-being is the primary moral driver, and that to achieve well-being it is necessary to foster an individual's capabilities (Nussbaum, 2003, Sen, 2005). Nussbaum (2003) delineated ten capabilities that are important to consider when there are questions of social justice. They include:

1. Having a normal, expected life span.
2. Being able to have good health and the elements that contribute to it such as food and shelter.
3. To be secure in movement and other abilities such as reproductive choice.
4. To be able to think, reason and imagine.
5. To be emotionally connected.
6. To have practical reason in order to critically evaluate one's life.
7. To have the ability to affiliate with others.

8. To live with and have concern for the earth, its animals and plants.
9. To be able to play and enjoy life.
10. To be able to control one's environment through political participation and property rights.

To achieve justice within this framework, it is necessary to promote acts that help achieve these ten capabilities. Many of the capabilities proposed by Nussbaum echo the nursing literature's emphasis of the bio-psycho-social care of the individual (Smeltzer, Bare, Hinkle & Cheever, 2010) and the self-care deficit concept of Orem's theory (Orem & Taylor, 2011).

It is important to remember that nurses make justice-based decisions daily, from triage in the emergency room to who receives the first or most care during a shift or in a clinic. Berlinger (2016) provides a compelling argument on the issues of justice in the workplace

1.5.6. Veracity

Another guiding ethical principle is that of veracity, or truth-telling. Truth is a difficult concept because there is little that is known to be absolutely true and so much is situational. Truth telling and its opposite, lying, are the center of a long history of debate. Many, but not all of the early philosophers, including Augustine and Aquinas, saw lying as a moral wrong and truth telling as the moral right (Bok, 1978). Later, Kant would say that there are no circumstances under which lying was acceptable (Kant, 1993). This would seem to be a statement with which many would initially agree. Yet there may be times when individuals lie and see it to be a moral good. In the famous example previously alluded to, it is posed to the reader that if you were hiding an innocent person in your house and a murderer came to the door, would you be justified in lying to the murderer? Many would argue that in this case, the lie was justified. Yet Kant would have disagreed. While extreme, this example demonstrates that an absolute statement against lying, or for truth telling, is not always desirable. It appears that not all lies are created equal. For as Grotius described it, an unacceptable lie could be defined as one that causes harm or violation of rights (Bok, 1978).

Sissela Bok, in her book *Lying*, describes four conditions in which lying could be justified, if justification is warranted (1978). These four conditions reflect the ethical principles of preventing harm, doing good, justice and veracity. First, Bok writes that it is acceptable to tell a lie if it will prevent harm, as in the example of the murderer seeking the innocent person. Second, it may be acceptable to lie if it promotes good. Not telling a dying patient the futility of treatment in order to maintain hope could be considered acceptable. Third, lies may be justified if it is known that the other party has already lied and it is seen as equalizing the situation. Fourth, one could justify a lie in order to protect a previous lie and so uphold the virtue of veracity. Yet even as these justifications are discussed, the possibility of abuse is real. It would be difficult to discern a clear line between a justified lie and one which was not. What if the person at the door was a policeman or a trusted friend, would you be justified in protecting the person who asked for refuge? As with all the principles, there is a continual struggle with what it means to hold veracity as an ideal.

1.5.7. Fidelity

Another important principle in bioethics is fidelity. Fidelity is generally more closely associated with the provider of care than with the recipient of care. Nurses have a commitment to their patients and to their employers as outlined in the ANA Code of Ethics (Fowler, 2015).

However, nurses rarely speak of patients in terms of fidelity unless it is in terms of fidelity to another principle, such as fidelity to truthtelling. Ross (1930) refers to fidelity as promise-keeping. Patients inherently want a professional relationship with providers. Lying, failing to deliver and other acts break the promise and threaten the relationship. It is promise-keeping in its broadest sense that ensures the relationship necessary for patient care. Nurses make a commitment to provide the care necessary because they are being paid to do so and because they see it as a societal/professional obligation.

As with veracity, there are situations in which the keeping of a promise is questioned. There are some who, like Kant and Aquinas may feel that a promise must be kept no matter what the consequences and there are other more moderate advocates, like Grotius who write that breaking a promise is acceptable if harm will result if the promise is not broken.

1.5.8. Privacy

Privacy is a cornerstone of bioethics. Patients expect that their private personal and medical information is confidential and only used for clinical matters (Moor, 1990). HIPAA has been the main mechanism through which privacy was assured.

The traditional notion of privacy is coming undone as technologies, technology companies, insurers and others rush to uncover as much information as possible in an effort to capitalize. The monetization of genetic and personal information is balanced by a real desire by scientists to create new knowledge based on the insights that big data provides. With this new porosity of information boundaries comes the threat of "…economic and social discrimination, hidden influence and manipulation, coercion or censorship…" (Acquisti, Brandimarte, & Loewenstein, 2015, p. 509).

Until recently individuals have had a reasonable expectation that their private information was not recoverable, nor accessible without permission. We have assumed our activities of daily living are private, for example grocery store purchases, driving routes and habits, fast food purchases and so forth. Yet all these seemingly innocuous bits of knowledge are collectable when we use loyalty cards, internet mapping and geo-tracking, credit cards and the internet and so forth. Even search engines collect information about our interests.

The second expectation about private information is that we have assumed that our information will not be made public without permission. In health care and research this is addressed through the informed consent process, in our private life we expect to be asked.

In privacy all Personally Identifiable Information (PII) is of concern. PII is contained in our personal characteristics such as education, marital status and so forth. We also have PII connected to our biometric data and other unique identifiers such as social security numbers. It is PII that facilitates the ties between the captured information and the individual. Several studies have shown the ability of computer scientists to uncover the individual within massive amounts of seemingly unrelated data (Narayanan, & Shmatikov, 2010). This ability to tie the individual to his or her private activities is troubling but as of the writing of this book there are no stringent controls in the United States. The European Union (EU) General Data Protection Regulations which went into effect in May 2018 provides some consumer protections for those in the EU (including all companies that do business or provide services to the EU):

> *"Companies must be clear and concise about their collection and use of personal data like full name, home address, location data, IP address, or the identifier that tracks web and app use on smartphones. Companies have to spell out why the data is being collected and whether it will be used to create profiles of people's actions and habits. Moreover, consumers will gain the right to access data companies store about them, the right to correct inaccurate information, and the right to limit the use of decisions made by algorithms, among others." (Tiku, 2018).*

Similar legislation in the US has met resistance from business and government. While HIPAA (HHS, accessed 2019) provides some protections, it is not sufficient in light of powerful computing and algorithms.

Privacy is a universal human need (Acquisti, Brandimarte, & Loewenstein, 2015) but can be assaulted in many ways. In some cases we give permission to invade our privacy. Privacy is challenged by context dependent permission which may or may not carry over to other use. Consider insurance companies that offer a discount for the installation of monitoring devices in cars and house alarm systems that include audio and visual communication connected to the web. In each case the company is collecting information which may or not benefit the consumer but is used for activities removed from its primary purpose. More troubling is the recent push by some health systems to monitor patients by RFID bracelets after discharge and in one case to propose implantation of monitoring microchips (Peirce, personnel communication 2017). This information shared with insurance companies, technology companies or others would present a very real threat to the individual's privacy. Dennet writes about this vanishing privacy where the "membranes protecting our lives and institutions have been permeated and secrets are almost impossible."(Dennet, 2017).

APRNs have a real (but sometimes unrealized) and significant involvement in protecting patients' privacy. All information collected should be scrutinized for relevance. Too often information is collected that has no connection to care, but is a matter of habit. All information collected should also be thoughtfully considered before it is entered into computers and websites with their connection to the internet. Patients should be advised about the vulnerability of data to exposure even though there are few protections that can be offered. Christians (2019) writes about the ethics of privacy and says the focus should be on the common good rather than professional standards while Richards and King (2014) propose that privacy should not be equated with secrecy but rather with regulation. APRNs should advocate for privacy regulations in the workplace and the government but still remember our role in promoting privacy as foundational to the common good.

1.6. NEUROETHICS

Ethics discussions in health care are generally based upon the ideal of rational thought; that there will be one best solution to a dilemma if enough information, time and resources are expended in its pursuit.

Neuroethicists are challenging the importance, as well as the feasibility of logically thinking through all decisions. As Greene et al. (2009) note, "There is a growing consensus that moral judgments are based largely on intuition –'gut feelings' about what is right or wrong in particular cases."

Kahneman (2011) writes that there are two primary decision making processes. One is the instinctive, and/ or intuitive; the second is the logical rational process. He refers to these two processes as system 1 and system 2. According to Kahneman, system 1 is fast, instinctive and tied to emotions while system 2 is slower, deliberate and logical. Some of the decisions within system 1 are based upon instinctive evolutionary development, such as the reaction to sudden loud noises while other more intuitive decisions develop as a result of deep experience.

Harris (2012) and others (Gazzaniga 2005, Greene, 2007, Greene, 2017, Conway, et al 2018) propose that genetic makeup, neurological systems and perhaps the effects of environment have a profound influence on ethical choices; making individuals more dependent on intuition and physics than rational thought and philosophy. These neuroethecists base their reasoning on recent studies which appear to show that some actions start to occur before the person is conscious of the need to make a decision. Soon and colleagues (2008) using a functional MRI, had participants make a choice about an ethical decision. They found that the unconscious brain was activated in advance of the conscious brain by up to ten seconds, indicating a bias against free will. In another study, Greene and Paxton (2008) examined patterns of brain activity in moral decisions related to honest and dishonest actions. They found that with subjects who faced a decision related to dishonest gain, the MRI revealed that neural activity more closely related to unconscious control than conscious control.

The so called Trolley Problem helps elucidate the presence of both the logical and intuitive in any given ethical dilemma. In the Trolley Problem, first proposed by Foot (1978), a switchman has the ability to throw a switch which will save five persons standing on the track but in doing so he will kill one standing off to the side. The dilemma illuminates the utilitarian versus deontological, in that it must be questioned if five lives are worth more than one if you have to consciously throw a switch to save them. The trolley problem then asks what if the only way to save the five is to throw a large man off the bridge. In general the response is different, most are reluctant to actively sacrifice one, while the switch in the earlier scenario is seen as passive and thus less ethically troubling (Edmonds, 2014).

Functional magnetic resonance imagery has shown that impersonal decision dilemmas such as throwing a switch to divert the trolley and personal decisions such as throwing the large man off the bridge activate different portions of the brain. The former activates the controlled reasoning areas while the later activates the area controlling emotions (Greene, 2001). See: https://www.youtube.com/watch?v=yg16u_bzjPE for a visual look at the trolley problem.

While the debate rages on over neuroethics, free will, biochemical responses and genetics in the moral landscape, nurses should consider that some, but not all ethical decisions may have an unconscious or automatic nature. Benner (1984) in fact has long linked intuitive thinking to the expert nurse. If this is true, then the mediating effect of the environment should be acknowledged as well as experience, thus strengthening collective support for individual decisions.

1.7. ETHICAL REASONING

The history of ethical thinking and some of the many principles that go into discussions surrounding ethics and specifically bioethics have been discussed. With this background, how does one make ethical decisions, if in fact one does? Some have asked why does one even need to make these decisions, don't people know instinctively what is right and what is wrong? (Richardson, 2018) None of the overarching ethical principles are absolutely adhered to without debate (Cahn-Fuller & Parent, 2017). Researchers believe that two main ethical decision making approaches exist; the automatic; including instinct and intuition and the reasoned (Hauser, 2008, Kahneman, 2011, Levy, 2011). Even if the neuroethics theory is accepted with its reliance on instinct and intuition, there will still be a need to review dilemmas, or to debrief about those decisions where instinct ruled.

Also, there are many questions that are not even asked because of prevailing world view. Just a few years ago, the mentally ill were institutionalized. This world view was not questioned, it was accepted. Now forced institutionalization is thought to be wrong and the mentally ill are housed in the community to the extent possible. Similarly, women and children have often been the recipients of decisions that may not have been in their best interest, because they were deemed incapable of self-determination. This world view continues in many parts of the world.

1.7.1. Instinct, Intuition and Ethical Decision Making

The instinctive response in decision making is helpful in times when reasoned judgment cannot occur, for example in times of a natural disaster. The instinct to help can override a more logical decision. The intuitive thought comes to mind quickly, without much reflection (Kahneman, 2002). There are many examples in the popular press of instances when someone has risked their own life to save another - not a logical decision - but one that feels right to most people none the less.

Klein (2004) writes that intuition is the way we translate experience into decisions using pattern recognition. Klein is not referring to uninformed decisions, but experience informed intuition or what he refers to as "recognition-primed decisions" (2004, p 27). Experts, who have more experience, also have more recognizable patterns of cues and what Klein calls action scripts (2004). He cites his own research and that of others showing that expert decision makers whether they be military, police, firemen or nurses rely on intuition 80-90% of the time in their decisions. Recent work is indicating that such adaptive decision making may be even more beneficial than previously thought (Klein, 2009, Kahneman, 2011). In fact, Klein (2009) has shown that many of our preconceived notions about good decision-making, such as checklist and rules, are not always accurate or helpful. He advocates listening to gut feelings, positing that they are often more right than a logically reasoned decision. Intuitive decision making reflecting the "gut feeling" about what is right and what is wrong in an ethical dilemma (Greene, 2003), may also be what Klein (2004) calls recognition-primed decision making.

1.7.2. Logical Reasoning

Does someone with a criminal history deserve the same consideration when it comes to a kidney transplant? What arguments could and should be used the determine this? Arguments for and against a transplant could be made on the basis of finance, justice, policy, adherence or a myriad of other factors. Health care professionals who use logical reasoning to solve health care dilemmas will consider each of these aspects and more in trying to come to the right decision.

Logical reasoning is the basis for the nursing process and therefore a very familiar and comfortable approach for nurses when considering ethical issues. In the logical approach, there is first the thoughtful identification of a problem, followed by the collection of relevant information, the development and implementation of a solution, and the evaluation of the outcome. For example, in the kidney transplant case a tremendous amount of information from pre-existing health to psychosocial status, will be collected to reach a logically derived decision. Information that may be collected includes social support, work history, age, co-morbidities, disease state, and ability to comply with medical regime. All these pieces of information and more will go into the decision about transplant status providing a reasoned, justifiable decision. In many cases it also provides the correct decision, but not always. The rational decision based upon logical reasoning assumes that all the factors that go into a decision are quantifiable. They may not be. Indeed, there is a subjective nature to at least some of the decisions made through logical reasoning.

Klein's work has identified factors where myths and misconceptions may lead us to either put more faith in the rational process than should be or to dismiss decisions made outside of the rubrics (2009). For example his research has shown that more information may not lead to a better decision or less uncertainty. Instead the additional information may serve to obscure a judicious decision. He also warns about the limitations that occur when roles are assigned, goals are set as the first step and ground rules are generated. All these seemingly rational steps in a thorough and thoughtful process can have the undesirable effect of shutting down creative problem solving by focusing on the process and not the outcome.

1.7.3. Religious Arguments

There are many cases in bioethics where there are profound moral disagreements which have a religious basis, of which the following are overt examples:

• The right of Jehovah Witnesses to refuse blood products.
• The right of Christian Scientists to use prayer for healing.
• The use of the" morning after" pill to prevent pregnancy.

A competent adult has the right to self-determination in any of these decisions as long as the decision is not illegal. The practitioner may disagree but it is the patient's right to do as he/she sees fit. Children fall into a different category and will be discussed in Chapter 6.

It should always be kept in mind that the patient's wishes, not what the family says the wishes are, are paramount. This may be particularly important in fundamentalist/patriarchal religions and cultures where the husband may see it as his right to make the health care decisions for both his wife and children. In these cases, a private conversation with the patient may ensure the patient's voice is heard.

An important cornerstone of much theology is the concept of choice, or free will. Free will is defined as the ability to choose among alternatives. Until recently, free will was considered essential for human morality (O'Connor &Franklin, 2018). Anyone could choose to make the right decision, and if they did not, their moral thinking was flawed. Sam Harris, in his book, *Free Will* (2012), proposes that human biochemistry may have more influence over our actions than does conscience thought. The notion of automatic decision making, not free will, is profoundly disturbing to many. But as Owen Jones (2012) has pointed out, one cannot will oneself out of many mental states, such as love and anger, so why should we see free as an absolute?

Pence (2004) notes that when there is a religious aspect to an ethical disagreement among professionals, it is sometimes helpful to try to steer it away from religion and into a more philosophical approach. He asks how do we know it is the deity's will ? If the answer depends on interpretation of religious writings, then many different interpretations are possible. Murder is considered morally wrong and there are many religious treatises that say just that. But if murder is wrong, what of war? What of cultures where it is permitted to murder a woman who marries against her parent's wishes? Most religions do not condemn war specifically. How is killing justified? If war is justified, what of civilians' deaths? Are the accidental killings of children during times of war morally defensible?

1.8. PHILOSOPHICAL TALKING POINTS AND THE ETHICAL DISCUSSION

There will always be discussion surrounding health care decisions. Sometimes the discussions seem minor in nature, and at other times, they have a feeling of critical significance. Regardless, all ethical decisions, large and small, are important. They are several philosophical talking points and argument strategies that all nurses should have in their ethical tool kits. They are discussed in the following paragraphs.

1.8.1. Reductio Ad Absurdum

Reductio ad absurdum is an attempt to reduce the premise of an argument to the absurd (Rescher, 2005). Nurses may recognize this as a common approach used in health care. Consider the following example:

The town is proposing to close the local hospital. One of the doctors argues if the hospital is closed no one in that town will receive the health care that they deserve.

That is an example of an argument to the absurd. If a hospital closes, people will find other ways to receive care. It may not be as convenient but it would be extremely unlikely that all people in a town would never have health care again. That would be absurd! When faced with this form of argument the best strategy is to point out its absurdity; not to treat the argument as rational.

1.8.2. Ad Hominem

Ad hominem, also known as argumentum ad hominem, is the attempt to undermine an argument by pointing out a negative characteristic or belief of the person supporting it (Goarke, 2017). Ad hominem decisions are made based upon the characteristics of the person, or family, involved. For example, the patient does not deserve a transplant because his family is a well-known crime family. Or a woman is homeless and therefore she should not be given certain medications that have to be taken at specific times. In both cases, a negative thought about crime families or homelessness carries over to the individual without any proof that it would impact the situation.

An ad hominem argument generally implies a negative halo effect that covers both the information and the person involved. A positive halo effect is also possible, although less common, in ethical arguments. This may be seen when a celebrity or politician is used to present an ethical argument.

1.8.3. Slippery Slope

Slippery slope is the argument that a small action will inevitably lead to major changes or effects (Beauchamp & Childress, 2002, 2013). It is a frequently used in health care. For example many believe that pain medication should be used sparingly because it inevitably leads to drug addiction. Others believe that if patients see their medical records they will use the information to sue the hospital. The slippery slope argument completely overlooks the middle ground and assumes that there is an inevitability that cannot be controlled. The fear of possible drug addiction may keep people who are in real pain from either asking for medication for fear of becoming addicted or from receiving the medication they need from providers who assume they will become addicts. The slippery slope argument is best countermanded by remembering that most situations are not extreme and that the middle ground/average is the norm.

1.8.4. Double Effect

Many times the ethical dilemma has to do with the double effect, where one act can have both a good and a bad outcome (Armstrong, 2007). The use of morphine for pain in the terminally ill has the benefit of alleviating pain but also the very real consequence of reducing respirations and hastening death. When making the decision to order or administer morphine, the nurse should consider four basic questions can be asked of any situation when there might be a double effect and where the answer as to what to do may not be clear (Beauchamp & Childress, 2013).

1. Is the act good in and of itself and not bad? In other words is ordering the morphine done for the reason of reducing pain and not to hasten death?
2. Is the good effect as immediate as the bad? Does the morphine reduce the pain as quickly as it might reduce respirations? If the answer is yes it is a very different decision than if you could expect the respirations to slow first followed by the reduction of pain.
3. Was only the good effect desired? Did the nurse want only to reduce pain? If the desired effect to reduce pain than it is good.
4. Is the reason for the act as important for the good effect as for the bad? In other words can pain reduction in the terminally ill be considered important enough to warrant its use?

1.8.5. The Active-passive Distinction

Acting in order to cause something to happen is generally held to a higher moral standard than not doing something or failing to take an action (Abronheim, Moreno, & Zuckerman, 2000). For example, giving a patient the wrong medication is often seen as 'more wrong' than failure to give a medication. Yet both may have equally dire consequences.

Nurses may argue that they are not the active decision maker but the passive recipient of a decision that they only carried out. For example, the APRN could be told by her employer to prescribe pain medication to a patient but not to perform the requisite pain assessment. This would be a wrong act and one that would be indefensible as the APRN knows that prescribing pain medication without a pain assessment does not meet the acceptable standard of care. The Nuremburg Trials provided very clear guidelines on this type of thinking; all people are responsible for their actions. It is not an acceptable legal or moral excuse to say one was just following orders.

1.8.6. Ordinary and Extraordinary Care Distinction

It may be difficult to distinguish ordinary from extraordinary care, but the distinction is important because there is a moral commitment to ordinary care but not necessarily to extraordinary care (Abronheim, Moreno, & Zuckerman, 2000). Ordinary care is generally thought of as simple, low risk, routine, beneficial, and low cost care that all patients can expect. Extraordinary care, on the other hand is high risk, expensive, complex, and may be of questionable benefit (Beauchamp & Childress, 2008) and patients do not have an absolute right to expect this level of care. Many devices and treatments that once were considered extraordinary, such as respirators and dialysis, are now considered routine making this distinction difficult as well as ever changing.

1.8.7. Withholding and Withdrawing Care Distinction

Withholding and withdrawing treatments provide some of the most difficult ethical decisions. On one hand treatment is never started (withheld) and on the other, treatment that has been started is stopped (withdrawn) (Beauchamp & Childress, 2013). Withholding and withdrawing treatment decisions generally, but not always, involve the end of life. A non-end of life example of withholding treatment could be parental decision not to have cochlear implants for a deaf child. An end of life decision might be to not start another chemotherapy regime for a child near death. Withdrawing treatment would involve stopping medication, therapies or nutrition.

Never starting a treatment or a medication can be distinguished from starting and then stopping the same. For example, beginning a course of chemotherapy and then stopping it is different than never starting it in the first place. Tube feeding provides another compelling situation. If tube feedings are never started it can be argued that it is not necessary to interfere with the natural process of dying, but if tube feedings are started and then stopped, there may be a sense of harm. These issues may be compounded by legalities involved. To start a treatment does not usually involve the legal system, yet its discontinuance may require a court order.

Levin and Sprung (2005) write that there are important moral distinctions between withholding and withdrawing, although others, such as the AMA do not see a difference (AMA Opinion 5.3). The AMA opinion notes that autonomy is the key ethical principle, so if a patient or the approved surrogate wants treatment not to start or to be

---

Box 1.1 - Principles of Withdrawing Life Support

1. The goal of withdrawing life-sustaining treatments is to remove treatments that are no longer desired or do not provide comfort to the patient.
2. Withholding life-sustaining treatments is morally and legally equivalent to withdrawing them.
3. Actions whose sole goal is to hasten death are morally and legally problematic.
4. Any treatment can be withheld or withdrawn.
5. Withdrawal of life-sustaining treatment is a medical procedure.
6. Corollary to 1 and 2: when circumstances justify withholding one indicated life-sustaining treatment, strong consideration should be given to withdrawing all current life-sustaining treatments.

Attributed to Rubenfeld, G.D. (2004). Principles and practices of withdrawing life-sustaining treatements. *Crit Care Clin,* 20:435_451 (used with permission from Elsivier).

stopped; it is within the patient's rights to do so. The AMA notes that they see no ethical difference between withholding and withdrawing treatment.

1.8.8. Killing and Letting Die Distinction

Patients die every day and although it is rarely discussed, many patients die without resuscitation or extraordinary measures. In many of these cases health care providers would say that these deaths are a good, natural and moral decision (Jackson, 2006). The patient is allowed to die and nature directs the time and circumstances of the death.

However, not all deaths are "natural". More and more providers are contemplating the role of assisted suicide and euthanasia in health care. The discussions about assisted suicide and euthanasia are relevant to APRNs who may be asked to participate by patients or providers. Assisted suicide is defined as giving a person the means with which to commit suicide, such as prescriptions of pain medications or sedatives. Euthanasia means actively helping the patient to die, for example by actually administering the medications to the patient (Benedict, Peirce, & Sweeney, 1998). Giving patients prescriptions with large enough dosages to take their own life is seen as fundamentally different from administering the medication. In one, the practitioner is helping the patient hasten death, in the other there is an active sense of killing the patient. This distinction has legal precedence.

The Supreme Court has distinguished between actions that actively bring about death and those that do not. The judges wrote," Everyone, regardless of physical condition, is entitled, if competent to refuse life-saving medical treatment; no one is permitted to assist suicide."(Vacco v. Quill, 117 S. Ct. 2293 [1997]). Yet the tide of thought about assisted suicide has been changing in this country.

As of the writing of this book, there are seven states, plus the District of Columbia which allow limited assistance with the accumulation of prescription medications that could be used for suicide: California, Colorado, District of Columbia, Hawaii, Montana, Oregon, Vermont, and Washington. The Oregon Death with Dignity Act withstood a 2004 and 2006 court challenge (Gonzales v Oregon 368 F. 3d 1118 (2004) affirmed by 546 U.S. 243 (2006). The debate about assisted suicide continues as other states have legislation under consideration and other courts have issued challenges.

1.9. NURSING AND ETHICAL DECISION MAKING

Ethical based decision making in the workplace may come through three primary venues; that of the individual practitioner, the ethics consultant and the ethics committee. All nurses should include themselves in bioethical discussions but this is particularly important for those with advanced preparation. Individually, advanced practice nurses make decisions on a daily basis that have ethical implications, from the simplest as to how to handle an unnecessary request for pain medications to the more complex of prescription shopping. Within teams and on ethics committees APRNs provide a unique perspective that must be included if the goal is good decision-making.

The philosophical underpinnings of ethical thought have led to several different approaches to logical ethical decision-making (Ahronheim, Moreno & Zuckerman, 2000, Beauchamp & Childress, 2013, Childress, 1997). Although often not clearly differentiated it is helpful to consider them separately as an individual who comes to ethics with a strong virtue–based approach may have fundamental differences with someone who is strongly rule adherent. Determining these differences can sometimes identify the root of the disagreement and refocus the argument to the patient. The main approaches are:

1. Deontology (rule adherence) approach. All ethical decisions should follow the prescribed, previously established rules. These may include policies and procedures, as well as regulations and laws.
2. Utilitarian approach. The ethical decision should be the one that does the least harm and brings about the greatest good.

3. Human rights approach. Ethical decision-making should be based upon human rights including free will, liberty, privacy and so forth.
4. Justice approach. All ethical decision should be fair and just, based upon the ideals of distributive and commutative justice.
5. Virtue approach. Ethical decisions should contribute to character by demonstrating or being consistent with the appropriate virtues such as kindness, loyalty, unselfishness and so forth.

1.10. ETHICS COMMITTEES, ETHICS CONSULTANTS AND ETHICAL DECISION MAKING PROCESSES

Hospital Ethics Committees (HEC) evolved in part from suggestions from the court in the Karen Ann Quinlan case (Aulisio, 2016). Almost all hospitals now have ethics committees as a result of state or organizational mandates but even if they don't JCAH requires that all hospitals have a mechanism to resolve ethical issues. In general, HECs are composed of physicians, nurses, clergy, attorneys, social workers, hospital administrators and others (see Peirce, 2004 about the importance of diversity in committee composition). HECs provide guidance and direction about ethical dilemmas, develop policies and provide ethics education and training. The assumption underlying the work of HECs is that the focus is on the patient and not that of the institution or workers, although that is not always true, nor desirable. It should be noted that HECs have quasi-legal standing and courts often defer to their decisions (Peirce, 2004).

Ethics consultants are clinical ethics experts who can be called upon when there are ethics questions. The consultant can lead the interested parties through a decision making process, helping to clarify issues and solidify decisions. The consultant can either be an individual or sometimes a subcommittee of a larger HEC.

Common issues that are generally considered by ethics committees (Romano et al, 2009)

1. Withholding or withdrawing treatment
2. Appropriateness of treatment, goals of care, or futility
3. Resuscitation
4. Legal-ethics interface
5. Competency or decisional capacity
6. Psychiatric

7. Family conflict
8. Staff or professional conflict
9. Discharge disposition
10. Allocation of resources

HECs, consultants and individuals may all use a rationally based step-wise process to resolve ethical dilemmas. To start with all relevant information must be gathered, not only from the person posing the dilemma, but from those representing alternate views as well. It may be necessary to review case law, institutional policies, relevant literature or other precedent cases. Baseline ethical principles should be identified in any case. Finally a written summary and recommendation should be provided.

Not all advanced practice registered nurses will work in places with HECs or consultants, but all nurses can use the same process by themselves or with interested others to more fully understand a dilemma before making a final decision. It also should be remembered that neuroethics may play a strong, previously unrecognized role in decision making. A decision made intuitively by an individual may represent the best decision at the time but when reconsidered by a group rational approach with knowledge of results and additional information a different decision may be considered the best.

A generic list of rationally based questions, culled from a variety of sources, is as follows (Ahronheim, Moreno & Zuckerman, 2000, Beauchamp & Childress, 2013, Childress, 1997):

1. What is the dilemma?
   a. A clear concise articulation of the problem is the first step.
2. What are the facts of the case?
   a. If it is a question regarding a patient, what is the current medical situation, treatment ramifications if relevant, and prognosis?
   b. Is the patient competent?
      i. What are the patient's wishes?
   c. For other situations consider who, what, when, where and how.
3. Who is concerned about the situation and why?
   a. Who else should have input into the decision?
   b. What does the family want?
   c. Are there religious considerations? If so is an appropriate clergy available?

4. Are there quality of life issues?
5. What ethical principles are relevant?
6. Are there legal issues?
   a. Are there laws governing the case?
   b. Are there advanced directives, living wills, power of attorney, guardianship or other legal documents to be considered?
7. Are there institutional policy issues to be considered?
8. Are there professional standards or codes of ethics to be considered?
9. Are there undue financial or social burdens involved?
10. If the conflict resolvable or is there an acceptable compromise?
11. What next steps are needed if no resolution is possible?

1.11. MICROETHICS

In recent years attention has turned from focus on the rare and unusual ethics event that may require referral to an ethics committee (macroethics), to the ethics of the everyday (Truog et al, 2015). These small ethical dilemmas have been labeled microethics. It is apparent that the everyday choices that APRNs make are ethically significant, be it who to see first when faced with two patients who require care to maintaining eye contact during difficult discussions (Komesaroff, 1995). In yet another example, Berlinger (2016) makes a compelling argument about the ethics of the common nursing practice of creating workarounds to compensate for lack of supplies and materials.

Microethics forces us to take the view from the inside rather than the view from the outside (Truog, et al, 2015); that is what are the individual ethical needs and wants as opposed to the traditional use of theory, decision analysis and standard principles. Truong et al (2015) emphasize that the two approaches are not contradictory but instead complementary. We would argue that as with much of health care it is important not to split the discussion into an either or, but to see ethics as a whole, from the major to the minor.

The role values play in ethical decision making are critical in both the provider and the patient and while this is certainly acknowledged in the health care literature it is not as well understood as might be expected. Truong et al (2015) suggest that microethics compels practitioners to help patients arrive at a decision that resonances with their core values. It thus becomes a hands on process rather than a hands off process, made all the more difficult by the need to not "nudge" the patient in a certain direction (Thaler & Sunstein, 2008).

1.12. SUMMARY

Ethics and ethical decision making is important and will become even more so in the future. Advanced practice registered nurses must make decisions regarding clinical care that are ethically as well as clinically defensible. Many avenues are available for support including ethics consultation, clinical ethics committees, moral case deliberation, ethics rounds, ethics discussion groups, and ethics reflection groups (Rasoal, Skovdahl, Gifford, & Kihlgren, 2017). This chapter provides the language and background needed to participate in discussions about ethical dilemmas. In the following chapters specific clinical populations with their particular issues will be considered.

1.13. WEBSITES

- **ANA Code of Ethics (2015):**
  https://www.nursingworld.org/practice-policy/
  nursing-excellence/ethics/code-of-ethics-for-nurses/
- **American Medical Association Code of Ethics:**
  https://www.ama-assn.org/delivering-care/ethics
- **Brain Toolkit:**
  https://www.neurocriticalcare.org/education/digital- education/brain-death-toolkit
- **The Stanford Encyclopedia of Philosophy:** www.plato.stanford.edu
- **National Academy of Medicine*:**
  https://nam.edu/human-genome-editing-science-ethics-and-governance/

*The Institute of Medicine (IOM) is now known as the National Academy of Medicine (NAM). Please note within this book that references may include both names (IOM/NAM) or just IOM or NAM dependent on the circumstances.

1.14. REFERENCES

ACOG Committee Opinion. Number 695. (April, 2017). Sterilization of women: Ethical issues and considerations. https://www.acog.org/-/media/Committee-Opinions/Committee-on-Ethics/co695.pdf.

Acquisti, A., Brandimarte, L. & Loewenstein, G. (2015). Privacy and human behavior in the age of information. *Nature* 347: 6221, 509-514.

Ad Hoc Committee of the Harvard Medical School (1968). A definition of irreversible coma—report of the Ad Hoc Committee of the Harvard Medical School to examine the definition of brain death," *Journal of the American Medical Association*, 205 (6): 337–40.

Ahronheim, J.C. Moreno, J.D. & Zuckerman, C. (2000). *Ethics in Clinical Practice*. Gaithersberg MD: Aspen.

AMA (accessed, 2019) Opinion 5.3- Withholding or withdrawing Life-Sustaining Medical Treatment. American Medical Association. https://www.ama-assn.org/delivering-care/ethics/withholding-or-withdrawing-life-sustaining-treatment.

Armstrong, A.E. (2007). *Nursing Ethics: a Virtue-Based Approach*. New York: Palgrave MacMillan.

Arras, J. (Winter 2016 Edition). Theory and Bioethics, *The Stanford Encyclopedia of Philosophy*, Edward N. Zalta (ed.), URL = <https://plato.stanford.edu/archives/win2016/entries/theory-bioethics/>.

Aristotle (1980). *The Nicomachean Ethics*. Ross, D. trans. Revised Ackrill, J.L. & Urmson, J.O. UK: Oxford University Press.

Ahronheim, J.C. Moreno, J.D. & Zuckerman, C. (2005). Ethics in Clinical Practice (2nd ed), Boston: Jones & Bartlett

Auslio, M.O. (2016). Why did hospital ethics committees emerge in the US? *AMA J Ethics*. 18(5): 546-553. doi: 10.1001/journalofethics.2016.18.5.mhst1-1605.

Baltzly, D. (Summer 2018 Edition). Stoicism, *The Stanford Encyclopedia of Philosophy*, Edward N. Zalta (ed), URL = <https://plato.stanford.edu/archives/sum2018/entries/stoicism/>.

Bartz, R. (2000). Remembering the Hippocratics: Knowledge, practice, and ethos of ancient Greek physician-healers. In Kuczewski, M.G. & Polansky, R. (eds). *Bioethics: Ancient Times in Contemporary Issues*. Cambridge MA: Bradford.

BBC (accessed 2019). Kant (https://www.youtube.com/watch?v=x_uUEaeqFog).

Beauchamp, T. (Winter 2016 Edition), The Principle of Beneficence in Applied Ethics, *The Stanford Encyclopedia of Philosophy*, Edward N. Zalta (ed.), URL = <https://plato.stanford.edu/archives/win2016/entries/principle-beneficence/>.

Beauchamp, T.L. & Childress, J.F. (2002). *Principles of Biomedical Ethics* (2nd ed). New York: Oxford University.

Beauchamp, T.L. & Childress, J.F. (2013). *Principles of Biomedical Ethics* (7th ed). New York: Oxford University.

Beauchamp, T. Walters, L. Kahn, J.P. & Mastroianni, A.C. (2008). *Contemporary Issues in Bioethics* (7th ed) Belmont CA: Thomson Wadsworth.

Benedict, S. & Kuhla, J. (1999). Nurses participation in the euthanasia programs of Nazi Germany. *Western Journal of Nursing Research*, 21(2): 246-63.

Benedict, S, Peirce, A & Sweeney, S (1998). Historical, ethical, and legal aspects of assisted suicide. *Journal of the Association of Nurses in AIDS Care*, 9(2): 34-44.

Benner, P (1984). *From novice to expert: Excellence and power in clinical nursing practice*. Menlo Park: Addison-Wesley, pp. 13-34.

Benthem, J. (1961). *The Principles of Morals and Legislation*. Garden City: Doubleday.

Berlinger, N. (2016). *Are Workarounds Ethical? Managing Moral Problems in Health Care Systems*. NY: Oxford University Press. ISBN: 978-0-19-026929-6.

Blackburn, S. (2001). *Ethics: a Very Short Introduction*. Oxford UK: Oxford University Press.

Bok, S. (1978). *Lying: Moral Choice in Public and Private Life*. New York: Vintage Books.

Bringsjord, S. & Govindarajulu, N.S. (Fall 2018 Edition), Artificial Intelligence, *The Stanford Encyclopedia of Philosophy*. Edward N. Zalta (ed.), URL = <https://plato.stanford.edu/archives/fall2018/entries/artificial-intelligence/>.

Bulger, R.E., Heitman, E., & Reiser, S.J. (2002). *The Ethical Dimensions of the Biological and Health Sciences* (2nd ed). Cambridge UK: Cambridge University Press.

Cahn-Fuller, K. & Parent B. (2017). Transplant Eligibility for Patients with Affective and Psychotic disorders: a Review of Practices and a Call for Justice. *BMC Medical Ethics* 78:17 http//:doi: 10.1186/512910-017-0235.4.

Carpenter, K. & Dittrich, D. (2011). Bridging the distance: Removing the technology buffer and seeking consistent ethical analysis in computer security research. 1st International Digital Ethics Symposium, Loyola University Chicago Center for digital Ethics and Policy. Google Scholar

Char, D.S., Shah, N.H. & Magnus, D. (2018). Implementing Machine Learning in Health Care-Addressing Ethical Challenges. *N Engl J Med* 378(11): 981-983.

Childress, J.E. (1997). *Practical Reasoning in Bioethics*, Bloomington IN: Indiana University.

Chitty, K.K. & Black, B.P. (2011). *Professional Nursing: Concepts and Challenges.* Maryland Heights MO: Saunders Elsevier.

Christians, C.G. (Accessed January 2019). The Ethics of Privacy, *Oxford Scholarship Online* DOI:10.1093/acprof:oso/9780195370805.003.0014

Cicero (1914). *De Finibus et Molorum.* H. Rackham, trans. NY: Macmillan.

Collins, K. (2007). Maimonides and the ethics of patient autonomy. *IMAJ*, 9: 55-58.

Conway, P., Goldstein-Greenwood, J., Polacek, D., Greene, J.D. (2018). Sacrificial utilitarian judgments do reflect concern for the greater good: Clarification via process dissociation and the judgments of philosophers *Cognition* 179, 241-265

Daniels, N. (Winter 2017 Edition), Justice and Access to Health Care, *The Stanford Encyclopedia of Philosophy*, Edward N. Zalta (ed.), URL = <https://plato.stanford.edu/archives/win2017/entries/justice-healthcareaccess/>.

Dennet D. (2017). Lunch with the FT: Daniel Dennett. Interview by J. Thornhill. *Financial Times Weekend*, 4-5, March 2017, Life, p. 3.

Driver, J/ (Winter 2014 Edition), "The History of Utilitarianism", *The Stanford Encyclopedia of Philosophy*, Edward N. Zalta (ed.), URL = <https://plato.stanford.edu/archives/win2014/entries/utilitarianism-history/>.

Drizis, T.J. (2008). Medical ethics in the writings of Galen. *Acta med-hist Adriat*, 6(2): 333-336.

Edmonds, D. (2014). *Would You Kill the Fat Man?: The Trolley Problem and What your answer Tells Us About Right and Wrong.* Princeton: Princeton University Press.

Engel, G.L. (1977). The need for a new medical model: A challenge for biomedicine. *Science*, 196: 129–136. doi: 10.1126/science.847460

Faden, R. & Shebaya, S. (Winter 2016 Edition), "Public Health Ethics", *The Stanford Encyclopedia of Philosophy* Edward N. Zalta (ed.), URL = <https://plato.stanford.edu/archives/win2016/entries/publichealth-ethics/>.

Foot, P. (1978). *Virtues and Vices and Other Essays in Moral Philosophy.* Oxford: Oxford University Press.

Fowler, MDM (2015). *The Code of Ethics for Nurses with Interpretive Statements: Development, Interpretation and Application (2nd ed).* American Nurses Association, Silver Spring MD: Nursebooks.org.

Frankena,W. (1988). *Ethics.* Englewood Cliffs NJ: Prentice Hall.

Franssen, M., Lokhorst, G.J. and van de Poel, I., (Fall 2018 Edition). Philosophy of Technology, *The Stanford Encyclopedia of Philosophy*, Edward N. Zalta (ed.), https://plato.stanford.edu/archives/fall2018/entries/technology/.

Fry, S.T. & Veatch, R.M. (2006). *Case Studies in Nursing Ethics* (3rd ed). Sudbury MA: Jones and Bartlett.

Gazzaniga, M.S. (2005). *The Ethical Brain.* New York: Dana Press.

Gert, B. & Gert, J. (Fall 2017 Edition),The Definition of Morality, *The Stanford Encyclopedia of Philosophy*, Edward N. Zalta (ed.), URL = <https://plato.stanford.edu/archives/fall2017/entries/morality-definition/>.

Gesundheit, B. (2011). Maimonides' appreciation for medicine. RMMJ, 2(1): 1-8.

Groarke, L. (Spring 2017 Edition). Informal Logic, *The Stanford Encyclopedia of Philosophy* Edward N. Zalta (ed.), URL = <https://plato.stanford.edu/archives/spr2017/entries/logic-informal/>.

Greene, J (2003). From neural 'is' to moral 'ought': what are the moral implications of neuroscientific moral psychology? Nature Reviews/Neuroscience. 4(October): 847-850.

Greene, J.D. (2007). Why are VMPFC patients more utilitarian? A dual process theory of moral judgment explains. *Trends in Cognitive Sciences*, 11(8): 322-323.

Greene, J.D., Cushman, F.A., Stewart, L.E., Lowenburg, K., Nystrom, L.E., & Cohen, J.D. (2009). Pushing moral buttons: The interaction between personal force and intention in moral judgment. *Cognition*. doi:10.1016/j.cognition.2009.02.001.

Greene, J.D., Morelli, S.A., Lowenberg, K., Nystrom, L.E., & Cohen, J.D. (2008). Cognitive load selectively interferes with utilitarian moral judgment. *Cognition*, doi:10.1016/j.cognition.2007.11.004.

Greene, J.D., & Paxton, J.M. (2009). Patterns of neural activity associated with honest and dishonest moral decisions. *PNAS*, 106(30): 12506-12511.

Greene, J.D. (2017) The Rat-a-gorical Imperative: Moral Intuition and the Limits of Affective Learning. *Cognition* 167: 66-77.

Grossman, C.L. (3 Jan 2014). *Family, ethics, medicine and law collide in Jahi McMath's life-or death*. Washington Post.

Harris, S. (2012). *Free Will*, NY: Free Press.

Hauser, M.D. (2008). The liver and the moral organ. *Soc Cogn Affect Neurosci*. 1(3): 214-220.

Held, V. (2005). *The Ethics of Care*. Oxford: Oxford University Press. doi:10.1093/0195180992.001.0001.

HHS (accessed 2019). Guidance Regarding Methods for De-identification of Protected Health Information in Accordance with the Health Insurance Portability and Accountability Act (HIPAA) Privacy Rule

https://www.hhs.gov/hipaa/for-professionals/privacy/special-topics/de-identification/index.html

Houchmandzadeh, B. & Vallade, M (2012). Selection for altruism through random drift in variable size populations. *BMC Evol*. Biol. 12(1), 61.

Hursthouse, R. & Pettigrove, G. (Winter 2018 Edition).Virtue Ethics, *The Stanford Encyclopedia of Philosophy*, Edward N. Zalta (ed.), URL = <https://plato.stanford.edu/archives/win2018/entries/ethics-virtue/>.

Ienca, M., Vayena, E & Blasimme, A. (2018). Big Data, and dementia: Charting the route ahead for research, ethics and policy. *Perspective5*:13, doi: 10.3389/fmed.2018.00013.

Jackson, J. (2006). *Ethics in Medicine*. Malden MA: Polity Press.

Jones, O. (2012). The end of discussing free will. *Chronicle of Higher Education*. http:// chronicle.com/article/Is-Free-Will-An-Illusion-131159.

Kahane, G., Everett, J.A.C., Earp, B.D., Caviola, L., Faber, N.S., Crockett, M.J., & Savulescu, J. (2018). Beyond sacrificial harm: A two-dimensional model of utilitarian psychology. *Psychological Review*, 125(2), 131-164. http://dx.doi.org/10.1037/rev0000093.

Kahneman, D. (2002). Maps of bounded rationality: A perspective on intuition, judgment and choice. Nobel Prize Lecture, December 8, 2002. http://www.nobelprize. org/nobel_prizes/economics/laureate/2002/kahnemann-lecture.pdf.

Kahneman, D. (2011). *Thinking Fast and Slow*. NY: Farrar, Straus and Giroux.

Kant, I. (1998) *Critique of Pure Reason*. Guyer, P., & Wood, A.W., trans-eds. Cambridge UK: Cambridge University Press.

Kant, I. (1993). *Grounding for the Metaphysics of Morals*. J.W. Ellington, trans. London UK: Hackett.

Klein, G.A. (2004). *The Power of Intuition*. NY: Currency Book.

Klein, G.A. (2009). *Streetlights and Shadows: Searching for the Keys to Adaptive Decision Making*. Cambridge, MA: MIT Press.

Komesaroff, P.A. (1995)."From Bioethics to Microethics: Ethical Debate and Clinical Medicine," in *Troubled Bodies: Critical Perspectives on Postmodernism, Medical Ethics, and the Bodied*. Durham, N.C.: Duke University Press.

Kuczewski, M.G. & Polansky, R. (eds) (2000). *Bioethics: Ancient Times in Contemporary Issues*. Cambridge MA: Bradford.

Levin, P.D. & Sprung, C.L. (2005). Withdrawing and withholding life-sustaining therapies are not the same. *Crit. Care 9*(3): 230-232.

Levy, N. (2011). Neuroethics: A new way of doing ethics. *AJOB Neurosci*. 2(2): 3-9.

Mappes,T.A., & Degrazia, D. (2001). *Biomedical Ethics* (5th ed.). New York: McGraw-Hill.

McConnell, T. (Fall 2018 Edition). Moral Dilemmas, *The Stanford Encyclopedia of Philosophy*, Edward N. Zalta (ed.), URL = <https://plato.stanford.edu/archives/ fall2018/entries/moral-dilemmas/>.

McGowan K. (2016) Our medical data must become free. *WIRED*. https://www.wired. com/2016/02/our-medical-data-must-become-free/.

McIntyre, A. (Spring 2019 Edition). Doctrine of Double Effect, *The Stanford Encyclopedia of Philosophy*, Edward N. Zalta (ed.), forthcoming URL = <https://plato. stanford.edu/archives/spr2019/entries/double-effect/>.

Meyers, H.S. (2006). Review of *Maimonides* (2005) by S.B. Nuland. NY: Schoken. JAMA 295(2): 217. doi: 10.1001/jama.295.2.217-a.

Mill, J.S. (1871). *Utilitarianism*. London UK: Longmans.

Moor, J.H. (1990). The ethics of privacy protection. *Library Trends* 39: 1-2, pp. 69-82.

Murphy, M. (Winter 2011 Edition). The Natural Law Tradition in Ethics, *The Stanford Encyclopedia of Philosophy* Edward N. Zalta (ed.), URL = <https://plato.stanford. edu/archives/win2011/entries/natural-law-ethics/>.

Morris, W.E. & Brown, C.R. (Spring 2017 Edition), "David Hume", *The Stanford Encyclopedia of Philosophy*, Edward N. Zalta (ed.), URL = <https://plato.stanford. edu/archives/spr2017/entries/hume/>.

Murphy, L.B. (1993). The demands of beneficence. *Philosophy and Public Affairs*, 22: 267–92.

Murphy, M. (Winter 2011 Edition), The Natural Law Tradition in Ethics, *The Stanford Encyclopedia of Philosophy*, Edward N.. Zalta (ed.), URL = <https://plato.stanford. edu/archives/win2011/entries/natural-law-ethics/>.

Narayanan, A. & Shmatikov, V. (2010). Myths and fallacies of "personally identifiable information". Communications of the ACM 53 (6): 24. doi:10.1145/1743546.1743558.

Neurocritical Care Society (accessed January, 2019). Brain Death Toolkit. https:// www.neurocriticalcare.org/education/digital-education/brain-death-toolkit.

NIH (accessed 2018). What is Big Data? https://datascience.nih.gov/bd2k/about/what.

NYSNA. New York State Nurses Assciation. (n.d.) Role of the registered professional nurse in ethical decision-making. NYSNA Position Statement. http:// www.nysna. org/practice/positions/position6.htm.

Nuland, S. (2008). *Maimonides*, NY: Schocken Books.

Nussbaum, M. (2003). Capabilities as fundamental entitlements: Sen and social justice. *Feminist Economics*, 9: 2-3:33-59.

O'Connor, T. & Franklin, C. (Fall 2018 Edition), "Free Will", *The Stanford Encyclopedia of Philosophy*., Edward N. Zalta (ed.), URL = <https://plato.stanford.edu/archives/fall2018/entries/freewill/>.

ORI (Office of Research Integrity) (accessed January, 2019). Nuremberg Code: Directives for human Experimentation. https://ori.hhs.gov/content/chapter-3-The-Protection-of-Human-Subjects-nuremberg-code-directives-human-experimentation.

Orem D.E., Taylor S.G. (2011). Reflections on nursing practice science: the nature, the structure, and the foundation of nursing sciences. *Nurs Sci Q*, Jan; 24(1): 35-41. doi 10.1177/0894318410389.

Paul, E.F., Miller, F.D. & Paul, J. (2002). *Bioethics*. Cambridge UK: Cambridge University.

Paxton, J.M., Greene, J.D., (2010) Moral reasoning: Hints and allegations. *Topics in Cognitive Science*. DOI: 10.1111/j.1756-8765.2010.01096.x

Paxton, J.M., Ungar, L. & Greene, J.D. (2011). Reflection and reasoning in moral judgment. *Cognitive Science*, doi: 10:1111/j.1551-6709.2011.01210.x

Paharia, N. Kassam, K.S., Greene, J.D. & Bazerman, M.H. (2009). Dirty hands, clean work: The moral psychology of indirect agency. *Organizational Behavior and Human Decision Processes*. doi: 10.1016/obhdp.2009.03.002.

Peirce, A.G. (2004). Some considerations about decisions and decision–makers in hospital ethics committees. *Online Journal of Health Ethics*.1:1. http://test2.ojhe.org/index.php/ojhe/article/viewarticle/14/17

Peirce, A.G. (2017). *The Words of Florence Nightingale: Lesser Saint, Philosopher, Social Activist, Political Reformer and Accidental Nurse*. Litchfield ME: Cobassee Press. ISBN:9781544982397.

Peirce, A.G. & Eckhart, P. (nd). 'Black Swan' nursing in times of evidence based practice. Unpublished manuscript.

Peirce, A.G. & Smith, J.A. (2008). The ethics curriculum for doctor of nursing practice programs. *Journal of Professional Nursing*. 24(5): 270-274.

Pellegrino, E.D., & Thomasma, D.C. (1993). *The Virtues in Medical Practice*. New York: Oxford University.

Pence, G.E. (2004). *Classic Cases in Medical Ethics: Accounts of Cases that have Shaped Medical Ethics with Philosophical, Legal and Historical Background* (4th ed). New York: McGraw-Hill.

Pearlman R.A. (2016, modified). Ethics in Medicine: Ethics Committees and Ethics Consultation. University of Washington School of Medicine. http://depts.washington.edu/bioethx/topcs/ethics.html

Prehn, K., Wartenburger, I., Mériau, K., Scheibe, C., Goodenough, O.R., Villringer, A, van der Meer, E, & Heekeren, H.R. (2007). Individual differences in moral judgment competence influence neural correlates of socio-normative judgments. *Soc Cogn Affect Neurosci*. 3(1): 33-46.

Rasoal, D., Skovdahl, K., Gifford, M. & Kihlgren, A. (2017). Clinical ethics support for healthcare personnel: an integrative literature review. *HEC Forum* 29(4): 313-349. doi:10.1007/s10730-17-9325.4

Rawls, J. (1971). *A Theory of Justice*. Cambridge MA: Belknap Press.

Rescher, N. (2005 revised). Reductio ad Absurdam. *Internet Encyclopedia of Philosophy*. www.iep.utm.edu/reductio/.

Richards, N.M. & King J.H. (2014). Big Data ethics. *Wake Forest Law Review* 49(2), 393-432.

Richardson, H.S. (Fall 2018 Edition). Moral Reasoning, *The Stanford Encyclopedia of Philosophy*, Edward N. Zalta (ed.), URL = <https://plato.stanford.edu/archives/fall2018/entries/reasoning-moral/>.

Robeyns, I. (Winter 2016 Edition). The Capability Approach, *The Stanford Encyclopedia of Philosophy*, Edward N. Zalta (ed.), URL = <https://plato.stanford.edu/archives/win2016/entries/capability-approach/>.

Rohlf, M. (Summer 2018 Edition). Immanuel Kant, *The Stanford Encyclopedia of Philosophy*, Edward N. Zalta (ed.), URL = <https://plato.stanford.edu/archives/sum2018/entries/kant/>.

Romano, M.E., Wahlander, B., Lang, B.H., Li, G. & Prager, K.M.(2009). Mandatory ethics consultation policy. *Mayo Clin Proc.*, 84(7): 581–585.

Roskies, A., (Summer 2016 Edition).Neuroethics. *The Stanford Encyclopedia of Philosophy* Edward N. Zalta (ed.), URL = <https://plato.stanford.edu/archives/spr2016/entries/neuroethics/>.

Ross, W.D. (1930). *The Right and the Good*. Oxford UK: Clarendon Press.

Roughgarden, J. (2012). Teamwork, pleasure and bargaining in animal social behavior. *J. of Evol. Biol*.25(7). 1454-62.

Rubenfeld, G.D. (2004). Principles and practices of withdrawing life-sustaining treatments. *Crit Care Clin*, 20:435–451

Sarbey, B. (2016). Definitions of death: brain death and what matters in a person. *Journal of Law and the Biosciences*, 3(3), 743-752. doi:10.1093/jlb/lsw054

Scheffler, S. (1997). Relationships and responsibilities. *Philosophy and Public Affairs*, 26: 189-209.

Schwab, K. (2016). *The Fourth Industrial Revolution*. NY: Crown Publishing Group.

Sen, A. (2005). Human rights and capabilities. *Journal of Human Development*, 6(2): 151-66.

Simonite, T. (2015). Probing the dark side of google's ad-targeting system. *MITS Technol Rev.* https://www.technologyreview.com/s/539021/probing-the-dark-side-of-googles-ad-targeting-system/.

Singer, P. (1972). Famine, affluence, and morality. *Philosophy and Public Affairs*, 1: 229–43.

Singer, P. (2011). *Practical Ethics* (3rd ed). Cambridge UK: Cambridge University Press.

Singer, P. (1999). Living high and letting die. *Philosophy and Phenomenological Research*. 59: 183–87.

Smeltzer, S.C., Bare, BG, Hinkle, J.L. & Cheever, K.H. (2010). *Brunner & Suddarth's Textbook of Medical-Surgical Nursing* (12th ed.). Philadelphia: Wolters Klower Health/Lippincott, Williams & Wilkes.

Soon, C.S., Brass, M., Heinze, H.-J. & Haynes, J.-D. (2008). Unconscious determinants of free decisions in the human brain. *Nature Neuroscience*, 11: 543-45. doi: 10.1038/nn2112.

Thaler, R.H., & Sunstein, C.R. (2008). *Nudge: Improving Decisions about Health, Wealth and Happiness*. New York: Penguin.

Tiku, A. (2018), Europe's new privacy laws will change the web, and more. *WIRED, https://www.wired.com/story/europes-new-privacy-law-will-change-the-web-and-more/.*

Truog, R.D. Berlinger, N., Zacharias, R.L. & Solomon, M.Z. (2018). What does dead mean? *Hastings Center Report*. https://www.thehastingscenter.org/publications-resources/special-reports-2/what-does-dead-mean/

Tuong, R.D., Brown, S.D., Brownin, D., Hundert, E.M., Rider, E.A., Bell, S.K. & Meyer, E.C. (2015). Microethics: The ethics of everyday clinical practice. *Hastings Center Report* 45: 1, 11–17. doi: 10.1002/hast.413.

Wilson, D.S. (2007). Rethinking the theoretical foundation of sociobiology. *The Quarterly Review of Biology*. 82(4): 1-43. doi: 10.1086/522809.

Zimmer, M. (2018). Addressing conceptual gaps in Big Data research ethics: An application of contextual integrity. *Social Media + Society*, April-June, 1-11.

Zsakó, L., & Szlávi, P. (2012). ICT competencies: Algorithmic thinking. *Acta Didactica Napocensia*, 5(2), 49-58. https://search-proquest-com.libproxy.adelphi.edu:2443/docview/1372344065?accountid=8204.

Zumpano-Canto, J. (1996). Nonconsensual sterilization of mentally disabled in North Carolina: An ethics critique of the statutory standard and its judicial interpretation. *Journal of Contemporary Health Policy Law*, 13(1): 79-111.

CHAPTER 2

Research Ethics

NANCY KING REAME

"The scientific research enterprise is built on a foundation of trust. Scientists trust that the results reported by others are valid. Society trusts that the results of research reflect an honest attempt by scientists to describe the world accurately and without bias. But this trust will endure only if the scientific community devotes itself to exemplifying and transmitting the values associated with ethical scientific conduct."
—On Being a Scientist (National Academy of Sciences, 2009)

2.1. INTRODUCTION

With the rapid developments in 21st Century health care, most doctorally-educated nurses, whether DNP or PhD prepared will be involved in either the discovery or translation of clinical care innovation. Research ethics, defined as "the ethics of the planning, conduct and reporting of research" (NAPRI, 2016), is a necessary cornerstone of training for all clinical scholars. To develop and integrate evidence-based practice requires a working knowledge of the responsible conduct of research and the elements of scientific integrity. Specifically, a foundation in research ethics is essential for several reasons:

1. To fully comply with the legal requirements for knowledge competency about the ethical treatment of human subjects, all participants at any level of the research team, from subject recruiter to lead investigator, including students, must be certified by their sponsoring institution.
2. To ensure the safety of patients serving as research participants, including their privacy and fully-informed consent to participate.
3. To protect students and researchers themselves from unsafe or unethical practices.

4. To appropriately guide the resolution of misunderstandings, disputes or research misconduct.
5. To preserve the public's trust and support of the national research agenda.

Clinical nurse specialists, clinical leaders, nurse navigators and others in specialty roles also require an understanding of research ethics, given their important role in patient advocacy and safety, and as valued members of the research team. Because the breadth and scope of content in research ethics has dramatically expanded in the last decade, this chapter serves as a general introduction to essential content for the ethical conduct of research involving human subjects. Additional readings and resources are provided for advanced study.

2.2. HISTORICAL CONTEXT FOR THE CONTEMPORARY MODEL OF RESEARCH ETHICS

A detailed discussion of the philosophical underpinnings of research ethics is beyond the scope of this chapter, but it is important to understand the historical context of the rules, regulations and moral codes that define the ethical conduct of contemporary research. Sadly, many of the regulations and laws that guide the American research enterprise today came about in response to terrible acts of misconduct and unethical practices of medical researchers over the last 70 years. Most infamously, the medical experiments performed on prisoners of war by Nazi doctors in the early 1940s served as the springboard for worldwide guidelines to prevent such atrocities ever again. The Nuremberg Code in 1949 was the first international code of ethics to specify rules for the humane treatment of research subjects. Although it had no force of law, key elements included mandates that:

- Human participation must be justified, and only after animal studies show promising results.
- There has been voluntary, informed consent, with the freedom (free will) to withdraw.
- The expected outcome holds promise of benefit to society.
- Subjects are protected from unnecessary physical and mental harm or injury, without any undue risk of suffering, disability or death.
- The experimenters are qualified.

The Declaration of Helsinki, created for physicians in 1964 by the World Medical Association, amplified the principles of the Nuremberg code to specifically address the use of patients as research subjects in the context of their care. It also expanded the limits of informed consent to allow for surrogate (proxy) consent when the potential research subject is incompetent, physically or mentally incapable of consenting, or is a minor.

2.2.1. Scientific Misconduct and Ethical Abuses in the U.S.

Despite these international reforms, it wasn't until the 1970s that the U.S. government responded with its own laws and regulations, after several alarming cases of abuses involving highly vulnerable populations were disclosed in the lay press (Truog, 2012). For example, in the early 1960s, researchers at the Willowbrook State School in New York intentionally infected disabled children with hepatitis to test a gamma globulin treatment. In a separate case at the same time, elderly patients at the Brooklyn Jewish Chronic Disease Hospital were injected with liver cancer cells without their knowledge and observed for tumor growth. Dr. Henry Beecher's exposure of these and dozens of other abuse cases in the New England Journal of Medicine (Beecher, 1966) forced the American public health community to confront the idea that blatantly unethical research was prevalent in the U.S., even in the wards of the most prestigious academic medical centers.

Probably the most notorious and consequential case of ethical abuses in biomedical experiments occurred in the Tuskegee syphilis study, which ran for 40 years from 1932–1972. Sponsored by the U.S. Public Health Service, medical researchers studied the effects of untreated syphilis in some 400 African-American men from impoverished farming areas near Tuskegee, Alabama. Although not deliberately infected with syphilis as is sometimes reported in error (Reverby, 2001), male residents of Macon County were recruited to undergo diagnostic lumbar punctures (called "back shots"), and then told they were being medically "treated" for "bad blood", a lay term of the time referring to a non-specific medical condition. Not only were subjects unaware of their participation in a research study, but they were intentionally deceived about the nature of their illness, and offered incentives for staying in the study including free health care (for conditions other than syphilis), exemption from the military draft, and life insurance coverage for funeral costs. Most troubling, the subjects were not given counseling on how to avoid spreading the disease to their partners, nor treated with penicillin once it became widely available by the late 1940s. It wasn't until a young investigator revealed the story to the New York Times in 1972, that the study was forced to close down. By that time, more than 100 affected individuals (including wives and children) had died.

As noted by Corbie-Smith (1999), the 40-year study became "the longest non-therapeutic experiment on humans in the history of medicine, and has come to represent not only the exploitation of blacks, but the potential for exploitation for any population that may be vulnerable because of race, ethnicity, gender, disability, age or social class". Although it would take another 25 years before an official Presidential apology was issued to the surviving victims and their families (Reverby, 2011), the Tuskegee scandal spawned a series of landmark regulations and rules of conduct that remain in effect today to help protect research subjects and researchers themselves from acts of deliberate or unintentional wrong-doing.

2.3. THE U.S. GOVERNMENT RESPONDS TO RESEARCH ABUSES: THE BELMONT REPORT

In 1973, the Department of Health, Education and Welfare (now Health and Human Services) drafted the first set of federal regulations on the protection of human subjects. Foremost was the mandate that all biomedical research studies funded by the government must be reviewed, approved and overseen by a local institutional review board (IRB) composed of scientists and the lay community for the purpose of protecting the rights of research participants. In 1974, the National Research Act was passed by Congress, which authorized federal agencies to systematically formalize (codify) regulations for the protection of human research subjects. The Act also created a national commission to examine the ethics of research with human subjects. It took 5 years for this same commission to publish its famous Belmont Report (named after the building where the meetings took place in Washington, DC) in 1979 that defined the key principles that serve as the foundation for the ethical conduct of research today. The Belmont Report laid out three fundamental rules of conduct as a framework for judging professional ethical practices in all aspects of research: respect for persons, beneficence, and distributive justice (https://www.hhs.gov/ohrp/regulations-and-policy/belmont-report/index.html).

2.3.1. Respect for Persons

Respect for persons is derived from the ethical principle of autonomy, or the right to self-determination. To be respectful of the autonomous individual, the Report's authors noted that researchers must respect the decisions that a competent person makes, including choosing not to participate in a research study, no matter how potentially worthy or beneficial to public health. Persons not capable of making a competent decision (diminished autonomy) are still entitled to participate in research, as long as special protections are in place. Individuals with diminished autonomy include children (where autonomy is not fully mature), prisoners with restricted freedoms, and persons with cognitive or emotional disabilities. The Report emphasized that autonomy can vary in different situations, such as during an incapacitating illness, and should be reevaluated over time. In the abuse cases noted above, this ethical guideline was the one most flagrantly violated (https://www.hhs.gov/ohrp/regulations-and-policy/belmont-report/index.html).

2.3.2. Beneficence

Beneficence refers to the ethical obligation to act for the benefit of, or promote the welfare of, others. The complimentary obligation is to prevent or remove possible harms, also known as maleficence (i.e., derived from the "Do No Harm" caveat of the physician's Hippocratic Oath). Beneficence is thus accomplished when one "maximizes the benefits while minimizing possible harms" for research participants (Belmont Report, 1979, retrieved from: https://www.hhs.gov/ohrp/regulations-and-policy/belmont-report/index.html). Because there is also an obligation for researchers to benefit society, the Report acknowledged that natural tensions and conflicts can arise between benefits to society and direct benefits to the individual research participant. In these cases, avoiding immediate risks to the individual subject "carries special weight" and takes priority, although the interests of others beyond the participant can be justified in some circumstances, providing the subject's rights are protected.

2.3.3. Distributive Justice

Distributive justice means that the benefits and burdens of research should be fairly distributed and equally shared. Publically-funded research that leads to new therapeutic innovations should not be made available only to those who can afford them, nor should the same research over-burden persons from groups unlikely to benefit directly from the research findings. It is worth noting the special emphasis placed on the need to prevent exploitation of vulnerable subjects. The authors of the Report cautioned:

> *"Certain groups, such as racial minorities, the economically disadvantaged, the very sick, and the institutionalized may continually be sought*

as research subjects, owing to their ready availability in settings where research is conducted. Given their dependent status and their frequently compromised capacity for free consent, they should be protected against the danger of being involved in research solely for administrative convenience, or because they are easy to manipulate as a result of their illness or socioeconomic condition." (https://www.hhs.gov/ohrp/regulations-and-policy/belmont-report/index.html).

The Belmont Report also provided examples of how the three ethical rules of conduct should be applied to the consent process and other research procedures (Table 2.1).

2.4. THE U.S. CODE OF FEDERAL REGULATIONS: THE COMMON RULE

Using the Belmont Report as the foundation, the Department of Health and Human Services (HHS) expanded and systematically organized (codified) a set of policy guidelines into the Code of Federal Regulations (CFR) in 1981. CFR Title 45 (Public Welfare), part 46 (Protection of Human Subjects) protects research participants involved in all types of research conducted or supported by the HHS. In another section of the CFR (Title 21, parts 51, 56), the Food and Drug Administration adopted similar rules for pharmaceutical and medical device research. In 1991, Subpart A of "45 CFR 46" was adopted by 14 other federal agencies (e.g., Department of Defense) as the common Federal Policy for the Protection of Human Subjects, and became known as "The Common Rule". The Common Rule for the first time defined and operationalized key functions and procedures of IRBs, and general requirements for informed consent for human subjects involved in all types of medical and behavioral research. These regulations remain in place today with additional revisions developed over time as new issues emerge. The latest revisions completed in 2018 were made to simplify IRB procedures and better protect the public in response to the new and evolving landscape around genomics research, precision medicine/health and the emergence of "big data" as a research tool (Menikoff et al, 2017). As of January 21, 2019 the new provisions are in place except for the rule concerning use of a single IRB (Revised Common Rule: Federal Register Volume 82, Number 12) for multi-site research which applies January, 2020 (Common Rule (2018), accessed January 2019).

To help implement the Common Rule, the Office for Human Re-

**TABLE 2.1. Translating the Belmont Report's Ethical Rules of
Conduct into "Best Practices in Research"
(modified from sections of the Belmont Report, HEW, 1979).**

Ethical Principle	Research Procedure Safeguards
Respect for Persons	Valid Consent Safeguards • adequate information to make an informed decision as to the purpose, procedures, full disclosure of risks and possible benefits, rights and responsibilities as a participant • understandable in lay terms • without undue pressure or inducement to diminish the voluntary nature of participation
Beneficence	Assessment of the Balance of Risks and Benefits: There must be a favorable balance in the nature and scope of the likelihood (risk) for harm vs. expected benefits (i.e., the risk-benefit ratio). • Important role for the IRB. • Risks and benefits to families and larger society must also be considered. All categories of risk must be assessed including: psychological, physical (e.g., pain or injury), legal, social, economic • Other options for using human subjects or alternative procedures for reducing risks have been considered • The use of vulnerable populations must be especially justified
Justice	Equitable Selection of Subjects: • Selection methods should be fair to ensure an equitable distribution of burdens and benefits so as not to over-burden some populations vulnerable to coercion with the riskiest or least beneficial studies. • Social justice requires that special populations such as children, institutionalized adults and prisoners are only selected under certain conditions.

search Protections (OHRP) was created within HHS to maintain regulatory oversight and provide guidance to IRBs and researchers on ethical and regulatory issues in biomedical and social-behavioral research funded by HHS. Over the years, the office has issued interpretative statements to help operationalize sections of the code. For example, OHRP interprets an "investigator" to be anyone involved in conducting human subject research studies, including any individual who assists the principle (lead) investigator, such as "physicians, scientists, nurses, administrative staff, teachers, and students, among others". This means that individuals considered to be investigators would also include any staff member who: obtains information about living individuals by intervening or interacting with them for research purposes; obtains identifiable private information about living individuals for research purposes; or studies, interprets, or analyzes identifiable private information or data for research purposes. In essence, all members of the research team (including students) share in the obligations and accountability for protecting research subjects (Common Rule, 2018).

2.4.1. Institutional Review Boards (IRBs): Purpose, Composition and Oversight Role

All US organizations engaged in human subjects' research, whether in the public or private domain, must operate under the ongoing oversight of an objective and unbiased IRB. Typically, unless certain criteria apply (as listed below), all active research studies must be approved by an IRB and reviewed annually or sooner if substantial changes are made to the protocol or unanticipated events occur. According to the Common Rule, an IRB committee must be composed of at least five regular members with the following characteristics:

- Sufficient scientific expertise and knowledge to "promote complete and adequate review of research activities commonly conducted by the institution";
- Relevant experience and diverse make-up in terms of gender, racial and ethnic diversity, and representativeness of community cultural attitudes;
- More than one discipline represented among committee members;
- Research experience or professional knowledge of the special needs of vulnerable populations, such as children and cognitively impaired persons, depending on the research focus of the institution;
- At least one member whose primary concerns are in nonscientific areas;
- At least one member who is not otherwise affiliated with the institution and who does not have an immediate family member affiliated with the institution; Ad-hoc members to provide specific knowledge or expertise, but who are not allowed to vote.

(See Common Rule, 2018)

Box 2.1 - HHS Policy for Protection of Human Research Subjects: Definition of Terms

Research means a systematic investigation, including research development, testing and evaluation, designed to develop or contribute to generalizable knowledge

Human subject means a living individual about whom an investigator (whether professional or student) conducting research obtains

(1) Data through intervention or interaction with the individual to use for research, or

(2) Identifiable private information or identifiable biospecimens to use for research.

Investigator is an individual performing various tasks related to the conduct of human subjects research activities, such as obtaining informed consent from subjects, interacting with subjects, and communicating with the IRB.

Intervention includes both physical procedures by which data are gathered (for example, venipuncture) and manipulations of the subject or the subject's environment that are performed for research purposes.

Interaction includes communication or interpersonal contact between investigator and subject.

Private information includes information about behavior that occurs in a context in which an individual can reasonably expect that no observation or recording is taking place, and information which has been provided for specific purposes by an individual and which the individual can reasonably expect will not be made public (for example, a medical record). Private information must be individually identifiable (i.e., the identity of the subject is or may readily be ascertained by the investigator or associated with the information) in order for obtaining the information to constitute research involving human subjects.

An identifiable biospecimen is one that can be readily linked to the identity of the research participant

Clinical Research includes:

- Patient-oriented research. Research conducted with human subjects (or on material of human origin such as tissues, specimens and cognitive phenomena) for which an investigator (or colleague) directly interacts with human subjects. Excluded from this definition are in vitro studies that utilize human tissues that cannot be linked to a living individual. Patient-oriented research includes: a. mechanisms of disease; b. therapeutic interventions; c. clinical trials, or d. development of new technologies.

- Epidemiologic and behavioral studies

- Outcomes research and health services research

Clinical trial is now defined as "a research study in which one or more human subjects are prospectively assigned to one or more interventions (which may include placebo or other control) to evaluate the effects of the interventions on biomedical or behavioral health-related outcomes"*.

Note that only clinical trials supported directly or indirectly by a federal government agency (vs private industry) are subject to this definition.

(continued)

Box 2.1 - HHS Policy for Protection of Human Research Subjects:Definition of Terms

In the 2018 revisions, the definitions of research requiring limited or no IRB oversight was expanded. Four categories of activities now classified as non-research include:

(1) Scholarly and research activities such as oral histories, historical and legal research, journalism and literary writing.

(2) Public health surveillance

(3) Collection and analysis of information, biospecimens or records for criminal investigation

(4) Certain activities in intelligence, homeland security, defense or for national defense

Exempted research (meaning research not involving IRB review) includes:

(1) Secondary research where consent is not required

    a. Research where HIPAA protection is in place such as using protected health information by covered entities for health care operations, public health and research. This reduces duplication between the Common rule and HIPAA. (see section on HIPAA below)

    b. Storage and maintenance of identifiable information or biospecimens where there is broad consent and the IRB conducts a limited review.

    c. Educational, benign behavioral interventions and surveys and interviews. A new ineligibility criterion applies when there is the possibility of adverse effects on students or educators.

(2) Exemptions are not permitted when there is:

    a. Research interventions

    b. Biospecimen collection

    c. Linkages to personally identifiable information

    d. Children are involved except with educational tests and some public observational studies.

Benign interventions are defined as being of short duration, noninvasive, painless, not embarrassing or offensive with no long lasting effects.

Minimal risk research (nonclinical studies, studies using benign interventions, and consumer preference research) no longer requires continuing IRB review. If a study is granted an expedited review it does not have to be reviewed if it only involves data analysis, or information obtained as clinical follow-up. If any of the conditions are met, the IRB must document why it is requiring review.

Retrieved from https://www.hhs.gov/ohrp/regulations-and-policy/regulations/finalized-revisions-common-rule/index.html) Accessed January 2019.

Common Rule revised in 2018 reference as above.

2.4.2. Quality Improvement\Evaluation Projects: A Subtype of Research?

In the past, quality improvement activities were typically exempt from IRB review as there was no expectation of publication or generalization to larger groups beyond the local hospital unit or agency. However, as clinical data management techniques and corresponding regulations have increased in complexity for most health care organizations, more quality improvement activities are considered a subtype of research and rise to the threshold of IRB review. To help distinguish research from quality control studies, Hauser (2011) recommends that IRB approval should be requested when the proposed activity meets any of the following conditions:

- Assigns people or lab specimens to groups for systematic comparison;
- Is being conducted in hopes of contributing to generalizable knowledge (and not for the sole purpose of improving a clinical process);
- Intentionally leads to publishable results or findings;
- Involves clinical procedures, interactions or observations (if patients) or work activities (if employees) that are not part of routine standard of care or employment;

Box 2.2 - When is Practice Really Research and in Need of IRB Approval? From: Boundaries Between Practice & Research (Part A, BELMONT REPORT, HEW 1979) https://www.hhs.gov/ohrp/sites/default/files/the-belmont-report-508c_FINAL.pdf, accessed 1/29/2019

"The distinction between research and practice is blurred partly because both often occur together (as in research designed to evaluate a therapy) and partly because notable departures from standard practice are often called "experimental" when the terms "experimental" and "research" are not carefully defined. For the most part, the term "practice" refers to interventions that are designed solely to enhance the well-being of an individual patient or client and that have a reasonable expectation of success. The purpose of medical or behavioral practice is to provide diagnosis, preventive treatment or therapy to particular individuals. By contrast, the term "research" designates an activity designed to test an hypothesis, permit conclusions to be drawn, and thereby to develop or contribute to generalizable knowledge (expressed, for example, in theories, principles, and statements of relationships). Research is usually described in a formal protocol that sets forth an objective and a set of procedures designed to reach that objective . . . the general rule is that if there is any element of research in an activity, that activity should undergo review for the protection of human subjects."

- Involves increased burden to the participants;
- Involves releasing protected health information or personal information to individuals other than for regulatory/accreditation purposes (adapted from Hauser, page 86).

2.5. INFORMED CONSENT

Designed to promote autonomy of a prospective research partici-pant, regulations governing the informed consent process are a cornerstone of the Common Rule and remain today at the heart of ethical research practices. Investigators may not ask individuals to participate as research subjects before obtaining (usually in writing) the legally effective, informed consent of the subject or a legally authorized representative. Specific types of information in understandable language (free of medical jargon) must be included that cover an essential set of elements about the study and risks, and any other relevant types of information as required by the approving IRB (Table 2.2). Other information that the IRB will often require includes the total number of subjects in the study, any costs to the subject, reasons why a subject might be withdrawn from the study by the investigators, and the subject's right to learn of any new findings while participating that might alter the decision to participate. Importantly, researchers must never ask subjects to waive their rights or release the investigators from liability for negligence.

The 2018 revisions to the Common Rule include a number of updates to the consent requirements to better promote an individual's ability to make an educated decision about whether to join a research study. These changes now include the following requirements:

1. Consent forms must now begin with a brief summary of "concise and focused" key information and be written in more understandable language that a reasonable person would want.
2. All consents under the 2018 Common Rule must:
   a. Explain purpose, procedures and reasonable and forseeable risks.
   b. State whether biospecimen may be used for profit and if it will be shared with subject.
   c. Note if and how any clinically relevent material will be returned to the subject ,
   d. Make explicit if biospecimens will, or have the potential to include whole genome processing

TABLE 2.2. Basic Elements of Informed Consent for the Protection of Human Subjects involved in Research (https://www.hhs.gov/ohrp/ regulations-and-policy/guidance/faq/informed-consent/index.html)

- A statement that the study involves research
- An explanation of the purposes of the research
- The expected duration of the subject's participation
- A description of the procedures to be followed
- Identification of any procedures which are experimental
- A description of any reasonably foreseeable risks or discomforts to the subject
- A description of any benefits to the subject or to others which may reasonably be expected from the research
- A disclosure of appropriate alternative procedures or courses of treatment, if any, that might be advantageous to the subject
- A statement describing the extent, if any, to which confidentiality of records identifying the subject will be maintained
- For research involving more than minimal risk, an explanation as to whether any compensation, and an explanation as to whether any medical treatments, are available, if injury occurs and, if so, what they consist of, or where further information may be obtained
- An explanation of whom to contact for answers to pertinent questions about the research and research subjects' rights, and whom to contact in the event of a research-related injury to the subject
- A statement that participation is voluntary, refusal to participate will involve no penalty or loss of benefits to which the subject is otherwise entitled, and the subject may discontinue participation at any time without penalty or loss of benefits, to which the subject is otherwise entitled

3. Broad consent is now permitted for unspecified future research when there is potential secondary use of identifiable private information or biospecimens. In such cases this is necessary to identify, and track agreements and refusals of consent. A template for broad consents is found at https://www.hhs.gov/ohrp/ sachrp-committee/recommendations/attachment-d-august-2-2017/ index.html.
4. New consent regulations about privacy and informational and genetic identifiers now call for all subjects to be given:
   a. Statements about the potential removal of identifiers from identifiable information or biospecimens.
   b. Information that the information or biospecimen could be shared in the future and no further consent will be obtained or if it will not, even if all identifiers are removed.

An example of a consent form template developed by the University of Michigan incorporating these revisions to the Common Rule can be found at https://research-compliance.umich.edu/informed-consent-guidelines. It is important to note that the 2018 revisions also allow for an IRB to waive the need for a consent form signature when: a) the prospective participant belongs to a distinct cultural group or community where signing forms are not the norm, or an alternative method for documenting consent is available. OHRP has developed an extensive set of FAQs for researchers to help them implement these new regulations about informed consent (see FAQs on the Common Rule at https://www.hhs.gov/ohrp/education-and-outreach/revised-common-rule/revised-common-rule-q-and-a/index.html#definitions).

2.5.1. Consent as a Dynamic, Continuing Process

Because so much emphasis is placed on the content of the written consent form, the idea that valid consent is a process, not just a signed document, sometimes gets forgotten. OHRP has developed a series of web-based educational materials, tips and FAQs designed to clarify and interpret the Common Rule's regulations for informed consent. Importantly, it emphasizes the prospective, dynamic, ongoing nature of the consent process that begins with the initial recruitment activities, and doesn't end until the study is completed. Much more than a piece of paper, "the informed consent process is an ongoing exchange of information between the investigator and the subject and could include, for example, use of question-and-answer sessions, community meetings, and videotape presentations. In all circumstances individuals should be provided with an opportunity to have their questions and concerns addressed on an individual basis." (Informed Consent, FAQs, OHRP:https://www.hhs.gov/ohrp/regulations-and-policy/guidance/faq/informed-consent/index.html).

2.5.2. Vulnerable Research Populations

In addition to the Common Rule (subpart A), added protections for specific vulnerable groups of subjects were defined in subparts B, C, and D of the code: pregnant women, human fetuses, and neonates (subpart B); prisoners (subpart C); and children (subpart D). These are summarized in Table 2.3

TABLE 2.3. Added Protections for Vulnerable Research Populations in 45 CFR 46, Subparts B-D. (summarized from http://www.hhs.gov/ohrp/humansubjects/guidance/45cfr46.html#46.102).

Vulnerable Group	Key Safeguards and Requirements
Subpart B: Pregnant Women or Fetuses	All of the following must be met:
	Where scientifically appropriate, preclinical studies on pregnant animals, and clinical studies on non-pregnant women, have been conducted and provide data for assessing potential risks to pregnant women and fetuses;
	(1) The risk to the fetus is caused solely by interventions or procedures that hold out the prospect of direct benefit for the woman or the fetus; or, if there is no such prospect of benefit, the risk to the fetus is not greater than minimal and the purpose of the research is the development of important biomedical knowledge which cannot be obtained by any other means;
	(2) Any risk is the least possible for achieving the objectives of the research;
	(3) If the research holds out the prospect of direct benefit to the pregnant woman, the prospect of a direct benefit both to the pregnant woman and the fetus, or no prospect of benefit for the woman nor the fetus when risk to the fetus is not greater than minimal and the purpose of the research is the development of important biomedical knowledge that cannot be obtained by any other means, her consent is obtained in accord with the informed consent provisions of subpart A of this part;
	(4) If the research holds out the prospect of direct benefit solely to the fetus then the consent of the pregnant woman and the father is obtained in accord with the informed consent provisions of subpart A of this part, except that the father's consent need not be obtained if he is unable to consent because of unavailability, incompetence, or temporary incapacity or the pregnancy resulted from rape or incest.
	(5) No inducements, monetary or otherwise, will be offered to terminate a pregnancy;
	(6) Individuals engaged in the research will have no part in any decisions as to the timing, method, or procedures used to terminate a pregnancy; and
	(7) Individuals engaged in the research will have no part in determining the viability of a neonate.
	Viable neonates. A neonate, after delivery, that has been determined to be viable may be included in research only to the extent permitted by and in accord with the requirements of subparts A and D.

(continued)

TABLE 2.3 (continued). Added Protections for Vulnerable Research Populations in 45 CFR 46, Subparts B-D. (summarized from http://www.hhs.gov/ohrp/humansubjects/guidance/45cfr46.html#46.102).

Vulnerable Group	Key Safeguards and Requirements
Research involving neonates	Additional safeguards for neonates of uncertain viability and nonviable may be found at §46.205 (www.hhs.gov/ohrp/humansubjects/guidance/45cfr46.html#46.102)
Subpart C: Prisoners	**Approved categories of Research involving Prisoners:** A. A study of criminal behavior and of the possible causes, effects, and processes of incarceration that presents no more than minimal risk and no more than inconvenience to the subjects B. A study of prisons as institutional structures or of prisoners as incarcerated persons that presents no more than minimal risk and no more than inconvenience to the subjects Research on conditions particularly affecting prisoners as a class (for example, vaccine trials and other research on hepatitis which is much more prevalent in prisons than elsewhere; and research on social and psychological problems such as alcoholism, drug addiction, and sexual assaults). C. Research on practices, both innovative and accepted, which have the intent and reasonable probability of improving the health or well-being of the subject. http://grants.nih.gov/grants/policy/hs/prisoners_categories_research.htm
Subpart D: Children	**In most cases, parents must provide permission for children under age 18 (varies by State) to participate in research** **When capable, a child's assent (agreement) is needed** **Research can be approved when these categories apply:** • where there is no greater than minimal risk (no greater than what is encountered in daily life or in routine medical practice) • greater than minimal risk is permitted, if there is a favorable benefit equal to that of alternative treatments • if there is no direct benefit, but the risk represents only a minor increase over minimal risk and the research can yield vital information about the child's specific condition/disorder • when not otherwise approvable but determined by the IRB and the HHS Secretory to hold promise of new findings about a serious health problem

2.5.3. Other Vulnerable Groups

In addition to pregnant women, fetuses, children and prisoners, the Common Rule also identifies mentally disabled persons and those who are "economically or educationally disadvantaged" as likely to be vulnerable to coercion or undue influence and thus in need of special safeguards to protect their rights and welfare when participating as research subjects. In 2009, the NIH commented on the special challenges to involving volunteers with questionable capacity to consent (Table 2.4).

Students and employees of the research organization are also considered "vulnerable" groups, whether justified or not, due to the potential of undue gains for research participation (e.g., pay raise for employees, or higher grades for students), or conversely, retaliation from supervisors in the case of refusal to volunteer.

2.5.4. Informed Consent: Issues to Consider

A wide variety of mental disorders, neurologic diseases (dementia, stroke), metabolic impairments, psychoactive medications, substance abuse, and injuries (head trauma) can impair a person's ability to understand and make an informed decision about research participation. Consent capacity in the same individual can vary depending on the complexity and nature of the research study.

TABLE 2.4. Research Participants with Questionable Capacity to Provide Informed Consent: Issues to Consider. (Office of Extramural Research, 2009; adapted from http://grants.nih.gov/grants/policy/questionablecapacity.htm#_ftn9).

- A wide variety of mental disorders, neurologic diseases (dementia, stroke), metabolic impairments, psychoactive medications, substance abuse, and injuries (head trauma) can impair a person's ability to understand and make an informed decision about research participation.
- Consent capacity in the same individual can vary depending on the complexity and nature of the research study.
- The ethical principle of equitable subject selection requires that persons with impaired cognition not be excluded from research, in order to advance the knowledge base in neurologic disease and brain injury. Indeed, those with the most severe impairments may be the most important participants.
- Rather than specific HHS requirements, each IRB can recommend on a case by case basis the nature of any additional safeguards, as well as state and local laws.

The ethical principle of equitable subject selection requires that persons with impaired cognition not be excluded from research, in order to advance the knowledge base in neurologic disease and brain injury. Indeed, those with the most severe impairments may be the most important participants. Rather than specific HHS requirements, each IRB can recommend on a case-by-case basis the nature of any additional safeguards, as well as state and local laws (Questionable Capacity, see Table 2.4 for reference, accessed, 2019).

2.6. OTHER SOCIAL INFLUENCES ON HUMAN SUBJECTS' PROTECTIONS

Beyond human subject abuses, another important force shaping the evolution of research ethics has been the huge societal shifts in attitudes and values about the individual's rights. As noted by Truog (2012), the patients' rights movement in the U.S. was spawned from the consumers' rights movement and the social gains for women and ethnic minority groups beginning in the 1960s. After a government audit revealed that most NIH research grants were singularly focused on men or used male animal models to study disease mechanisms, Congress passed the NIH Revitalization Act (PL103-43) in 1993, which mandated that women and ethnic minorities be included in all clinical research studies. Critics of the bill argued that such action was unnecessary and costly, believing (erroneously) that most scientific findings observed in white men could be directly applied to women and men of non-white ethnicities. Moreover, they viewed studies using women as too complex because of the issue of menstrual cycle hormones. At the same time, many researchers still believed that women of childbearing potential should be automatically excluded from medical studies because of possible harm to the fetus. As a result of the collective reforms over the last few decades of the twentieth century, medical paternalism was slowly replaced with a shared decision-making model that re-positioned the locus of authority from the physician to the patient. In turn, this paradigm shift has also transformed the relationship between investigator and research volunteer. Increasingly, with the advent of community-based, participatory research, where the community is actively engaged in all aspects of the research process including identification of the study question and design, research participants and the community itself are viewed as co-researchers or research partners.

2.6.1. Role Conflict

Sometimes tensions and conflicts are created for the clinician-researcher who must occupy two distinct roles: clinician and scientist. As noted by Resnick (2009), "As a clinician, the investigator has duties to provide the patient with optimal care and undivided loyalty. As a scientist, the investigator has duties to follow the rules, procedures and methods described in the protocol." (p. 1). Consider the following real case concerning pregnant women as a vulnerable research population.

A clinical investigator writes a NIH grant application for the study of perinatal stress effects on maternal-fetal/newborn health outcomes in a sample of low SES minority patients. The application receives an outstanding score, but the NIH reviewers request the addition of a urine toxicology test to the prenatal screening assessment of the eligible research participants. The grant is funded and the investigator presents the revised research proposal for final approval to the local Institutional Review Board (IRB) where the study will be conducted. Before approving, the Committee wants to know from the investigator, "What will be done if the urine toxicology is positive?" The investigator would like to simply withdraw anyone from the study with a positive result without disclosing to the volunteer the true reason for the protocol failure. In that way, the subject's confidentiality would be protected, but the researcher worries about the potential harm to the fetus, if there was no follow-up referral to the obstetrical care provider. She wonders if the IRB will approve this strategy.

In the end, an acceptable plan for handling a positive drug screen was approved by the IRB, which provided for an alert in the consent form that urine drug screens will be conducted during the study and the provision for follow-up disclosure of a positive test to the volunteer's provider. The case also prompted a collaborative commentary on the ethical challenges of clinical care studies (Rohan et al., 2011).

2.7. THE HIPAA "PRIVACY RULE"

The HIPAA Privacy Rule is the common term for the federal regulation that protects the privacy of personal health information (PHI) of individuals either living or deceased. It was established as law under the Health Insurance Portability and Accountability Act (HIPAA) of 1996, became effective in 2003 for most "covered entities" (see definitions below, Box 3) and continues to undergo refinements in scope. In terms of research, the "Privacy Rule" specifies the conditions under which researchers can gain access to PHI. Its goal is to balance an individual's interest in keeping health information confidential with other social benefits, including health care research. According to the HIPAA NIH website https://www.hhs.gov/hipaa/for-professionals/covered-entities/index.html, covered entities include health plans, health care clearinghouses, and health care providers that transmit electronic health information for the purpose of certain defined HIPAA transactions, such as claims or eligibility inquiries. Researchers are not themselves covered entities, unless they are also health care providers and engage in any of the covered electronic transactions. Nonetheless, investigators may be

---

Box 2.3 - HIPAA Privacy Rule: Relevant Definitions for Research (http://privacyruleandresearch.nih.gov/dictionary.asp)

Research—A systematic investigation, including research development, testing, and evaluation, designed to develop or contribute to generalizable knowledge. This includes the development of research repositories and databases for research.

Covered Entity—A health plan, a health care clearinghouse, or a health care provider who transmits health information in electronic form in connection with a transaction for which HHS has adopted a standard.

Health Information—Any information, whether oral or recorded in any form or medium, that (1) is created or received by a health care provider, health plan, public health authority, employer, life insurer, school or university, or health care clearinghouse; and (2) relates to the past, present, or future physical or mental health or condition of an individual; the provision of health care to an individual; or the past, present, or future payment for the provision of health care to an individual.

Individually Identifiable Health Information—Information that is a subset of health information, including demographic information collected from an individual, and (1) is created or received by a health care provider, health plan, employer, or health care clearinghouse; and (2) relates to the past, present, or future physical or mental health or condition of an individual; the provision of health care to an individual; or the past, present, or future payment for the provision of health care to an individual; and (a) that identifies the individual; or (b) with respect to which there is a reasonable basis to believe the information can be used to identify the individual.

Protected Health Information—PHI is individually identifiable health information transmitted by electronic media, maintained in electronic media, or transmitted or maintained in any other form or medium. PHI excludes education records covered by the Family Educational Rights and Privacy Act, as amended, 20 U.S.C. 1232g, records described at 20 U.S.C. 1232g(a)(4)(B)(iv), and employment records held by a covered entity in its role as employer.

indirectly affected by the" Privacy Rule" if covered entities (e.g., hospitals) supply their data.

2.7.1. Impact of HIPAA on Research

Because researchers frequently make use of medical records and other types of personal health information, HIPAA permits access to these important data sources under specific conditions explained in the following box.

Individually identifiable health information—Information that is a subset of health information, including demographic information collected from an individual, and (1) is created or received by a health care provider, health plan, employer, or health care clearinghouse; and (2) relates to the past, present, or future physical or mental health or condition of an individual; the provision of health care to an individual; or the past, present, or future payment for the provision of health care to an individual; and (a) that identifies the individual; or (b) with respect to which there is a reasonable basis to believe the information can be used to identify the individual.

2.7.2. De-identifying Protected Health Information Under the Privacy Rule

The "Privacy Rule" specifies 18 types of information that must be removed from a patient/medical record before PHI can be used for research (Table 2.5).

Box 2.4 - How can Researchers Obtain PHI?

The Privacy Rule allows access to patient data as long as the information is uncoupled to the individual in any identifying manner, and written authorization has been obtained from the individual. Required authorization can be waived in the following circumstances:

- for the creation of a limited data set with a data use agreement;
- to conduct a preliminary feasibility assessment (but not the actual removal of records) in preparation for research;
- when individuals are deceased.

In all three instances, documented approval by an IRB must be obtained.

(modified from: How Can Covered Entities Use and Disclose Protected Health Information for Research and Comply with the Privacy Rule? http://privacyruleandresearch.nih.gov/pr_08.asp#8i) accessed 1/28/2019)

See also https://www.hhs.gov/hipaa/for-professionals/special-topics/research/index.html for updates.

TABLE 2.5. The 'Safe Harbor' 18 HIPAA-Mandated Data Elements that Must be Removed from an Individual's PHI Record Prior to Research Use.

1. Names.
2. All geographic subdivisions smaller than a state, including street address, city, county, precinct, ZIP Code, and their equivalent geographical codes, except for the initial three digits of a ZIP Code if, according to the current publicly available data from the Bureau of the Census:
   a. The geographic unit formed by combining all ZIP Codes with the same three initial digits contains more than 20,000 people.
   b. The initial three digits of a ZIP Code for all such geographic units containing 20,000 or fewer people are changed to 000.
3. All elements of dates (except year) directly related to an individual, including birth date, admission date, discharge date, and date of death; and all ages over 89 and all elements of dates (including year) indicative of such age, except that such ages and elements may be aggregated into a single category of age 90 or older.
4. Telephone numbers.
5. Facsimile numbers.
6. Electronic mail addresses.
7. Social security numbers.
8. Medical record numbers.
9. Health plan beneficiary numbers.
10. Account numbers.
11. Certificate/license numbers.
12. Vehicle identifiers and serial numbers, including license plate numbers.
13. Device identifiers and serial numbers.
14. Web universal resource locators (URLs).
15. Internet protocol (IP) address numbers.
16. Biometric identifiers, including fingerprints and voiceprints.
17. Full-face photographic images and any comparable images.
18. Any other unique identifying number, characteristic, or code, unless otherwise permitted by the Privacy Rule.

(http://privacyruleandresearch.nih.gov/pr_08.asp#8i, accessed June 26, 2012, accessed 1/23/2019). See also https://www.hhs.gov/hipaa/for-professionals/special-topics/research/index.html for updates.

Table 2.5, Figure 2.1 and Figure 2.2 elucidate the de-identification methods for HIPAA. Table 2.5 lists the 18 types of identifiers that must be addressed in the "Safe Harbor" approach to de-identification. Figure 2.1 is a flow chart of the two methods. Figure 2.2 shows the Expert Determinatiuon methodology.

All investigators are required to undergo periodic institutional training in order to make their research HIPAA-compliant. In general, researchers should assume that anytime a patient participates as a research subject in an IRB-approved study protocol, a signed HIPAA authorization to release medical information must also be obtained. As noted on the website of Columbia University Medical Center's HIPAA Training Program, "Consent is permission to participate in a research protocol. Authorization is permission to use the data collected during the study". (ttps://www.rascal.columbia.edu/courses/tc0019/index.html) accessed 1/29/2019.)

Table 2.6 lists the 10 key elements, written in plain language, that must be included in a HIPAA Clinical Research Authorization form. Once signed by the research participant, and a copy provided to the participant, it must be kept by the lead investigator for 6 years.

2.7.3. HIPAA and HITECH

In response to the massive expansion of the use and exchange of electronic data and the increasing potential for confidentiality and pri-

TABLE 2.6. Required Elements of the HIPAA Clinical Research Authorization Form (Form A). (From: Columbia University Institutional Review Board Policy on the Privacy Rule and the Use of Health Information in Research

1. The PHI information you intend to use with specific details about all the health information that will be needed.
2. The people/organizations that may use or disclose the information (e.g., the PI and research team).
3. The people/organizations who will receive the information (e.g., study sponsor, central laboratories, IRB, FDA).
5. The purpose of the use or disclosure (study description), including the possibility of future research if applicable, and the identity of possible future recipients of the PHI.
6. Expiration date (e.g., anticipated end of study).
7. Right to revoke the authorization for subsequent use or disclosure of PHI, which must be done through a statement of withdrawal in writing
8. Whether or not there the authorization includes conditions for treatment, payment, eligibility or enrollment for benefits.
9. Whether or not the PHI will be disclosed to another party – such as the funding sponsor- and if so, a statement that the PHI will no longer be covered under the HIPAA privacy rule.
10. The individual's signature and date (HIPAA requires subjects be provided with a signed copy of the HIPAA authorization).

(https://research.columbia.edu/sites/default/files/content/HRPO/ HIPAAandResearchPolicy2017.docx, accessed 1/29/2019) vacy breaches, the Health Information Technology for Economic and Clinical Health (HITECH) Act was signed into law as part of the sweeping reforms of the American Recovery and Reinvestment Act in 2009 (HITECH, accessed 2019). Part D of the Act dramatically increased the penalties and fines for privacy violations (up to $1.5 million) as a way

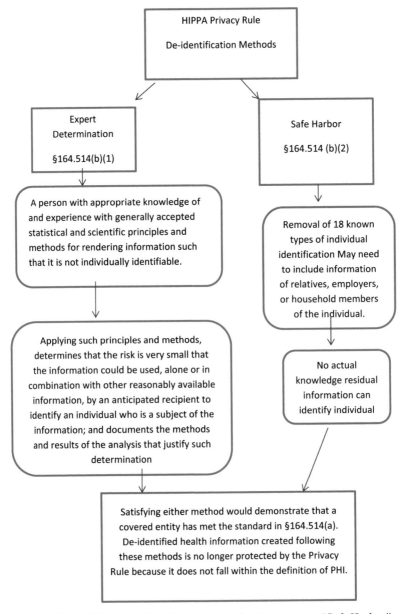

FIGURE 2.1. *HIPAA De-Identification Methods: Expert versus "Safe Harbor".*

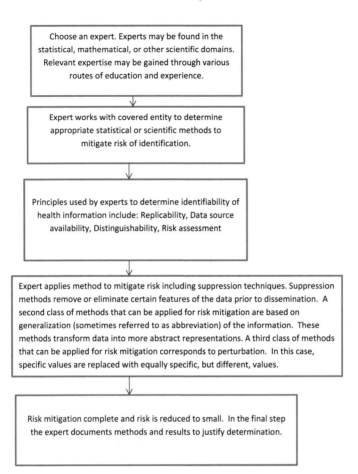

FIGURE 2.2. *Both Figure 2.1 and 2.2 are modified from http://hhs.gov/hipaa/fpr-professionals/privacy/special topics/de-identification/index.html. (Section 164.514 Table 1 and Text).*

to encourage institutions, both public and private, to develop their own internal set of strict compliance programs. It also mandated that entities report data breaches involving 500 or more individuals to HHS and the media as well as to the affected individuals. In response, health care and research institutions have amplified the security training of their employees, students and faculty members. Most now require that all investigators use only encrypted (password-protected) desktop and portable devices (laptops, cell phones, USB drives) for storing, sending and retrieving clinical data. Institutional email systems should only be used to send PHI internally within the institution, and never used to send data external to the organization. External document storage sites, Wikis, blogs, or web-based calendars should never be used to store research subject files.

Two case studies are presented below.

2.7.4. HIPAA Case Studies

2.7.4.1. HIPAA Case Scenario #1: Converting Patient Records to a Clinical Database

Dr. Jenna Smith, DNP is a nurse-midwife who also occasionally engages in clinical research. Dr. Smith has kept all of the outcome data from her obstetrical patients for the last 20 years and frequently consults the database for interesting trends that could form the basis of research. Since Dr. Smith has documentation on all of the postpartum patients' consents granting their permission to use their PHI for research, she assumes she has the right to keep her own research database of her patient's data. When she queries the University's HIPAA compliance officer, she is told she may keep a separate research database providing certain measures are taken. Dr. Smith will need to submit a protocol and obtain IRB approval to maintain a research database. The protocol must indicate that all of Dr. Smith's patients contributing data after April 14, 2003 (when HIPAA went into effect) will sign an IRB-approved HIPAA authorization which gives her permission to use their medical information for her research (from the files of N. Reame, Columbia University School of Nursing)

2.7.4.2. Case Scenario #2: Data Management and the Use of Electronic Records

You are the study coordinator for an NIH-funded trial of the effects of exercise on morbidly obese women. The project is still in the screening phase and your recruitment goal is 100 participants meeting all eligibility criteria. The PI has asked you on Friday to prepare a preliminary report of the demographics for the first 60 respondents to the study flier placed in a weight loss clinic. She needs them by Monday to add to an abstract for a poster presentation which is due at midnight. Because you will be recruiting on Saturday morning at the weight loss clinic and will be entering data directly into an electronic spreadsheet on your laptop, you can work at home on Sunday to develop the preliminary data tables. You send the raw data at 6 PM Sunday evening by email attachment to the PI's home email address to make sure she gets them in time. About a month later, one of the research volunteers reports that her son "Googled" her name for a 4th grade class project and discovered that all of her identifying information, including her reproductive history and other sensitive information, were posted on the world-wide web as part of the study file. You wonder how this could have happened. (from the files of N. Reame, Columbia University School of Nursing)

2.7.5. Patient-Centered Outcomes Research

The HITECH Act of 2009 also established the Office of the National Coordinator for Health Information Technology (ONC) as a way to advance person-centered health, while transforming health care delivery. ONC's primary goal is to enhance the nation's health IT structure, including electronic health records (EHRs) and private and secure electronic health information exchange (https://searchhealthit.techtarget.com/definition/HITECH-Act, accessed 1/29/2019). In terms of its research agenda, ONC has played a central role in the creation of the rapidly advancing data infrastructure to support patient-centered outcomes research (PCOR). The PCOR initiative, funded as part of The Affordable Care Act of 2010, is designed to actively recruit patients as research partners in studies of healthcare decision-making and incorporate their responses into research through an integrated electronic environment. PCOR studies focus on studying "the effectiveness of prevention and treatment options informed by the preferences, values, and questions patients face when making healthcare choices" (https://www.healthit.gov/topic/scientific-initiatives/building-data-infrastructure-support-patient-centered-outcomes-research, accessed 1/30/2019). In parallel with these federal initiatives came the launch in 2010 of an independent, non-profit, non-governmental organization, the Patient-Centered Outcomes Research Institute (PCORI) with a focus on comparative effectiveness research and specifically health outcomes important to patients (https://www.pcori.org/about-us/our-story).

2.7.6. Community Engagement in Research

A key feature of all of these research initiatives is the emphasis on the concept of community engagement (CE), a model proposed first by the CDC in 1997, and defined as "the process of working collaboratively with groups of people who are affiliated by geographic proximity, special interests, or similar situations with respect to issues affecting their wellbeing" (https://www.cdc.gov/learning/continuing-education/index.html CDC, 1997, p. 9). By 2010, the definition had evolved to emphasize a more balanced power relationship between the research investigator and the study subjects. As defined by Ahmed and Palermo (2010), community engagement in research is "a process of inclusive participation that supports mutual respect of values, strategies, and actions for authentic partnership of people affiliated with or self-identified by geographic proximity, special interest, or similar situations to address issues affecting the well-being of the community of focus". As observed by Bromley et al (2015), community-engaged research (CER) is now understood to be "with the community" rather than "for" it.

2.7.7. Ethical Principles to Guide CER

It has been argued that central to community engagement is the ethic of reciprocity-the ongoing process of exchange with the aim of establishing and maintaining equality between parties (Maiter et al, 2008). Other analysts have noted its grounding in the principles of community organization: fairness, justice, empowerment, participation, and self-determination (McCloskey et al, 2011). To better apply to ethical community-engaged research, Bromley and colleagues (2015) have proposed that the original principles of the Belmont Report (respect, autonomy, justice) should be re-conceptualized as:

- embodying ethical action (ie acting with the highest ethical standards in all community interactions through mutuality, equity, and shared responsibility, as a way to compensate for past indignities in the community).
- respecting all participants (ie not just study patients, but in all research roles) to build trust in the team and community
- generalizing beneficence (ie beyond the research volunteers, to across the community, while mitigating harms (such as undue expectations or work burden for community partners)
- negotiating justice (i.e. fair and non-exploitive research ideally determined in collaboration with the community)

2.7.8. Unique Ethical Challenges of Community-Engaged Research

Not only do health research sponsors today assume research participants are involved in the data collection phase of a study, but many agencies expect community members to be involved in research design, execution, and dissemination (Wallerstein & Duran, 2010). For example, engaging communities in research is a key goal of the NIH National Center for Advancing Translational Science (NCATS). Bromley and colleagues (2015) observed that this shift—from research subject to research participant—places community partners in multiple roles, such as board member, volunteer, advocate, or research team member, of varying intensities and durations over the course of the project. Additional responsibilities can include consensus-building activities, shared control of data, and long-term partnerships that extend well beyond the endpoint of data collection for a particular study.

Thus it is no surprise that a number of "lessons learned" are beginning to emerge about the ethical challenges faced by academic investigators and research partners when conducting CER within traditional models of clinical research. As part of a study to examine the utility of translating the protections of the Belmont Report to those for research-engaged communities, Bromley and colleagues (2015) identified unique ethical dilemmas incurred as a research participant.

- Multiple roles for participants beyond providing data complicated maintaining confidentiality.
- Processes that generate benefits for participants (e.g., leadership or advocacy roles for community members) also carried risks (e.g., work burden, inadequate training).
- unanticipated risks due to unique stressors faced by community partners acting as data collectors or research assistants

In a qualitative study of the quality of the experience of community research participants involved in research with impoverished, ethni-

---

BOX 2.5 Examples of Ethical Challenges Experienced by Community Researchers Involved in Community-Engaged Research (From: Salway, Chowbey, Such, & Ferguson, 2015)

- *"I did feel a bit cheeky about that, especially with the poorer communities because obviously most of these people aren't working or ... or part-time or low paid. It's ... to ask them to give their time for free ... yeah, I did feel a bit cheeky doing all that especially when I knew that I was being paid for it, so ... the most you could ... be able to offer them was a cup of tea." (pages 8-9 of 21).*
- *"There was nothing that I could do to help them ... They [community members] thought it's good that I can put their points across and I thought it was good that they thought that, "Because she's Pakistani, because she speaks the language, maybe our problems will get solved and she can do something." (Page 8 of 21)*
- *I remember going home and saying to my wife that, you know, I've met this guy with a kidney problem ... normally we wouldn't discuss work, but I'm saying, "I think, you know what, I'm thinking of asking him to come and spend weekends, you know, just on the day, not sleeping over, but just come and sit by us and, you know, with the kids around" and, you know, and I'm thinking, you know, "Where am I going with this?" (page 8 of 21)*

cally diverse residents of London (Salway et al, 2015), the investigators reported there were considerable benefits for community researchers (e.g .personal empowerment, being an "insider", helping neighbors) but also unexpected or adverse consequences. Some of these included conflict between the role of participant vs researcher, knowing too much about the lives of other residents, frustration by the limited impact of the research at the local level, and guilt for being compensated as an interviewer while participants were not. Some expressed feelings of inadequacy and distress for not maintaining their role after study completion. The investigators concluded by providing practical strategies for mitigating the risk-benefit trade-offs for CER participants across the full spectrum of the research process.

2.7.9. CER Issues for the IRB

Some analysts (McCloskey et al, 2011) have called for greater attention by the IRB to the unique ethical challenges posed by CER and to address such questions as:

- Should there be a process for evaluating the level of trust among community research collaborators, and if so, should this be performed by the IRB?
- Is the current IRB system adequate for providing oversight of all forms of community-engaged research?
- Should there be continuing input from the community partners (beyond the official letter of support) at the time of each annual review?
- What protections are in place for community partners resulting from negative findings that may cause harm to the community?
- Should communities like individuals be informed of their risks and benefits and have the right to consent to research?

2.8. GENOMIC RESEARCH

In 2003 the international scientific community announced the human genome had been decoded. Since that time there have been astronomical leaps and bounds in understanding and usage of "omics" technologies—those approaches used for determining the actions and roles of molecules at the cellular and subcellular level. With this unfolding of knowledge have come the inevitable ethics questions and dilemmas. Many professional organizations as well as the Federal agencies have set out guidance in regards to genomic research. However, it is not stat-ic and all nurse researchers must keep current in order to provide the best protection for subjects and their families.

The basic ethical framework that protects all research subjects remains critically important in genomic research but it is not sufficient. The elements of privacy, justice, harm and autonomy must be expanded and revised.

2.8.1. Privacy

The information provided by genomic research is critical to understanding health and illness and so there is a push to expand the access to all genomic information (Roberts & Middleton, 2018). However, this may also mean that the assumption of privacy is easily violated. Its sequence has important ethical ramifications for the subject but also the family because of the shared information between family members. Critical to concerns about privacy is the fact that the DNA sequence is a unique and permanent individual identifier.

Among the privacy issues with genomic research are that:

1. Genetic materials last indefinitely.
2. Information found may exceed what was asked
3. Genomic information may not be well understood at the time of discovery
4. Understanding of genetic information changes over time
5. There is ever growing commercial use of genetic materials and information with no clear understanding of the role of the subject in profit sharing
6. Storage and access issues abound: genomic data is commonly stored online making it easy to share but also to access without consent
7. There are difficulties in harmonization of genomic information for research because of differing rules and regulations across jurisdictions
8. Increasing linkages between clinical and research genomic data make privacy difficult

Privacy in the non-genomic world was predicated on the assumption of anonymity. With genomic information guaranteed anonymity is not presently possible, so different and innovative privacy protection measures are being developed.

2.8.1.1. Family Members

Because genomic research is concerned with heredity, families are also at risk for privacy violations. With whole genomic sequencing (WGS) information obtained from a family member can be used to identify other family members. There is also the real possibility that genomic information may reveal important genetic information about disease. The duty to warn about genetic predilection to disease can be in direct conflict with the privacy of the subject.

2.8.1.2. Identifiable Groups or Populations

Because of shared ethnicity, close geographical proximity of racial groups or persons with rare genetic conditions or diseases, there privacy issues in WGS that can cause group disruption and distress. Some more formal groups, such as Native Americans, have Tribal mechanisms to assist their members with genetic research questions.

2.8.1.3. Clinical Sample (Biospecimen)Usage

Medical specimens such as tissue and blood samples, as well as newborn blood spots have proven a rich source of genetic material for researchers. As defined by the NIH official ONC website (HealthIT. gov), biospecimens can comprise subcellular structures, cells, tissue (e.g., bone, muscle, connective tissue, and skin), organs (e.g., liver, bladder, heart, and kidney), blood, gametes (sperm and ova), embryos, fetal/placental tissue, and waste (urine, feces, sweat, shed epithelial cells, hair and nail clippings). In many cases these biospecimens have been de-indentified by the usual approaches, such as removal of name, address, and so forth. However, it is easy to identify the individual with a second sample or even a family member sample when DNA is involved.

2.8.2. Protections in Genomics

2.8.2.1. GINA

The Genetic Information Nondiscrimination Act (GINA, 2008) was put in place to protect the genetic privacy of the public. It makes it illegal for insurers, employers or others to discriminate on the basis of genetic information.

2.8.2.2. Certificates of Confidentiality

The National Institutes of Health (NIH) provides a protective mechanism when there is the potential that genetic (or other) information will be requested by legal or other entities and where employability, insurability, and so forth can be damaged. The Certificates ensure some measure of privacy as only the researcher and their institution can release the information, it cannot be subpoenaed.

2.8.2.3. HIPAA and Genomic Research

The Privacy rule was updated (2013) to capture research on genomic information. It is now required that genetic information be included as protected information and cannot be disclosed for underwriting purposes.

2.8.2.4. Other Protective Regulations

Newborn Screening Saves Lives Reauthorization Act was signed in 2014 and added the provision that parental permission is needed for researchers to use newborn blood spots in research activities.

2.8.2.5. NIH Genomic Data Sharing Policy

The NIH implemented the Genome-Wide Association Studies (GWAS, accessed 2019) which requires NIH funded genomic research to deposit WGS information in a central repository called the Genotype and Phenotypes database (dbGaP). The NIH recognizes that access to genomic data is critical for research, but that privacy is at stake. The NIH Genomic Data Sharing Policy (2015) now states that access to data bases, be consented or re-consented. These NIH data banks can only be accessed through written request to the Data Access Committee or data base curators.

2.8.2.6. Informed Consent

The Presidential Commission (2012) on *Privacy and Progress in Whole Genome Sequencing* notes informed consent should include:

1. Information about genomics; sequencing and analysis.
2. Clearly state how the DNA will be used in the research, as well as how it may be used in the future,

3. Explain who controls the information, and any role the subject may play in that control
4. While risks and benefits may be clear at the time of research the subject should understand that the future is unknown and it is probable understanding will change as time goes on.
5. Review how and when information and data will be returned to the subject, if at all.

2.8.2.7. General Considerations with WGS

The consent for WGS research should specify how the genomic bio-specimen will be used. Examples include use only for clinical application but not for ancestry, or the opposite the materials can only be used for ancestral reasons and not for clinical purposes or genomic research is limited to one disease. In all cases subjects should be apprised of any commercial use, present or future and be able to decline or accept as they see fit. They should also be made aware if they will receive any of the profits from commercial enterprise (See Common Rule, 2018).

If the genomic information is tied to family history, it might be necessary to consent appropriate family members because of the shared genomic information. In consent, the right to withdraw from the study has been sacrosanct but in genomic research there are limits when materials have been shared with other laboratories. Consent forms should lay out the difficulties with, and limits of withdrawal. Storage of genomic information is also of issue and must be clearly spelled out as to how and where, including laboratory location.

The consent should also outline whether the genomic information obtained in the research will or can be shared with the subject. The Federal laws governing disclosure of individual information are not current with WGS, having been last updated in 1988 (CLIA ,1988). If researchers plan to share the WGS information, how and what will be shared needs to be made clear as part of the consent form. Also to be considered is who will disclose as some information may be upsetting and require counseling.

The Presidential Commission is important and provides important guidance but relevant only to what was known prior to 2012. While informed consent in genomic research is subject to the rules and regulations surrounding all research it carries with it nuanced differences that are still evolving. For this reason the National Human Genome Research Institute suggests flexibility in approach to consent (NHGRI, Informed Consent for Genomics Research, accessed January 20, 2019). Subjects must be given enough time and enough comprehensible information to make a reasonable decision. And because of the dynamic nature of genomic information there are those that advocate revisiting consent over the subject's life time as understanding and usage evolves. Perishability of consent while problematic at this point has no clear cut solutions (Townsend, 2018). Among the proposed solutions include coupling " block chain" and other technological innovations with patient portals for ongoing consent (Townsend, 2018).

2.8.2.8. Broad Consent

Any genomic studies can use the so called "broad consent" that allows for the storage and future, unspecified use of biospecimens (see Common Rule, 2018)

See also the World Medical Association recommendations titled, WMA Declaration of Ethical Considerations Regarding Health Databases and Biobanks, for the international perspective (2016, revised). The Declaration begins:

"The Declaration of Helsinki lays down ethical principles for medical research involving human subjects, including the importance of protecting the dignity, autonomy, privacy and confidentiality of research subjects, and obtaining informed consent for using identifiable human biological material and data".

2.8.2.9. Precision Medicine and Precision Health

Building on the advanced technologies of genomics medicine, the infrastructure of Big Data, and the framework of community engagement, the Precision Medicine Initiative was launched in 2016 to revolutionize biomedical research in the United States. Precision medicine is "an emerging approach for disease treatment and prevention that takes into account individual variability in genes, environment, and lifestyle for each person" (NIH website), rather than "one-size fits all". In parallel, the NIH National Institute for Nursing Research (NINR) has adopted the term, precision health, to include conditions beyond illness to guide its 2016 strategic plan and research priorities. A key feature of this national initiative is the promise to "develop appropriate regulatory frameworks, that ensures consumers have access to their own health data–and to the applications and services that can safely and accurately analyze it –" (White House press release, 2015). Central to this concept is the use of public-private partnerships that engage private sector organizations, including the pharmaceutical industry, and patient groups to expand such efforts as cancer genomics, and the voluntary million-person cohort for research participation. Designed to promote social justice, The *All of US* program (https://allofus.nih.gov/) aims to recruit more than 1 million people to reflect the rich diversity of the US. In so doing, the NIH hopes to engender trust through treating volunteers as partners and sharing data with participants through secure systems.

2.8.2.10. CASE STUDY: Disclosure of Secondary Findings: Genomics Research*

"Dr. Jacqui is a psychiatrist interested in the molecular basis of several different anxiety disorders. Accordingly, she requested institutional approval to collect blood samples from a large population of both affected and unaffected individuals. The plan is to identify unusual genes that occur in the affected population. After receiving approval, numerous individuals, including staff and colleagues from Dr. Jacqui's medical center, were enrolled after signing the requisite consent form. Along with many other pieces of information, the form specifically (a) notifies the volunteer that he/she will be told at the end of the study whether or not they carry the genes in question and (b) prompts the volunteer to ask any questions they might have. The blood samples are then collected. In the process of testing and refining methodology, one of Dr. Jacqui's postdocs runs a "negative control" by screening the samples for the presence of a rare gene he has recently identified in a collaborative project with another laboratory studying breast cancer. Surprisingly, this gene is detected in one of the samples. Evidence to date is that this gene carries a small, but significant, increased likelihood of developing several different forms of metastatic cancer, and an estimated 70% likelihood for developing breast cancer. If known, the individual would increase their chances for long-term survival by prophylactic mastectomy and frequent check-ups. However, these measures would only decrease, not eliminate, the risk of developing cancer. The postdoc reports these findings to Dr. Jacqui. A quick look through the records allows Dr. Jacqui to identify the carrier of this gene as a clerk working in hospital admissions. Dr. Jacqui debates whether or not to tell the clerk what has been found. After some deliberation, she decides against telling the clerk because (a) the gene does not guarantee that the clerk will get

*This case was contributed by Dr. Michael Kalichman (kalichman@ucsd.edu) of the University of California, San Diego., ©1999.

cancer and (b) the clerk's wishes about whether or not she would like this information are not known.

2.8.2.10.1. Question

1. Consider the roles of Dr. Jacqui, the institutional review board, the postdoc, and the clerk in this case. Given the information pro vided, have any of them erred by acts of commission or omission?

From the ethics website at University of California, San Diego (ethics.ucsd) Resources for Research Ethics Education Human Subjects, Case Study #1 available at: research-ethics.org/topics/human-subjects/#discussion.

2.9. BIG DATA

The NIH Big Data to Knowledge Program (BD2K) was launched in 2013 to help make research on Big Data "FAIR": Findable, Accessible, Interoperable and Reusable. The use of Big Data in research is challenging the boundaries of ethical norms. Big Data is large volumes of information that is captured across a variety of information-rich sources ranging from social media messages to gas pump receipts. The ability to analyze Big Data is possible because of the speed of super computers and the use of algorithms and in some cases, artificial intelligence. Because of the challenge to norms of research, each of the major notions of human subjects protection must be re-calibrated for research with Big Data. To date there is some nascent guidance for human subjects protection, but it is not adequate leaving many questions unanswered.

2.9.1. Anonymity/Confidentiality

At present the access to Big Data information is porous, with no proven barriers. This porosity is leading to a reconceptualization of anonymity. Researchers have shown that it is not difficult to reconstruct data such that the individual is identified from seemingly innocuous information (Choudhury et al 2014). The standard de-identification of information do not hold up with super computers, algorithms and artificial intelligence.

Another recently voiced concern is the effect of Big Data research on the group rather than the individual (Choudhury et al 2014; Docherty,

2014). When data is grouped and responses are categorized according to those groups, there is a good chance that the group may be stigmatized or somehow singled out.

2.9.2. Harm

The research community is in agreement that research should not harm subjects. However, we now face a conceptual gap in how to define harm when using Big Data. This form of data does not seem to be about the individual but rather the collective with little or no connection to physical harm. Salero, Knoppers, Lee, Hlaing and Goodman (2014) note major avenues of harm. They include loss of privacy to the individual, analytic linkages which jeopardize the rights of groups, and the loss of data control.

Zimmer (2018) proposes that dignity based theory of privacy harm may be relevant. In this view having the individuals private data collected from multiple sources and used without knowledge or permission is a threat to dignity. The individual loses the ability to control the narrative.

In another approach Carpenter and Dittrich (2011) refer to the problem as human harming research which they attribute to the distance between the individuals and the researcher. The researcher has no conception of who is in the research pool and so the individual can be harmed.

2.9.2.1. Privacy

A good percentage of the information collected for Big Data research has been till now considered public and therefore not under rules protecting privacy. For example, Facebook, Twitter, and Instagram all have been considered public. Individuals who use these and other social media outlets sign agreements giving up rights to privacy but in reality there is often an assumption by the individual that the information will only be available to those with permission, such as friends or contacts. This thinking has recently been challenged using Nissembaum's (2004) work around the theory of privacy as contextual integrity. When context is stripped form the data collected it loses its normative anchor.

2.9.3. Consent

Consent as we now conceptualize it is not adequate for Big Data research. As Mittelstadt and Floridi (2016) note in this form of research consent in the traditional form is generally not possible as the future of the disposition of data provided by individuals cannot be known. Sometimes it is possible to have broad, open ended consents such as seen in hospitals but these tend to diminish the subjects autonomy. There is also some use of tiered consents which allow for some but not all uses as well as the possibility of re-consent in the future. Re-consent carries with it its own difficulties as it is not always possible to locate individuals at future times. The issue of consent is of concern in the European Union where the General Data Protection Regulations (Regulation (EU) 2016/679), went into place May of 2018. The regulations are meant to provide privacy and protection for individual's information. Issues have arisen and as they do, solutions are being proposed. Unfortunately, it is too soon to see how it will affect research.

There are another instances where traditional methods of consent may be abandoned in favor of new, and sometimes more realistic, yet unproven approaches. Prainsack and Buyx (2013) suggest that consents be focused on solidarity, seeking cooperation in the name of the greater good rather than the traditional individual focus. It becomes more contractual than consent (Prainsack & Buyx, 2013). This is similar to the Framework for Responsible Sharing of Genomic and Health Related Data proposed by the Global Alliance for Genomics and Health (www.genomicsandhealth.org) with its emphasis on human rights with a focus both on the sharing of data as a human right as well as the need for protections.

2.9.4. Justice

The issues surrounding justice and Big Data echo those found in all research. Researchers need to consider who's data is collected and why. Consider if the data collected is from such sources as credit card purchases, supermarkets and social media usage. The results from the collected information may systematically eliminate some groups from consideration. Even the ability to do Big data research may not be fairly distributed as it requires access to large data bases, which may be expensive to acquire and supercomputing ability which is also expensive and not accessible to many researchers. As a result the studies may only represent the views of those who have access and preclude the research of those who do not.

2.9.5. Ownership

In all research the subject is presumed to own their own data, which is only shared with permission. It is not assumed that the researcher has the right to the information, yet in Big Data acquisition of data may be out of the individual's control. The data is often "scraped" from existing sources, such as medical records and social media without the individual's knowledge. The internet information flow is also used and exploited by many companies who collect information and either use it or sell it to others.

As with any research the individuals involved should know what information is collected from them, how it is used, how it is stored and for how long and who can access it.

The International Medical Informatics Association Code of Ethics (2016) provides 7 principles regarding ethics and information. They are:

1. Principle of Information-privacy and disposition
   a. All have the right to privacy, including the control over collection, storage, access, use, communication, manipulation, linkage and disposition of data about themselves.
2. Principle of openness
   a. Individuals should be informed about their information in a timely manner
3. Principle of security
   a. Guards must be in place against loss of information, unauthorized use, destruction, manipulation, linkage, modification or communication.
4. Principle of access
   a. Individuals whose information is collected have the right to access that information as well the chance to correct it.
5. Principle of legitimate infringement
   a. Only a free, responsible and democratic society can infringe upon the rights of the individual
6. Principle of least intrusive alternative
   a. Any infringement should be the least intrusive
7. Principle of accountability
   a. Any infringement must be justified in a timely manner.

2.10. INTERNATIONAL RESEARCH: ABUSES, REGULATIONS AND GUIDELINES FOR GOOD CLINICAL PRACTICES

Unfortunately, cases of exploitation and ethical abuses of vulnerable populations are still coming to light and prompting additional protections for participants in medical research (Friedan and Collins, 2010). As recently as 2010, the Obama administration issued a formal apology for an international scandal dating back to the 1940s. In a two-year study conducted in Guatemala of the effects of different penicillin regimens as treatment for venereal diseases, the U.S. Public Health Service deliberately infected some 700 individuals. Funded by grants from the NIH, and approved by the U.S. Surgeon General, the researchers used female sex workers, institutionalized mentally-disabled patients, prisoners and soldiers as research subjects (http://www.hhs.gov/1946inoculationstudy/).

In response to the disclosure by Wellesley College Professor Susan Reverby, a Presidentially-appointed bioethics commission conducted an investigation and issued a set of 14 recommendations in 2011 to enhance accountability and study ways to compensate subjects injured during research (Presidential Commission for the Study of Bioethical Issues, 2011). Currently, the U.S. is one of the few developed nations that does not require researchers or sponsors to provide treatment, or

TABLE 2.7. The Time Course of US Federal Government Actions and Policies in the context of Human Subject Abuses (adapted from Friedan and Collins, 2010, page 264).

Year	Event
1932–1971	Tuskegee Syphilis Study
1946–1948	Guatemalan STD inoculation studies
1956–1971	Hepatitis studies at Willowbrook State School for the Retarded
1963	Jewish Hospital cancer study
1964	Declaration of Helsinki
1966	U.S. Surgeon General policy on human subject oversight by IRB
1971	NIH Office for Protection from Research Risks
1974–1978	National Commission for the Protection of Human Subjects
1974	National Research Act
1979	Belmont Report
1981	HHS 45 CFR and FDA 21 CFR 50, 56 regulations enacted
1991	45 CFR 46 becomes "Common Rule" across agencies
1993	NIH Guidelines for inclusion of women and minorities in clinical research
1995	WHO Guidelines for Good Clinical Practice
1996	Health Information Portability & Accountability Act (HIPAA)
1997	Presidential apology for Tuskegee syphilis study
1997	HIV drug studies in pregnant women in Africa
2010	Presidential apology for Guatemala inoculation study
2011	Presidential Commission to Study Bioethics recommends 14 safeguards
2018	45 CFR 46 updates in place

compensation for treatment, for injuries suffered by research subjects. The commission also cited the lack of a unified federal research database or cohesive system of documentation. In closing remarks, the lead commissioner noted that "our nation vigorously and rigorously protects people who volunteer for research studies. However, the Guatemala experiments remind us to never take ethics for granted. We must never confuse ethical principles with burdensome obstacles to be overcome or evaded. Good science requires good ethics, and vice versa." (Gutmann, 2011). In 2013, it is expected that new laws will mandate a change in the U.S. policy permitting compensation for research subjects injured while participating in research. The time line of some of the most serious cases of human subject abuses and subsequent legislative reforms in U.S. research policies are summarized in Table 2.7. As emphasized by Beauchamp and Childress in their epic text, Principles of Biomedical Ethics (2009), the utilitarian principle that "the end justifies the means" should never take precedence over autonomy to rationalize the mis-treatment of research participants.

2.10.1. A Global Agreement for Good Clinical Practices

Rules and regulations for global protections of human subjects have also continued to evolve as the international research enterprise has expanded to include the conduct of multi-site clinical trials that transcend national borders. A number of leading medical organizations have developed standards for good clinical practices. In 1990, the International Conference for Harmonization of Technical Requirements for Registration for Pharmaceuticals was launched by the U.S., Japan and countries of the European Union. Composed of members of both regulatory agencies and pharmaceutical industries of each country, its mission is to better "harmonize" (standardize) the approval and authorization procedures needed to ensure quality, safety and efficacy of new medicinal products across countries (http://www.ich. org/). The E6 guideline for Good Clinical Practice (GCP), finalized in 1996, is". . . an international and scientific quality standard for designing, conducting, recording, and reporting trials that involve the participation of human subjects" (ICH report, 1996, accessed January 2019 (http://www.ich.org/fileadmin/Public_Web_Site/ICH_Products/Guidelines/Efficacy/E6_R1/Step4/E6_R1Guideline.pdf and see also https://www.ich.org/products/guidelines/quality/article/quality-guidelines.html).Based on 14 ethical principles of the World Health Organization, The GCP guideline describes procedures for the monitoring, reporting and conduct of clinical trials, including the roles of the IRB, sponsor, and investigator (https://www.ich.org/products/guidelines/quality/article/quality-guidelines.html, accessed January 2019). As noted in the introduction, "Compliance with this standard provides public assurance that the rights, safety, and well-being of the trial participants are protected . . . and that the data are credible." (page 1). The U.S. Food and Drug Administration collaborated on the development of the document and has adopted the GCP guidelines as official FDA guidance.

2.10.2. Special Protections for Vulnerable International Populations

In 1992, the Council for International Organizations of Medical Sciences (CIOMS, accessed 2019), in partnership with the World Health Organization (WHO), published guidelines for the rights and welfare of research subjects from "underdeveloped communities" as a way to minimize their exploitation in international clinical trials. The most important sanction developed was against the use of subjects from underdeveloped/developing countries if the research could be carried out reasonably well in developed countries. A related guideline was that international studies must offer the potential of actual benefit to the residents of the developing country involved in the research. Specifically, inhabitants of the country where the research was carried out must have access to any products or interventions developed, even if the cost is substantial.

2.10.2.1. The AZT Trials in Africa

Despite these international safeguards, controversial clinical trials continue to be carried out seemingly at odds with the spirit of the existing international guidelines. As described on the website of the Kennedy Institute of Ethics at Georgetown University, the AZT studies in Africa in 1997 is one such example.

"The AZT studies in South Africa in 1997 created a public outcry when American and African researchers, funded by a grant from the Centers for Disease Control (CDC), gave a placebo, rather than the effective agent AZT, as a control treatment to pregnant women who were infected with HIV and were participating in clinical trials. The researchers argued that "standard" treatments for AIDS for these women were no treatments at all. (The AZT regimen studied in the U.S., for example, was too expensive for women and governments in poor countries, costing between $800–$1000 per person.) The researchers were evaluat-

ing lower and fewer doses of AZT in the African studies to see if low doses might be effective. Such doses might be affordable and accessible for the African women (and other poor women around the world). The researchers argued that placebo controls were appropriate, that they constituted the local "standard" therapy, and that they would provide answers faster than would other types of controls."

As to this case, some people argue that it is unethical to use different standard treatments for rich and poor women. Others say that western researchers should not impose "ethical imperialism" on women in other countries and that each country should determine its own standards for what is ethical in research. Still others argue that, because placebo trials end more quickly than do trials in which different doses of AZT are compared and because placebo trials use fewer subjects than do other trials, in the long run, more children would be saved through placebo trials. Still others counter that no person should be a means to an end, however positive that end might be." (adapted from Kennedy Institute of Ethics, Georgetown University http://highschoolbioethics.george-town.edu/units/cases/unit3_8.html)

2.10.2.2. The Concept of Clinical Equipoise

An essential ethical condition for comparing two drugs or treatments in a randomized controlled trial is that there is no evidence that one is more effective than the other. Known as clinical equipoise, investigators must be in a state of genuine clinical uncertainty about differences in therapeutic benefit when deliberately exposing study participants to experimental interventions. Although investigators may hope or even expect one agent may be safer, more effective or even just faster-acting, there should be no solid or well-accepted evidence one way or the other of a superior benefit. If that was the case, some of the research subjects would be intentionally assigned to receive the less effective intervention. Moreover, if evidence already existed of a known benefit, then repeating the same comparisons would be wasteful and of little scientific merit.

In the case of the AZT trials in South Africa, the concern that fewer children would be saved without the efficient use of placebo-controlled trials created an ethical dilemma for worldwide policy makers. In 2002, the Declaration of Helsinki language was revised to clarify the justified use of placebo control groups: 1) on a case-by-case basis for compelling scientific reasons to determine a drug's efficacy or safety; or 2) for minor conditions when no further harm is anticipated. In 2004, a further revision added the mandate that research subjects have post-trial access to procedures identified as new or alternative medical care. The current version was ratified by the WMA's General Assembly in 2013 and replaces all earlier versions (https://www.wma.net/policies-post/wma-declaration-of-helsinki-ethical-principles-for-medical-research-involving-human-subjects/.

2.11. THERAPEUTIC MISPERCEPTION

According to the Alliance for Human Research Protection, a national citizens' watchdog organization, some 15 million Americans are recruited every year into clinical trials (www.ahrp.org). Despite the many safeguards now in place to protect research subjects from harm, a large body of evidence has demonstrated a variety of flaws in the process to ensure truly informed consent in clinical research. For example, subjects often misunderstand the purpose of the research, and its true risks and benefits, or fail to make unbiased decisions due to illness, emotional duress, or socioeconomic and cultural barriers (Resnick, 2009). One of the most common ethical challenges to gaining valid consent is the widespread misperception that participation in a research study guarantees benefit for the patient-volunteer. As noted by Resnick (2009), "patients/subjects who are under the influence of the therapeutic misconception tend to overestimate the potential benefits of research and underestimate risks. . . . (it) is difficult to dispel, even when patients/subjects receive ample information about the research and are well-educated, because many patients enter clinical studies hoping to find a cure for their disease" (p. 4).

2.12. ETHICAL CODES GUIDING NURSES INVOLVED IN RESEARCH

2.12.1. ANA Code of Ethics for Nurses: The Moral Framework for the Nurse's Role In Research

The ANA Code of Ethics for Nurses with Interpretive Statements (ANA, 2015), first formulated in 1950, is the old set of guidelines that provides the fundamental ethical guidelines for all new members of the nursing profession, regardless of level of education. Because "the Code" is a living document, provisions are revised and re-interpreted regularly by ANA committees in response to emerging ethical issues in health care. Last revised in 2015, it currently has nine provisions grouped according to relations between the nurse and the patient, the profession and society at large, and serves as both a general guide for the profession's members and as a social contract with the public (available at: https://www.nursingworld.org/practice-policy/nursing-excellence/ethics/code-of-ethics-for-nurses/.

In its most recent rendition, the Code expands the definition of "patient" to encompass not only individuals, but families and relevant communities (Fowler, 2015). Noteworthy is the emphasis on consultation with the community to "help ensure enhanced protection, ..benefits, legitimacy and shared responsibility for members of the community through all phases of the research process " (ANA Code of Ethics, 2015, p. 27). By virtue of the advanced training and expanded roles in contributing to the generation of evidence-based practice, the doctorally-prepared nurse carries special obligations to adhere to its rules of conduct

2.12.2. Evolution of Nursing Guidelines for Research Practice

As far back as the "Nightingale Pledge", nursing practice codes have made mention of the expected behaviors of the nurse when involved in research-related activities. More recently, the ANA's Commission on Nursing Research published Human Rights Guidelines for Nursing in Clinical and Other Research in 1985 for the protection of research subjects. It included for the first time a dedicated guideline to the nurse's participation on institutional review boards. As the role of the nurse in research further evolved, these codes of conduct were integrated into contemporary provisions of the ANA Code, and were accompanied by relevant interpretative statements.

As described in the latest guide for applying the ANA Code to contemporary dilemmas (Fowler, 2015), both Provision # 3 and # 7 specifically include explanatory statements that outline the expected ethical behaviors for nurses involved in research. These expectations derive not only from the central role of the nurse as the patient's advocate (Provision 3), but also from the nurse's duty to develop the profession (Provision 7). As noted in the accompanying guide (Fowler, 2015), the participation by nurses in research has increased dramatically in recent years—not only as providers of care for research volunteers, but as members of research teams, and as scientific investigators. Moreover, the expanded research activity across all health care settings now demands a greater role for the primary nurse in the informed consent process for patients under their care who may be exposed to research opportunities. The relevant guidelines for research, summarized in Table 2.8, provide a moral framework for nurses at all levels of professional education, and across all patient care settings. Importantly, they specially address the rights of research

TABLE 2.8. ANA Code of Ethics Provisions and Interpretations for Research Conduct and Practices (modified from Fowler, (2015).

Provision 3. The nurse promotes, advocates for, and protects the rights, health, and safety of the patient.

Statement 3.1. The nurse safeguards the patient's rights to privacy and confidentiality

- Privacy and confidentiality are based on the bedrock of trust in the nurse-patient relationship

- Given the rapid and evolving advances in health information technology, there is a critical need for the nurse to safeguard patient secrets or prevent the disclosure of information without patient authorization.

- The nurses' duty to maintain confidentiality of both personal and clinical patient information extends off duty and in all venues

- When using social media, the Code specifically cautions the nurse to maintain vigilance against the intentional or unintentional breach of patient confidentiality through the use of un-approved postings, images, recordings or commentary.

Statement 3.2. Protection of Human Participants in Research

- The term "human participants" includes not only patient-volunteers involved in research, but also members of the research team, students and nurses..

- These principles are applied to human-participant research through informed consent, assessment of risks and benefits, and a just selection of subject participation

- This interpretive statement also addresses whistleblowing in research; that is, reporting researchers, research projects, or clinical trials that violate patient or participant's rights. Whistleblowing refers to the disclosure of wrongdoing.

Provision 7. The nurse, in all roles and settings, advances the profession through research and scholarly inquiry, professional standards development, and the generation of both nursing and health policy.

Statement 7.1. Contributions through Research and Scholarly Inquiry

- Although not all nurses must do research, as an obligation to society, the nurse must participate in the advancement of the profession through the use of research in the application to practice, especially new knowledge that advances one's own area of practice.

- Participants in nursing research must be shown respect and must be protected from potential harm.

- Inherent in this respect is the need to conform to ethical standards at every step of the research process including:

(continued)

TABLE 2.8. (continued) ANA Code of Ethics Provisions and Interpretations for Research Conduct and Practices (modified from Fowler, (2015).

- significant and feasible aims
  - — a soundly-constructed study design
  - — review and pre-approval by an IRB of all study procedures (including consent)
  - — dissemination of results at study completion

  The 2015 revision of the Code requires nurses to be in compliance with national and international standards for research; the ANA website contains links to training in human subjects' protections

  The patient/participant' welfare must never be secondary to the significance or outcomes of the research. "The nurse's primary allegiance is always first and foremost to the patient"

subjects to privacy, dignity and protections from harm. Notably, they emphasize the nurse's duty to question, to report and to refuse to participate in research deemed morally objectionable.

2.12.3. Application of the ANA Code of Ethics to Genetics Research

2.12.4. The International Society of Nurses in Genetics (ISONG) is the Subspecialty of Genetics Nurses Whose Mission is:

"To serve both the nursing profession and the public. ISONG fosters and advocates for the scientific and professional development of its members and the nursing community, in the discovery, interpretation, application, and management of genomic information, for the promotion of the public's health and wellbeing. ISONG advocates for public understanding of genomic health and use of genomic information." (https://www.isong. org/ accessed 2/1/2019).

Grounded in the ANA Code of Ethics, ISONG has developed a number of position statements "regarding ethical implications of genetics nursing. (see https://www.isong.org/page-1325072, accessed 2/1/2019). Of special relevance to research, are those related to expected roles and responsibilities of the nurse for protecting privacy and confidentiality of genetic information, and genetic biobanking for research. Updated in 2018 to be in line with ANA revisions that explicitly cover genetic information (ANA Position Statement on Privacy and Confidentiality (2015), the ISONG statement on privacy and confidentiality now includes a specified role of the nurse in relation to GINA, HIPAA and other relevant state laws, beyond his/her moral obligations (ISONG Position Statement: Privacy and Confidentiality: The Role of the Nurse, May, 2018) As summarized in Box 2.6, biobanking of genetic tissue for current and future research carries special ethical challenges related to confidentiality issues, informed consent, disclosure of future findings and data ownership for which the nurse must assume specific ethical duties.

2.12.5. Ethical Dilemmas in Genomic Nursing

Commentaries by ISONG members have recently highlighted how the ANA Code of Ethics can be applied to the expanding ethical dilemmas of genomic nursing (also known as omics nursing). Tluczek and colleagues (2018) contend that the revised Code coupled with the rapid application of genomic technologies to healthcare creates moral obligations and a distinct ethical responsibility for nurses to remain competent in genetics knowledge in order to participate in sound ethical research.

BOX 2.6. Summary of ISONG Recommendations for Ethical Conduct of Nurses Involved in Genetic Biobanking for Research (Modified from The ISONG Position Statement: Genetic Biobanking for Research (ISONG,2013).

"The Professional Nurse should:

- be knowledgeable about genetic biobanking research practices and related ethical issues;
- advocate for the protection of human subjects;
- ascertain that potential participants provide informed and voluntary consent for use of their biospecimen and clinical data;
- contribute to the development of standardized genetic biobanking procedures and protocols for the safe collection, management, storage, and dissemination of genomic, genetic, and corresponding clinical data,
- educate the public regarding the purposes, benefits, and risks associated with genetic biobanking research.

Nurse Educators should:

- include information about genetic biobanking research in the research curriculum.

Nurses who are prepared at an advanced level should:

- be involved in legislation and policy formation regarding genetic biobanking for use in future genomic and genetic research and consider generating research through use of genetic biobank data to advance the understanding of diseases and biobehavioral human responses to these conditions. "

Additionally they point out that the consent process needs to address two ethical issues unique to genetic/genomic research: 1) findings with potential health relevance that extends to family members; and 2) the chance that genetic results can include incidental or unintended findings that may or may not be treatable. Moreover, In research studies that involve genetic testing with members of a particular racial/ethnic group, such as among Native American tribal groups or international populations, investigators are advised to partner with community leaders in order to: a) assure relevance to community needs; b) incorporate culturally competent consent processes, c) avoid therapeutic misconception regarding study benefits.

Although still in its infancy, omics nurse scientists have already identified the need for a re-examination of conventional codes of bioethics in order to meet the evolving ethical challenges inherent in omics research. Williams and Anderson (2018) analyzed the literature regarding human subjects' protections' policies in light of pending revisions to the Common Rule, the Belmont Report and the ANA Code of Ethics to identify unresolved issues in omics bioethics research. Using the principles of respect, justice and beneficence, 11 concerns were raised (see Table 2.9).

2.12.6. Case Study

Grady and Edgerly (2009) present a case study of how the nurse as patient advocate can play an important role in resolving the ethical dilemma of therapeutic misconception.

2.12.7. Nursing Code of Ethics Case Study

"Alice is a 42-year-old woman with an aggressive cancer that has not responded to previous therapy. She is offered participation in a phase one clinical trial with a promising new investigational agent. Alice's nurse knows that the purpose of the trial is to evaluate the safety of the drug and that the possibility that Alice might benefit in terms of tumor shrinkage or an increase in the length or quality of her life is very small. The nurse is concerned that the principal investigator (PI) has not made this clear enough to Alice, and is concerned that Alice is not well informed about what alternatives are available to her. Respecting Alice's right to make her own decision about study participation, the nurse feels strongly that Alice's informed consent may be compromised. When the nurse raises these concerns, the PI expresses apprehension about confusing Alice. The nurse suggests that a multidisciplinary discussion of the options available for Alice and a plan for assuring she understands

TABLE 2.9. Bioethics Issues in Omics Research Practices (modified from Williams and Anderson, 2018)

Respect for persons requires:

- Understandable informed consent in the context of complex omics information and health literacy, with potential for disclosing findings at a future time;
- Summary of key points in the consent form that are personally meaningful to the individual, and thus not standardized;
- Personal utility (emotional, cognitive, behavioral or societal value) of participating;
- Broad consent for use of research samples for unknown future research purposes and by unknown investigators, including long-term tracking of refusal or withdrawal.

Justice (fair distribution of research burden and equal opportunity to participate) requires:

- Trust: between clinicians, patients, researcher to avoid therapeutic misconception, cultural mis-communication
- Equal opportunity to maximize benefit beyond volunteers from European white ancestry
- Equity in access to genetic health care and application of research findings across groups
- Inclusion of environmental and sociocultural factors as potential confounds of biologic findings

Beneficence requires:

- Privacy protections of clinical and research data to avoid violations and
- Confidentiality procedures to avoid breaches in data security that may carry special risks for insurance, employment or societal discrimination
- A plan for return of omics results, including incidental findings (now or in the future) and how they may or may not be relevant to medical care should be made and included in the consent

the options would be helpful for everyone. The PI agrees. The nurse organizes a patient care conference to include the PI, medical fellow, relevant nursing staff, social worker, spiritual counselor, and bioethicist. All agree that it would be helpful if the nurse spent additional time reviewing information about the study with Alice. After a lengthy and engaging discussion with Alice about the study and her options, the nurse asks Alice to explain in her own words what the study is about, what is likely to happen during the study, and what other choices she has besides participation. Much more confident that Alice has a better understanding of the study and is making an informed choice about participation, the nurse offers continued discussion with Alice throughout the study." (Grady & Edgerly (2009).

2.12.8. Applying the Big Data Approach to Nursing Research

As presented in Fig 2.3, Bakken and Reame argue that symptom science research (a 2016 NINR research priority) is especially conducive to Big Data methods, given the complementary data streams now available through traditional sources (eg demographics, health questionnaires), omic information (eg genetic mutations) and the public's growing use of consumer-generated data obtained from mobile apps and biosensors.

2.13. INTERNATIONAL NURSING RESEARCH

An international code of ethics for nurses was first adopted by the International Council of Nurses in 1953. It has been revised and reaffirmed at various times since, most recently in 2012 (ICN, accessed 2019). As part of Element 3: Nurses and Profession, an expected behavior of the nurse is to develop "a core of research-based professional knowledge that supports evidence-based practice".

FIGURE 2.3. Big Data: data streams for symptom management research.
Note: SNP= single nucleotide polymorphism; *consumer available.
From Bakken & Reame 2016, Annual Review of Nursing Research, Special Ethics edition. Reprinted with permission from Springer Publishing Company ©2016

BOX 2.7 Strategies for Reducing Ethical Challenges when Using Big Data Techniques with Underserved Communities: A Case Study

As part of a Big Data study of health characteristics of primarily Latino immigrant residents of a New York City community, Bakken and Reame (2016) described additional steps researchers undertook to promote autonomy, beneficence and justice in a community often underrepresented in research, with significant levels of health disparities, and historically low levels of participation in biobanks. In addition to data streams obtained from individual interviews and the clinical record, the study made use of omics data such as DNA from biospecimens, and quantified "self" data, obtained from cell phone apps. To promote autonomy over use of their data, participants were offered "opt-in/opt-out" strategies in the consent process for each level of data collected. For example, volunteers could opt to permit the use of surveys with or without linkage to electronic clinical data from a research data warehouse, or decide whether to allow use of biospecimens by the study team specifically to study cardiovascular biomarkers, but not for other uses (like genetic mutations), or use by other researchers. In addition to the use of advanced security systems for data storage to promote beneficence of the individual volunteers, aggregated findings were shared with local community-based and health care organizations to inform program development and community outreach. Beneficence was also promoted nationally through the incorporation of valid and reliable instruments including Patient-Reported Outcome Measures (PROMIS) symptom scales recommended by the NIH to better compare findings across studies. To support justice in the fair and equitable selection of research participants, multiple recruitment strategies beyond traditional sampling techniques were used to enrich the representativeness of the Latino groups, especially for females, where health disparities are high.

In 1999 at the University of Surrey in the UK, a cohort of international nursing scholars established a worldwide association of university research and teaching centers to address issues of morality, professional ethics, philosophy of care, cultural and religious values, law and accountability (www.surrey.ac.u/fhms/research/centres/ic). Known as the International Centre for Nursing Ethics (ICNE), it empaneled a working group to identify key ethical principles that should guide international nursing research (Olsen, 2003). Beyond the conventional bioethical principles of respect for persons, beneficence, and justice, the ICNE panel also emphasized respect for community, and contextual caring (not just professional obligation) as especially relevant for research across national boundaries. Based on these five principles, ICNE proposed three fundamental conditions and related assumptions under which international nursing research would be ethical (Box 2.8).

To broaden its focus to health and social care, ICNE was re-established in 2014 as the International Care Ethics Observatory (ICE), also at the University of Surrey (https://www.surrey.ac.uk/international-

---

Box 2.8 - Conditions for the Ethical Conduct of International Nursing Research. (adapted from Olsen, 2003, pp 127–129)

(1) "the local community has an early opportunity and an ongoing mechanism to provide input into the purposes, goals and methods of the research;

(2) the research design generates knowledge that has the potential to benefit the community or population providing the participants;

-This implies that any intervention that may be shown to be successful is affordable and practical in the local milieu. Although this stipulation is often applied to drug research, much nursing research involves testing person-to-person interventions, which can also be economically costly and may need to be implemented or administered by personnel with training that is largely unavailable in the local community.

(3) there is an ethically justifiable reason to target the population from which participants will be recruited. One of the following justifications should apply:

a. the phenomenon under consideration is biologically unique to that group or relates to a phenomenon that is biologically unique to that group (e.g., thalassemia, sickle cell anemia);

b. the phenomenon, although culturally mediated, is widely known to be group specific (e.g., the effect of local diet or sexual practices);

(4) there is an empirically demonstrated rationale for targeting a specific group (e.g. there is a demonstrated difference in incidence rate of detection or recovery);

(5) extensive normative data exist that do not include the targeted population—if it is reasonable to believe that the targeted population may vary from the general population described by the data;

(6) comparative data between groups would be helpful to mutual understanding or in designing treatment, service delivery or education (e.g., efforts to understand differences in ethical concepts cross-culturally)."

---

care-ethics-observatory). ICE publishes the renowned journal, *Nursing Ethics*, promotes research, sponsors international conferences and presents the prestigious international Human Rights and Nursing Award for humanitarian service.

2.14. SPECIAL ETHICAL CHALLENGES FOR NURSES IN RESEARCH

It has been argued that nurse researchers face distinct ethical considerations compared to scientists from other disciplines because of their key role as patient advocate and status as a developing academic science (Table 2.10). According to Fouka and Mantzorou (2011) the very nature of nursing may create heightened role conflict for the nurse investigator/practitioner who must protect the best interests of the patient while adhering to sound research practices. For example, to maintain scientific rigor of an intervention trial, the nurse researcher must exclude willing participants who do not meet eligibility criteria from potentially beneficial therapies, or assign some volunteers to a "wait list" control group, potentially delaying optimum patient care. Although a common circumstance faced by all clinical investigators, nurses in research may feel especially compelled to resolve such dilemmas with the best interests of the patient in mind. In addition, Grady and Edgerly (2009) note that patients may have difficulty distinguishing between the nurse's role as caregiver versus researcher, given the nurse's more direct contact with individual research participants than other members of the research staff. This role confusion for patients may be confounded by the three distinct nursing roles in clinical research, each with its own unique ethical challenges:

(a) the nurse as bedside care provider to the patient-participant involved in a research study; (b) the nurse as study coordinator, case manager or other research team member involved in such functions as recruitment, screening, and obtaining informed consent; and (c) the nurse as principal investigator of a research study who directs and oversees the conduct of all study procedures. (Grady & Edgerly, 2009)

Judkins-Cohn and colleagues (2014) contend that the informed consent process in nursing research may be especially daunting for nurses in the dual role of care provider and researcher. Using the ANA Code of Ethics as a framework, they argue that it is the nurse's duty to serve as patient advocate, respect dignity and preserve patient rights, while maintaining the integrity of the consent process. To avoid a potentially heightened risk of therapeutic misperception, there should be an emphasis on the likelihood of no clinical benefit to the individual and the quality of the informed consent (eg. level of understanding of risks and benefits, impact on clinical care) should be evaluated, using evidence-based strategies.

2.14.1. Qualitative Methods and Internet

2.14.1.1. Research Approaches

As noted by several nurse scholars (Robley, 1995; Morse, 2007, Grady and Edgerly, 2009), ethical guidelines established for the traditional scientific method are not adequate for qualitative research methods, in which unintended consequences and unanticipated implications for research participants emerge spontaneously as the data are collected. There is greater risk for the development of a therapeutic relationship during the interview and role confusion for both parties. Because human protection guidelines for qualitative research may be less prescriptive, there is more need for ongoing ethical audits beyond annual progress updates. Moreover, the common use of verbal agreements rather than formalized written consent procedures may pose documentation challenges. Robley (1995) noted that the use of case studies as data points makes it difficult to ensure findings are anonymous, thus increasing the vulnerability of subjects to breaches of confidentiality, privacy and psychological or social harms. With the expanding use of the Internet for on-line focus groups, interviews and analysis of social network electronic conversations, the United Kingdom's Royal College of Nursing (RCN), in its research ethics guide, recommends special protections for maintaining confidentiality, gaining informed consent and determining the identify of research participants when "using cyberspace as a research environment" (Royal College of Nursing, 2009). The RCN report notes that no policies for Internet research currently exist, but recommends that nurses follow the ethical guidelines of the Association of Internet Researchers (https://aoir.org/ethics/, accessed 2/2/2019). The two case studies below emphasize different issues relevant to decisions regarding the need for research consent.

2.14.2. Case Studies in Consent: When to Seek IRB Approval

2.14.2.1. Case Study #1: Is Pilot Testing a Simple Online Tool OK without IRB Approval?

You are a PhD student who is designing a new web-based risk assessment tool to prevent falls in the elderly. Your study population will be community-dwelling home-owners, age 65 and older and living alone. From the adult learning literature and in consultation with your advisor, you have devised a set of audiovisual and graphic tools that requires the user to make appropriate responses using a desktop computer. A focus group of research volunteers will first be tested for overall user acceptability, comprehension of the instructions, and voice preferences. Before you launch the focus group, you plan to ask your 74-yr-old grandfather and 3 of his friends who live on the same floor in an assisted living facility to try out the software and work out any "kinks' in the system to help fine-tune the study protocol. You simply want to see if they can understand the audio commands, read the screen accurately and follow

TABLE 2.10. Do Nurse Researchers have Special Ethical Challenges? Food for Thought. (Adapted from the Statement on Ethics of Nursing Research, Nursing research section, New Zealand Nurses' Organization. http://www. nzno.org.nz, accessed January 2019)

1. Because patient advocacy is central to nursing's code of ethics, the general research population at large—and not just special groups such as the mentally ill or children—should be considered vulnerable.
2. The potential for physical harm resulting from nursing research is generally small, there may be a tendency to underestimate other forms of risk, such as the chance of psychological harm.
3. Of the trust and intimacy inherent in the nurse-patient relationship, nurses have privileged access to multiple sources of formal and informal personal information, which may place them at special risk for breach of confidentiality.
4. As a relatively young academic discipline, there is a critical need to develop the science, yet the pool of experienced nurse researchers is still relatively small, making optimal training not always readily accessible.
5. In the public arena, the professional status of nursing has been ambiguous, and nursing research is still in the process of developing a distinct identity. Thus, the public may not yet have clear expectations for nurses in the researcher role.
6. While the future of nursing research depends upon its success in attracting funding, obtaining research grants is increasingly competitive. Given the current practice to adopt the same strategies which have been successful for other disciplines, nurse investigators may be exposed to the same social pressures and incentives for breaches in scientific integrity and ethical abuses.

the instructions written at the 6th grade reading level. Because you do not plan to actually assess their fall risk level or use any of their data, you assume that you do not need IRB approval for this pre-pilot test.

2.14.2.2. Case Study #2: Consent to Study Identified

2.14.2.2.1. Bio-banked Samples

Your first assignment as a part-time research assistant is to obtain 500 donated blood samples from the hospital bio-bank for a genetic bio-markers study. The samples are coded with identifiers to allow future contact and matching with clinical information. You know that your hospital includes standardized language on the admission form that says, "This is a teaching and research institution, and any specimens remaining after your care is complete may be used for teaching and research purposes". When you arrive at the bio-bank facility, the technician tells you that even though the desired blood samples are coded so as to make them unidentifiable to you, you still must have the express permission of each patient in order to gain access to the samples. This seems like a "Catch 22". Is he correct?

2.15. SCIENTIFIC INTEGRITY AND RESPONSIBLE CONDUCT OF RESEARCH

Although scientific integrity is fundamental to the ethical practice of research, it has only been since the 1980s that professional standards for the responsible conduct of research have been comprehensively promulgated by the scientific community. *On Being a Scientist*, now in its third edition (2009), describes the essential behaviors and values for fostering research integrity in early career researchers. First published by the National Academies Press (www.nap.edu, accessed January 2019) in 1989, the goal of these guidelines are to keep up with the ethical challenges faced by researchers that arise from the pace and complexity of 21st Century science. At the heart of the guidelines, however, are the same moral values that serve as the ethical foundation of everyday life: honesty, fairness, objectivity, openness, trustworthiness, and respect for others. In the context of research, these values translate to practices such as sharing research materials, fairness in reviewing grant proposals and manuscripts, respect for one's colleagues and students, honesty in reporting research results, and the disclosure of potential conflicts of interest.

2.15.1. Research Misconduct

In the 1980s, cases of scientific fraud and negligence in data acquisition, management and reporting prompted the federal government to establish policies for the investigation, review and punishment of the most serious violations of professional standards known as "research misconduct." Overseen by the HHS Office of Research Integrity (ORI), research misconduct includes the intentional or reckless acts of "fabrication, falsification, and plagiarism in proposing, performing, or reviewing research, or in reporting research results." (Box 2.9). Other types of standards violations are considered to be "questionable research practices" such as mistakes caused by negligence due to haste, carelessness or inattention. In keeping with ORI policies, all research institutions that receive federal funds must have policies and procedures in place to investigate,

Box 2.9 - Definitions of Research Misconduct

- **Fabrication** is making up data or results and recording or reporting them.
- **Falsification** is manipulating research materials, equipment or processes or changing or omitting data or results such that the research is not accurately represented in the research record.
- **Plagiarism** is the appropriation of another person's ideas, processes, results or words without giving appropriate credit.

As expressly noted in the CFR (42 CFR Part 93.103), research misconduct does not include honest error or differences of opinion (minutes of the Secretary's Advisory Committee on Human Research Protections, July 19, 2011,pg 20, https://wayback.archive-it.org/3919/20150824191216/http://www.hhs.gov/ohrp/sachrp/mtgings/mtg07-11/july2011minutes.pdf.pdf) accessed January 2019).

report and manage research misconduct, and anyone who is aware of a potential act of misconduct must follow these policies and procedures. Although primarily emphasizing ethical dilemmas confronted by "bench scientists", the ORI has become increasingly active in the education and training of students in avoiding research misconduct, offering on-line video case studies for resolving ethical challenges and clarifying responsible conduct (http://ori.hhs.gov/thelab).

2.16. MENTORSHIP IN ETHICAL RESEARCH PRACTICES

The NIH places special emphasis on the importance of mentorship as part of the obligation to train the next generation of responsible scientists. The NIH specifically recommends that all research fellows and trainees receive both formal and informal instruction in the responsible conduct of research that involves a variety of formats throughout the entire training experience. Specifically, the NIH notes that "while on-line courses can be a valuable supplement to instruction in responsible conduct of research, online instruction is not considered adequate as the sole means of instruction." http://grants1.nih.gov/grants/guide/, accessed 2019. In addition, other federal requirements regarding training for investigators must be met, such as the National Institute of Health's (NIH) requirement for the training of key personnel in NIH-sponsored or -conducted human subjects research. Ultimately, it is the principle or lead investigator who is accountable for the training of the research team in ethical practices. Topics covered typically include data acquisition and management, research misconduct, responsible authorship and avoiding conflicts of interest.

2.16.1. Case Study: Mentorship and Responsibilities of the Investigator

You're a DNP student who has just been hired as a part-time research assistant to help start up a new clinical study. The study is designed to identify early cancer bio-markers in individuals considered healthy and without overt clinical evidence of disease. The Principle Investigator, a molecular biologist, has already demonstrated elevated concentrations of a plasma protein produced in the liver in mice who develop spontaneous hepatomas. The animals with a specific genetic polymorphism in the protein's DNA remain healthy. This polymorphism is also present in humans in approximately 20% of the population. The next phase of the study will be to retrieve archived blood samples from the hospital's bio-bank to conduct research assays, DNA genotyping and characterize patient samples with and without the polymorphism. In the last phase of the project, a subset of the former patients in both groups will be contacted to participate in a detailed work-up of liver function. The PI is not a clinician and is relying on your clinical expertise and training to help carry out the recruitment and conduct of the clinical protocol, once patients are involved. You tell him you have already completed all the online training required by your university, and therefore can proceed with the studies.

In addition to going against the NIH recommendation to include more than online web-based training in research ethics, what's wrong with this approach?

2.17. PROMOTING OBJECTIVITY AND DICLOSING CONFLICTS OF INTEREST IN RESEARCH

"In academic research, the relationships between researchers and industry are critically important for the healthy exchange of ideas, opportunities and resources. These relationships can give rise to significant discoveries and to the translation of those discoveries into useful products. . . . The financial incentives that accompany such relationships, however, may lead to financial conflicts of interest that have the potential to create real or apparent bias in research. Conflicts of interest may affect research integrity, and in the case of human subjects research, may place research subjects at additional risk . . .

even the appearance of the conflict of interest may reduce confidence in the research enterprise generally, and in Columbia in particular." (Training Course TC0094, Financial Conflicts of Interest, Office of Research Compliance and Training, Columbia University, accessed 1/27/2019).

As noted on Columbia University's website on research compliance and training (http://www.columbia.edu/cu/compliance/docs/conflict_interest/index.html, accessed January, 2019), a conflict of interest (COI) exists when a researcher's outside employment or personal activities could improperly affect, or give the appearance of affecting, the researcher's primary responsibilities supported by her academic institution and research sponsor(s). Due to a growing concern that academic scientists were being unduly influenced by the pharmaceutical industry and other for-profit business opportunities, the Public Health Service issued the regulation "Responsibility of Applicants for Promoting Objectivity in Research for which PHS Funding is Sought" in 1995 (42 C.F.R. Part 50, Subpart F). Its purpose was to provide transparency to the public about potential and real conflicting financial interests of individuals and institutions applying for federal grants. Such interests were defined as stocks or other interests in companies, royalties or license fees, or directorships and management roles. The rule defined the nature of financial interests to be disclosed, and called for each institution to develop a management plan, including public disclosure procedures, enforcement mechanisms and sanctions. (An example of a public access website for COI disclosures used by the Columbia University Medical Center can be found at: https://www.rascal.columbia.edu/public/coi, accessed 1/27/2019).

Investigators are responsible for updating their financial disclosures annually and within 30 days when circumstances change substantially. Typically, a special Conflict of Interest Review Committee, separate from the IRB, oversees and reviews disclosures. Because the relevance of financial interest may vary with research proposals, investigators must also submit an updated, protocol-specific COI disclosure each time a new or continuing application to the IRB for human subjects research is submitted. In 2011, the PHS rule was amended to expand disclosure rules to cover financial interests of investigators, including student-investigators (and their immediate families) related to all "institutional responsibilities" (clinical care, education, committees), in addition to research. The level of "significant" financial interest was lowered from $10,000 to $5,000, and now covers payments for travel, as well as consulting and honoraria. Although the rule extends to relationships with non-profit groups, investigators do not have to include (1) salary paid by the institution or (2) income from seminars, lectures, teaching, service on advisory committees or review panels sponsored by a Federal, state or local government agency, a U.S. institution of higher education, an academic teaching hospital, a medical center, or a research institute affiliated with a U.S. institution of higher education (HHS Office of Extramural Research http://grants.nih.gov/grants/policy/coi/index.htm, accessed January, 2019). As of November 30, 2018, a training tutorial with printable certificate of successful completion on the NIH Financial Conflict of Interest (FCOI) policy for promoting objectivity in research can be found at: https://grants.nih.gov/grants/policy/coi/tutorial2018/story_html5.html, accessed January, 2019.

Box 2.10 - Example of a Statement of Speaker's Disclosure and Resolution of Vested Interests. (modified from a Speaker's Form for Disclosure of Potential Conflicts of Interest, Montefiore Hospital Nursing Research Committee/Nursing Department, New York, NY, 2012.)

A. Is there a financial, professional, or personal relationship that could potentially bias the content of the educational activity?

If yes, please list the companies and type of relationship (e.g., Research Support, Speaker's Bureau, Consultant, Shareholder, Other Support, Other):

If yes, you must disclose this information during your presentation. How will you do this? (e.g., Information provided in handouts, audiovisuals (slides, overhead, etc.)

If verbal disclosure is made, there must be a written verification on the part of the sponsor who was in attendance, which attests that a verbal disclosure did occur and that identifies the contents of the verbal disclosure).

B. How have you resolved this potential conflict of interest?

• The conflict has been discussed with the individual who is now aware of and agrees to our policy.
• Presenter has signed a statement that says s/he will present information fairly and without bias.
• An RN with minimum of a baccalaureate degree will monitor session to ensure conflict does not arise.
• Other. Please describe:

C. Disclosure of Unlabeled Use

Is there intent to discuss the use of a product/medication for a purpose other than that for which it was approved by the FDA? If yes, you must disclose this information during your presentation. How will you do this?

The signature is required (faxed, scanned, handwritten, or a digitally verified signature are acceptable)

Signature   Date

2.18. THE NURSE EXPERT AS CONSULTANT

Advanced practice nurses and nurse scientists participate in a variety of scientific meetings, continuing education programs and consultancies to report on research findings or provide expert opinion and knowledge on best practices. Most professional organizations, hospitals and other public or private institutions now require that speakers/consultants disclose in advance any potential or real conflicts of interest, including financial, professional or personal relationships that could influence or bias their remarks. An example in Box 2.10 provides a typical Speaker Disclosure Form for information about the nature and management of potential conflicts.

2.19. ETHICAL PRACTICES FOR SCIENTIFIC WRITING

Because of the weight given to academic publishing as a measure of investigator success, peer recognition, and worthiness for promotion and tenure, beginning scholars may need specific training in professional writing standards. The HHS Office of Scientific Integrity has developed a web-based tutorial for recognizing and avoiding questionable writing practices ("Avoiding plagiarism, self-plagiarism, and other questionable writing practices: A guide to ethical writing" by Miguel Roig 2015, revised. The resource offers a set of definitions, guidelines and training exercises for the practice of ethical scientific writing. Of Professor Roig's 26 guidelines, those most relevant for the doctorally-prepared nurse writing data-based, research reports are the following:

- "For authorship (including order of authors) should be in place at the start of research collaborations with the designated contributors aware of their roles and responsibilities that are based on well-accepted guidelines. Faculty mentors must apply the same authorship rules for student collaborators, taking great care to responsibly award authorship where credit is due.
- In the spirit of honesty and openness, researchers have an ethical obligation to disclose sufficient details of the study design and methodologies so that others can independently replicate the findings.
- To avoid the appearance of misrepresentation of the quality and volume of data-based papers, authors should avoid publishing complex research findings in serial publications or publishing reports that contain primarily old data with a few new data points included.

- Study results should be published in the context of the originally proposed data analysis plans; alternative statistical approaches used in the course of data analysis (e.g., the elimination of outliers) must be well-described and justified.
- Investigators have an obligation to consider alternative interpretations of their findings, to report and reconcile evidence that contradicts their hypotheses, and alternatively, to use only methodologically sound evidence to support their findings."

2.19.1. Unacceptable Writing Practices

Professor Roig (2015, revised)also notes a series of unethical writing practices including: "assignment of authorship as a courtesy to administrators/employers or study funders with no other role; use of professional "ghost" authors where the work is credited solely to the investigator; (and the) inappropriate assignment by mentors of credit to students or (alternatively) failure to acknowledge student work" (These ethical guidelines have been modified from M. Roig, 26 Guidelines at a Glance at: http://ori.hhs.gov/plagiarism, accessed 1/27, 2019).

It is important to read carefully the author's instructions prior to submitting a research study to a particular journal, as required content varies from journal to journal. For example, the authors' guidelines for the journal, Nursing Research (https://journals.lww.com/nursingresearchonline/Pages/informationforauthors.aspx, accessed January, 2019) recommends the use of the following scientific standards and ethical practices for the submission of manuscripts for publication:

- De-identification of authors in the body of the manuscript to aid the reviewers in an anonymous review.
- Guidelines for avoiding plagiarism (e.g., see the AJN plagiarism policy on the AJN Web site (http://www.editorialmanager.com/ajn/ accessed 1/27/2019).
- The CONSORT guidelines for reporting a randomized controlled trial (RCT) (http://www.consort-statement.org accessed 1/27/2019).
- The PRISMA (Preferred Reporting Items for Systematic Reviews and Meta-Analyses) guideline (http://www.prisma-statement.org/) for reporting a systematic review and meta-analysis.
- An explicit statement in the manuscript affirming the status for

institutional review of human or animal subjects. (http://edmgr.ovid.com/nres/accounts/ifauth.htm)

2.19.2. Authorship and the Allocation of Credit

For beginning nurse researchers, determining the composition and order of authorship in academic work is perhaps one of the thorniest issues to manage. Although students' scholarship may reflect their own independent work in collaboration with their advisor, in general, other individuals should be included as a co-author if they "make a substantial intellectual contribution to the design of the research, the interpretation of the data, and the drafting of the paper" (Committee of the NAS, NAE, IOM, https://www.nap.edu/ 2009).

As pointed out by the authors of the well-respected report, On Being A Scientist (Committee of the NAS, NAE, IOM, https://www.nap.edu/2009), there are two reasons for determining authorship: fairness in recognition, and responsibility for the content. However, as more and more research is conducted in multidisciplinary teams, with diverse research perspectives and journal policies, the level of incongruity and disagreement about authorship rules may rise. The report's authors go on to observe that "the distribution of accountability can be especially difficult in interdisciplinary research. Authors from one discipline may say that they are not responsible for the accuracy of material provided

TABLE 2.11. Definitions for Determining Level of Contributor Role in Data-based Reports (from: Uniform Requirements for Manuscripts Submitted to Biomedical Journals: Ethical Considerations in the Conduct and Reporting of Research: Authorship and Contributorship at: http://www.icmje.org

Authors must fulfill all 3 criteria:

- Contributed substantially to the conception and design of the study, the acquisition of data, or the analysis and interpretation;
- Drafted or provided critical revision of the article;
- Provided final approval of the version to be published.

Acknowledged contributors:

Individuals contributing to the manuscript but who do not meet the criteria for authorship

Note: Because readers may infer their endorsement of the data and conclusions, these persons must give written permission to be acknowledged.

Box 2.11 - Example of Language and Content for the Acknowledgments Section of a Research Report.

Authors' contributions

NN led the study, developed initial interpretations of the data and drafted and revised the manuscript. MG reviewed initial data analysis summaries and made substantial revisions to draft versions of the manuscript. CA conducted the interviews, assisted with the data analysis and reviewed versions of the manuscript. All authors read and approved the final manuscript.

Acknowledgements

We are indebted to the patients who served as research volunteers. We also thank the Institutes of Health Research (grant number) for funding for this project. Staff member X kindly provided assistance with subject recruitment and the IRB approvals. Professor Y served as scientific advisor and critically reviewed the study proposal. Nurse Colleague collected clinical data and cared for study patients. First Author is supported by a New Investigator Award from the Institute of Health Policy Research. The sponsors' support of this work should not imply endorsement of the conclusions, for which the authors retain sole responsibility.

Box 2.12 - Case study on Authorship and the Allocation of Credit

Dr. Ima Leader, PhD is a nationally-known nurse-scientist who directs the Biobehavioral Nursing Research Laboratory, an NIH-funded research center, at Renowned University School of Nursing. Her program has its own policy about authorship, which Leader discusses with each new member who joins her lab: (1) only those who have made a significant intellectual contribution to a project will be included on any paper; and (2) Leader is the final authority, should a disagreement arise, on what is defined as a significant intellectual contribution. Although not explicitly stated, it is common knowledge that Leader will be included as last (senior) author on any paper that results from research done in her program.

You are a third-year PhD nursing student being mentored by Dr. Leader. Your dissertation study aims to adapt a novel self-management approach for menopause symptoms in Hispanic breast cancer survivors that applies biobehavioral stress concepts using social networking. The project is funded as a small pilot study from several federal funding sources, including an RO1 (investigator initiated project), a Training Grant to support pre- and postdoctoral fellows, and pilot studies funds from the NIH Center program grant to Dr. Leader, who is the principal investigator on all projects. You work with several other trainees more senior to you, a postdoctoral fellow, and several junior nursing faculty, all involved in varying ways with the project.

Based on social networking principles, you have adapted an "off-the-shelf" model of a healthy lifestyle program for an intervention protocol in a way that has never been done (to your knowledge). Your dissertation study is a pilot test of the feasibility of the design and protocol in the target population.

(continued)

Box 2.12 (continued)- Case study on Authorship and the Allocation of Credit

In the weekly lab meetings you meet with the entire Center personnel to discuss your project, along with the other projects under Dr. Leader's direction. The discussions tend to be informal, with opportunities to trouble shoot problems with study design or challenges to progress. Two individuals are particularly encouraging with ideas on how to proceed in your research. Assistant Professor Dr. Colab Orator, PhD, an informatician, has sent you three articles on informatics, with lengthy emails from which you have gleaned a number of insights about alternative interpretations of the data that ultimately made it into the discussion section of your first poster presentation. Dr. Pearla Wisdom, RN, MS, PhD , is a 2nd year postdoctoral fellow who understands the research planning process. She usually gives you insights on how to navigate the system to complete the IRB applications, progress reports, and get to the right people for quick answers. This is always in hallway discussions after the meeting or during open dialogue on the agenda items.

Dr. Nancy Nurse, DNP directs a community nursing practice where patients will be recruited. She is a seasoned clinician who has worked with Dr. Leader for many years as a consultant on clinical issues. She has worked very closely with you on facilitating recruitment of study participants, doing most of the troubleshooting and optimization of procedures for your intervention protocol.

Ms. Bea Quik, BSN is a first year graduate student who is currently doing a six-week rotation through Leader's lab. She assists you in a highly focused, state-of-the-science literature review of data mining applications for cell phone-delivered health care interventions. While conducting the review, she uncovers new insights from the literature that suggested that this approach would be a good model for protocol testing.

Dr Leader encourages you to submit the systematic review for publication as quickly as possible. You do the writing, give the paper to Leader for review, and then present the findings at the lab meeting the following week. Following the meeting, Dr Orator sends an email to you, asking if she can be the "senior" author on your paper, as it would strengthen her CV in a needed area of expertise in time for her upcoming promotion review. You are a bit surprised as you had not planned on including her at all as a co-author. Your plan was to include Ms Quick as second author and Dr Leader as the last author on the paper since the work was done in her lab and supported by funds from her program.

(This hypothetical vignette is adapted from a case study for engineers by Daniel Vallero found at the website http://www.onlineethics.org/Resources/Cases/Chaos.aspx . It has been tailored to authorship practices relevant to those encountered by practice and research faculty in schools of nursing, students and other research team members).

Discussion Questions:

1. What should be the order of authorship for this manuscript?
2. Who should receive an acknowledgment? Omitted completely?
3. To whom or where would you go to seek authorship advice?

by authors from another discipline. A contrasting view is that each author must be confident of the accuracy of everything in the paper—perhaps by having a trusted colleague read the parts of the paper outside one's own discipline. One obvious but often overlooked solution to this problem is to add a footnote accompanying the list of authors that apportions responsibility for different parts of the paper."

The International Committee of Medical Journal Editors is the recognized body that sets the standard requirements for manuscripts submitted to biomedical journals. Most journals, including those in nursing, follow their suggested guidelines for distinguishing recognized from acknowledged contributors (Table 2.11).

A suggested format for the content and language of the acknowledgements section of a research report is provided in Box 2.11.

2.20. GENERAL RESOURCES

Belmont Report: Ethical Principles and Guidelines for the Protection of Human Subjects of Research. The National Commission for the Protection of Human Subjects of Biomedical and Behavioral Research, HEW, 1979 http://www.hhs.gov/ohrp/humansubjects/guidance/belmont.html accessed 1/31/2019.

Committee on Science, Engineering, and Public Policy, National Academy of Sciences, National Academy of Engineering, and Institute of Medicine. On Being a Scientist: A Guide to Responsible Conduct in Research, 3rd Edition. 2009. Washington DC: National Academies Press. https://www.nap.edu/catalog/12192/on-being-a-scientist-a-guide-to-responsible-conduct-in accessed 1/31/2019.

Informed Consent – FAQs. https://www.hhs.gov/ohrp/regulations-and-policy/guidance/faq/informed-consent/index.html, accessed 1/31/2019.

The International Committee of Medical Journal Editors. Recommendations for the Conduct, Reporting, Editing, and Publication of Scholarly work in Medical Journals. Updated December, 2018. http://www.icmje.org/recommendations/ accessed 1/31/2019.

Resources for Research Ethics Education. Website of the National Advisory Panel on Research Integrity (http://research-ethics.net/)

TRAINING IN RESEARCH ETHICS Collaborative Institutional Training Initiative. CITI is a subscription service providing research ethics education to all members of the research community. To participate fully, learners must be affiliated with a CITI participating organization.

2.21. WEBSITES

- **HHS.gov: The Common Rule:**
  https://www.hhs.gov/ohrp/regulations-and-policy/regulations/finalized-revisions-common-rule/index.html

- **NIH National Human Genome Research Institute: Highlights of Revisions to the Common Rule:**
  https://www.genome.gov/27568212/highlights-of-revisions-to-the-common-rule/
- **NIH Human Genome Research Institute:**
  https://www.genome.gov/27561533/human-subjects-research-in-genomics/
- **The National Human Genome Research Institute's (NHGRI) Ethical, Legal and Social Implications (ELSI) Research Program:**
  https://bioethicsarchive.georgetown.edu/pcsbi/sites/default/files/Privacy-Progress508_1.pdf
- **The International Society of Nurses in Genetics (ISONG):**
  http://www.isong.org
- **Clinical Laboratory Improvement Amendments of 1988 (CLIA), Public Health Services:**
  https://wwwn.cdc.gov/clia/Regulatory/default.aspx
- **Presidential Commission for the Study of Bioethical Issues (October 2012). Privacy and Progress in Whole Genome Sequencing:**
  https://bioethicsarchive.georgetown.edu/pcsbi/sites/default/files/Privacy-Progress508_1.pdf
- **NIH Big Data to Knowledge Program (BD2K):** https://commonfund.nih.gov/bd2k
- **The IMA Code of Ethics for Health Information Professionals (2016):** https://www.imia-medinfo.org/new2/pubdocs/Ethics_Eng.pdf
- **Global Alliance for Genomics and Health:** www.genomicsandhealth.org
- **Framework for Responsible Sharing of Genomic and Health Related Data proposed by the Global Alliance for Genomics and Health:** www.genomicsandhealth.org
- **University of Michigan site for researchers:** https://research-compliance.umich.edu/

2.22. REFERENCES

45 CFR 46 (accessed, January 2018) https://www.hhs.gov/ohrp/regulations-and-policy/regulations/45-cfr-46/index.html#46.102.

Ahmed, S.M., & Palermo, A.G. (2010). Community engagement in research: frameworks for education and peer review. *American Journal of Public Health*, 100(8), 1380-7.

ANA (American Nurses' Association) (1985). *Human Rights Guidelines for Nurses in Clinical and Other Research*, Kansas City, MO.

ANA (American Nurses' Association). (2015). *Code of Ethics for Nurses with Interpretive Statements*. Silver Spring, MD. Retrieved from

Anderson, E.E. (2010). The role of community-based organizations in the recruitment of human subjects: ethical considerations. *The American Journal of Bioethics* 10:3 20–21.

Appelbaum, P.S., Lidz, C.W. & Grisso, T. (2004). Therapeutic misconception in clinical research: frequency and risk factors. *IRB: Ethics and Human Research* 26: 1–8.

Bakken S. and Reame N. The Promise and Potential Perils of Big Data for Advancing Symptom Management Research in Populations at Risk for Health Disparities

(2016). *Ann Rev Nursing Research* (S. Gibbons and M Shafer, eds). Special ethics edition. Ch 13, pp 247-260, 2016. PMID: 26673385.

Beauchamp, T.L. and Childress, J.F. (2009) *Principles of Biomedical Ethics*, 6th ed. New York: Oxford University Press.

Beecher, HK (1966). Ethics and Clinical Research. *New Engl J Med* 274: 1354-1360.

Belmont Report: https://www.hhs.gov/ohrp/regulations-and-policy/belmont-report/index.html.

Bromley, E., Mikesell, L., Jones, F., & Khodyakov, D. (2015). From subject to participant: ethics and the evolving role of community in health research. *American Journal of Public Health*, 105(5), 900-8.

Carpenter, K., & Dittrich, D. (2011). Bridging the distance: Removing the technology buffer and seeking consistent ethical analysis in computer security research. *1st International Digital Ethics Symposium*, Loyola University Chicago Center for Digital Ethics and Policy.

Choudhury, S., Fishman, J.R., McGowan, M.L. & Juengst, E.T. (2014). Big data, open science and the brain: lessons learned from genomics. *Front. Hum. Neurosci.*, 16. doi.org/10.3389/fnhum.2014.00239.

CIOMS (Council for International Organizations of Medical Sciences (accessed January 2019). https://cioms.ch/

CLIA (Clinical Laboratory Improvement Amendments of 1988), Public Health Services. https://wwwn.cdc.gov/clia/Regulatory/default.aspx

Common Rule (2018). https://www.hhs.gov/ohrp/regulations-and-policy/regulations/finalized-revisions-common-rule/index.html

Corbie-Smith, G. (1999) The continuing legacy of the Tuskegee Syphilis study: Considerations for Clinical Investigation. *Am. J. Med. Science* 317: 5–8.

Covered Entities (accessed, 2019). How Can Covered Entities Use and Disclose Protected Health Information for Research and Comply with the Privacy Rule? http://privacyruleandresearch.nih.gov/pr_08.asp#8i) accessed 1/28/2019). As the prior web site is under construction see also https://www.hhs.gov/hipaa/for-professionals/special-topics/research/index.html for updates.

Docherty, A. (2014). Big Data: Ethical Perspectives. *Anaesthesia*, 69(4), 390-391.

FAQs on the Common Rule: (accessed, January 2019). https://www.hhs.gov/ohrp/education-and-outreach/revised-common-rule/revised-common-rule-q-and-a/index.html#definitions.

FAQs on Informed Consent (accessed, January, 2019): https://www.hhs.gov/ohrp/regulations-and-policy/guidance/faq/informed-consent/index.html.

Friedan, T.R. & Collins, F.S. (2010). Intentional infection of vulnerable populations in 1946-1948: Another tragic history lesson. *JAMA* 304: 2063–64.

Fouka, G. & Mantzorou, M. (2011). What are the major ethical issues in conducting research? Is there a conflict between research ethics and the nature of nursing? *Health Science J.* 5(1): 3–14.

Fowler M.D.M.(2015). *Guide to the Code of Ethics for Nurses: Interpretation and Application*. Silver Spring, MD: American Nurses Association.

Global Alliance for Genomics and Health www.genomicsandhealth.org

Grady, C. and Edgerly, M. (2009). Science, technology and innovation: nursing responsibilities in clinical research. *Nurs. Clin. North Am.* 44: 471–481.

Guttman, A. (2011). "Ethically Impossible" The Blog, for *The Huffington Post*, posted 9/14/2011. http://www.huffingtonpost.com/amy-gutmann/guatemala-syphilis_b_963035.html, accessed 1/31/2019.

GWAS (Genome-Wide Association Studies) (accessed, January 2019). https://www.genome.gov/20019523/

Haigh, C. & Jones, N. (2005). An overview of the ethics of cyberspace research and the implication for nurse educators. *Nurse Education Today* 25: 3–8.

Hauser, J. (2011). Legal and regulatory considerations in research. In: *Nursing Research: Reading, Using and Creating Evidence*, 2nd ed, pp. 53–99. Boston: Jones and Bartlett Publishers.

HIPAA (accessed, 2019). https://www.hhs.gov/hipaa/for-professionals/covered-entities/index.html.

HITECH, (Health Information Technology for Economic and Clinical Health) (accessed, 2019). https://searchhealthit.techtarget.com/definition/HITECH-Act

ICE (International Care Ethics Observatory), University of Surrey (https://www.surrey.ac.uk/international-care-ethics-observatory

ICN (International Council of Nurses) (2012). The ICN code of Ethics for Nursing. Retrieved from https://www.icn.ch. Accessed January 2019.

IMA (The International Medication Association) (2016). *The IMA Code of Ethics for Health Information Professionals.* https://www.imia-medinfo.org/new2/pubdocs/Ethics_Eng.pdf

INSONG The International Society of Nurses in Genetics (INSONG). http://www.isong.org.

ISONG The International Society of Nurses in Genetics (2103). Position Statement on Privacy. \https://www.isong.org/resources/Documents/ISONG%20Position%20Statement_Privacy%20and%20Confidentiality%20of%20Genetic%20Information%20approved%20May%201%202018.pdf, accessed 2/1/2019.

Judkins-Cohn T., Kielwasser-Withrow K., Owen M. & Ward J.(2014). Ethical Principles of Informed Consent: Exploring Nurses' Dual Role of Care Provider and Researcher. *J Contin Educ Nurs* 45(1) 35-42. doi: 10.3928/00220124-20131223-03.

Lipworth, W., Mason, P.H. & Kerriidge, I. (2017). Ethics and Epidemiology of big data. *Bioethical Inquiry*, 14: 485-488.

Maiter S., Simich L., Jacobson N., & Wise J. (2008). Reciprocity: an ethic for community-based participatory action research. *Action Res.* 6(3): 305–25.

McCloskey D.J., McDonald, M.A., Cook, J., Heurtin-Roberts, S., Updegrove, S., Sampson, D., Gutter, S., & Eder, M (2011). Definitions and Organizing Concepts from the Literature Ch 1 In: *Principles of Community Engagement*, 2nd ed.

Menikoff, J., Kaneshiro, J. & Pritchard, I. (2017). The Common rule Updated. *NEJM* 376: 7. 613-615.

Mittelstadt, B.D. & Floridi, L. (2015). The ethics of big data: current and forseeable issues in Biomedical Contexts. *Sci Eng Ethics* 22: 303-341. Doi 10,1007a/s11948-015-9652-2.

Morse, J.M. (2007). Ethics in action: ethical principles for doing qualitative health research. *Qual Health Research* 17: 1003–05.

NAPRI (National Advisory Panel on Research Integrity) (2016) http://research-ethics.net/introduction/NAPRI/#overview accessed 1/31/2019.

NHGRI (The National Human Genome Research Institute's).(accessed January 20, 2019). *Ethical, Legal and Social Implications (ELSI) Research Program.* https://bioethicsarchive.georgetown.edu/pcsbi/sites/default/files/PrivacyProgress508_1.pdf

NIH Big Data to Knowledge Program (BD2K). https://commonfund.nih.gov/bd2k

NIH Genomic Data Sharing (2015). https://osp.od.nih.gov/scientific-sharing/genomic-data-sharing/. Accessed, January 2019.

NIH National Human Genome Research Institute (accessed January 2019). Highlights of Revisions to the Common Rule. https://www.genome.gov/27568212/highlights-of-revisions-to-the-common-rule/

NIH publication No. 11-7782. https://www.atsdr.cdc.gov/communityengagement/pdf/PCE_Report_Chapter_1_SHEF.pdf, accessed 1/30/2019

NIH Human Genome Research Institute (accessed January 20, 2019). https://www.genome.gov/27561533/human-subjects-research-in-genomics/

Nissenbaum, H. (2004). Privacy as contextual integrity. *Washington Law Review*, 79, 119–157.

Noble-Adams, R. (1999) Ethics and nursing research. 1: Development, theories and principles. *Br. J. Nurs.* 8(13):888–92.

NOH (2003). Protecting Personal Health Information in Research: Understanding the HIPAA Privacy Rule. NOH Publ # 03-5388. http://privacyruleandresearch.nih.gov/HIPAA_Booklet_4-14-2003.rtf; accessed 1/31/2019.

Olson, D.P. (2003). Working Group for the Study of Ethical Issues in International Nursing research. Ethical considerations for international nursing research: A report from the international centre for nursing ethics. *Nursing Ethics* 10: 122–137.

ORI (Office of Research Integrity) (2019, accessed). *The Lab: Avoiding Research Misconduct.* See http://ori.hhs.gov/thelab.

Prainsack, B. & Buyx, A. (2013). A solidarity-based approach to the governance of research biobanks. *Medical Law Review*, 2: 1, 71-91. doi: 10.1093/medlaw/fws040

PCORI (Patient-Centered Outcomes Research Institute) (accessed 2019). https://www.pcori.org/about-us/our-story

Presidential Commission for the Study of Bioethical Issues. (September 2011) "Ethically Impossible" STD Research in Guatemala from 1946 to 1948. Washington, DC, September, 2011. www.bioethics.gov

Presidential Commission for the Study of Bioethical Issues (October 2012). *Privacy and Progress in Whole Genome Sequencing. https://bioethicsarchive.georgetown.edu/pcsbi/sites/default/files/PrivacyProgress508_1.pdf*

Questionable Capacity (accessed, 1/29/2019). Office of Extramural Research, 2009; adapted from http://grants.nih.gov/grants/policy/questionablecapacity.htm#_ftn9).

Resnik, D.B. (2009. The clinical investigator-subject relationship: a contextual approach. *Philosophy, Ethics, and Humanities* in Medicine 4: 16.

Reverby, S. (2001). More than fact and fiction: Cultural memory and the Tuskegee Syphilis Study. *Hastings Center Report* , Sept/October: 22–28.

Reverby, S. (2011). The art of medicine: listening to narratives of the Tuskegee Syphilis Study. *Lancet* 377:1646–47.

Roberts, J. & Middleton A. (2018). Genetics in the 21st Century: Implications for patients, consumers and citizens {version 2; referees: 4 approved] *F1000Research 6*: 2020 doi: 1012688/f1000reearch.12850.2)

Robley, L.R. (1995). The ethics of qualitative nursing research. *J. Prof. Nursing* 11: 45–48.

Rohan, A., Monk, K., Marder, K. & Reame, N.E. (2011) Prenatal toxicology substance abuse screening in research: codes and consequences. *Substance Abuse* 32: 159–164.

Roig, M. (2015, revised). Avoiding Plagiarism, Self-plagiarism, and Other Questionable Writing Practices: A Guide to Ethical Writing. https://ori.hhs.gov/avoiding-plagiarism-self-plagiarism-and-other-questionable-writing-practices-guide-ethical-writing, accessed January, 2019.

RCN (Royal College of Nursing) (2009). *Research Ethics: RCN guidance for nurses. Revised edition. Page 11.* Retrieved from: https://www.rcn.org.uk/professional-development/publications/pub-003138 accessed 2/2/2019.

Salerno, J., Knoppers, B.M., Lee, L., Hlaing, W.H., & Goodman, K.W.. (2017). Ethics, big data and computing in epidemiology and public health. *Annals of Epidemiology* 27:297-301.

Salway, S., Chowbey, P., Such, E., & Ferguson, B. (2015). Researching health inequalities with community researchers: Practical, methodological and ethical challenges of an 'inclusive research approach. *Research Involvement and Engagement*, 1 Retrieved from http://ezproxy.cul.columbia.edu/login?url=https://search.proquest.com/docview/1772419193?accountid=10226

Tluczek, A.; Twal, M.E.; Beamer, L.C.; Burton; C.W.; Darmofal, L.; Kracun, M.; Zanni, K.L.; & Turner M. (2018). How American Nurses Association Code of Ethics informs genetic/genomic nursing. *Nurs Ethics*, Jan 1:969733018767248. doi: 10.1177/0969733018767248

Townsend, D. (2018). Conclusion: Harmonization in genomic and health data sharing for research: An impossible dream? Human Genetics 137: 657-664.

Truog, RD (2012). Patients and doctors: the evolution of a relationship. New Eng. J. Med. 366:581–85.

U.S. Dept of HHS Office of Scientific Integrity. Guidelines for Avoiding Plagiarism and Other Questionable Writing Practices. http://ori.hhs.gov/plagiarism-0 accessed 1/31/2019.

Wallerstein, N. & Duran, B. (2010). Community-based participatory research contributions to intervention research: the intersection of science and practice to improve health equity.

Am J Public Health. 100, Suppl 1:S40-6. doi: 10.2105/AJPH.2009.184036. Epub 2010 Feb 10.

White House https://obamawhitehouse.archives.gov/the-press-office/2015/01/30/fact-sheet-president-obama-s-precision-medicine-initiative.

Williams, J.K., & Anderson, C.M. (2018, July-August). Omics research ethics considerations. Nursing Outlook 66(4), 386–393. https://doi.org/10.1016/j.outlook.2018.05.003.

WMA (World Medical Association General Assembly) (2013). Declaration of Helsinki, Ethical Principles for Medical Research Involving Human Subjects. October 2013. Retrieved from: https://www.wma.net/policies-post/wma-declaration-of-helsinki-ethical-principles-for-medical-research-involving-human-subjects/ Accessed 1/31/2019,

WMA (World Medical Association General Assembly) (2016, Revised). WMA Declaration of Taipei on Ethical Considerations Regarding Health Databases and Biobanks: https://www.wma.net/policies-post/wma-declaration-of-taipei-on-ethical-considerations-regarding-health-databases-and-biobanks/

Zimmer, M. (April-June 2018). Addressing conceptual gaps in Big Date research ethics: an application of contextual integrity, Social Media + Society, 1-11. doi: 10.1177/2056305118768300

CHAPTER 3

Ethical Guidelines Particular to Practice

COURTNEY REINISCH

Clinical care is guided by knowledge, competency, and the maintenance of ethical standards. Maintenance of ethical standards is necessary by all care providers across disciplines. Attention should be paid to the following ethical tenets: autonomy, beneficence, nonmaleficence, justice, veracity, and confidentiality. Avoiding paternalism is a goal for providers to optimize outcomes for individuals and families. Providers who demonstrate a thorough understanding of ethical principles best serve individuals, communities, and populations by strengthening trust with adherence to ethical standards.

3.1. AUTONOMY

Autonomy allows an individual to make decisions in their own perceived best interest: free from deceit, duress, constraint or coercion. Individuals are to be informed participants in the decision-making process. Autonomy respects personal freedom for the individual, family, and community in receipt of care. Respect for autonomy enhances the professional relationship between provider and humans engaged in a clinical encounter.

Inherent to the principle of autonomy is the concept of informed consent. Individuals have the right to be properly informed of their state of health, be it illness or wellness. Risks and benefits of any procedures that will be used to assess and treat a human should be clearly described. This facilitates the individual, family, or community's decision-making regarding care. Discussions regarding treatment options, risks, and benefits are necessary to educate recipients of care. This allows the individual to provide informed consent.

When discussing risk and benefits of treatment, the APRN should speak in a manner which is understandable to the individual. This may present a challenge when an individual or family's native languages is different from the APRN. The use of professional translation services is necessary to ensure the humans involved understand the implications of the discussion. It is not acceptable to put the burden of translation on individuals who are not trained professional. Interpretation services must be employed to confirm consent is truly informed.

Individuals and families with limited literacy pose a significant challenge in the process of risk, benefit discussions. APRNs need to proceed with caution when dealing with individuals or populations with low literacy levels. It is imperative to minimize risk for coercion when dealing with vulnerable populations.

When providing written information to individuals, forms must be written at an appropriate literacy level. The Joint Commission recommends patient educational materials be written at or below a fifth grade reading level (TJC, 2010). In cases of low literacy, information should be read to the individual to ensure comprehension. Health information and forms for consent should be available in the individual's native language to ensure understanding.

Health literacy includes the reading and math skills which allow an individual to function in the health care environment. Limited health literacy can increase risk for hospitalization, and in-adherence with medications and treatment plans. The APRN needs to deliver necessary health education in clear, concise, and understandable terminology when speaking with humans. Older adults are at greater risk for limited health literacy skills as they deal with declines in cognition and senses.

The APRN who respects the principle of autonomy respects the individual's freedom to make their own decisions. For example, an 89 year old female presents to her internist as she is preparing to travel with her family. The individual lives in the community with an aide due to Alzheimer's dementia. She is forgetful at times regarding appointments, keys, and pots on the stove. She no longer drives or cooks, as these tasks are completed by the assistant. At the time of consultation, the individual is oriented to person, place, and time. She knows the names of all her family members.

The individual advises the provider she will be traveling with her daughter's family to a location at 5000 feet elevation. The APRN understands the concern for the effects of altitude and possible anxiety associated with air travel. However, the APRN respects the individual's autonomy. She asks the individual, "Do you want to go on this trip?" The 89 year old individual confirms that she wants to travel with her family. Although this individual has Alzheimer's dementia, she is able to articulate her desires. Understanding the risks, the APRN develops a plan to support the individual's health so she may travel with her family.

3.2. BENEFICENCE

Beneficence is defined as the principle of doing "good". It involves doing as much good as possible in order to benefit another. It may consist of a positive action which removes or prevents the individual's problem. Beneficence strives to promote the very best.

Doing "good" sounds like a reasonable charge; however, this may be a challenge for the practicing APRN. When evaluating a 69 year old obese male individual for right leg pain who presents to the emergency department due to a fall, the APRN determines that the individual has no fractures or thrombosis. The individual has a history of chronic back pain, and recurrent lower extremity cellulitis. This individual is unable to ambulate during this ED admission. The APRN calls the individual's primary care provider to discuss the case. The APRN believes this patient may require a 23 hour observation or admission to the hospital for physical therapy evaluation and potential sub-acute placement. In the APRN's opinion, it is not safe to discharge this individual to home as he lives alone and is unable to care for himself. The APRN is acting utilizing the principle of beneficence.

The APRN respects the individual's autonomy and discusses the proposed plan with the individual. The individual verbalizes understanding of the issues and the reasons for admission. He agrees that this seems like a reasonable plan. However, when the APRN speaks to the individual's primary care physician, she is met with resistance. The PCP suggests to the APRN the individual is not telling the truth, and that the individual could walk if he so chose. The APRN advocates for the individual and the ultimately individual was admitted for observation and PT evaluation. Although doing "good" seems a reasonable goal for the APRN, it may be a challenge.

3.3. NONMALEFICENCE

Nonmaleficence is defined as "do no harm nor inflict damage to another". Nonmalficence is embodied in the principle of Primum Non Nocere. It is reflected in the Hippocratic Oath as "physician—do no harm". Treatment for a particular individual's diagnosis may not balance the risks associated with the treatment when a risk-benefit analysis is considered. Ergo, a provider may choose to not perform a procedure or intervention if there is an increased risk of doing harm.

When considering any treatment, the prudent APRN will consider both the risks and the benefits to the individual. For example, a 23 year old individual with end-stage leukemia requests to enroll in a clinical trial to appease her parents' request for her to not resign herself to hospice or palliative care. In the parents' view, accepting hospice care would be "giving up." The APRN must balance the individual's desire to please her parents with the chance of futility from treatment. The risks associated with the clinical trial include side effects of the medications, additional complications, and no benefit from treatment to slow or stop the progression of the individual's disease. The risk of death is inherent in the case, as the individual is extremely debilitated from her cancer. The possible benefits for the individual could be an improvement in her condition and eradication of her disease.

When considering care for this individual the concepts of autonomy, veracity, and beneficence must be considered in this type of decision making. The APRN wants to respect the autonomy of the 23 year old individual with leukemia to make her own decisions. The APRN is truthful about the risks and benefits of the treatment being considered.

Evidence-based treatment guidelines need to be employed when considering a risk benefit analysis. Treatment within guidelines provides benefit to the majority of the individuals with a syndrome or disease. Providers use guidelines to provide benefit to most individuals. Consideration for cultural and family preferences need to be included in decision making processes.

3.4. JUSTICE

Justice includes the concepts of fairness and entitlement. Fairness encompasses the distribution of goods and services as well as equitability amongst a society. Fairness evaluates who receives benefits and to what degree. Individuals deserve to be treated in a fair and equal manner regardless of ethnicity, social status, religious beliefs, sexual orientation, or any other social or personal uniqueness.

The APRN may serve justice in the system by utilizing evidence-based guidelines which have been shown to provide positive individual outcomes. By following guideline-based care for individuals with diabetes, the APRN may optimize the individual's glucose levels. This may then prevent future, costly complications to the individual and the health care system at large.

The APRN who respects health care resources as limited and valuable understands distributive justice. Distributive justice is important when considering health care services as a right for all or when considering a social system of health care services. The APRN who is able to deliver high quality care at an affordable price will be a key player in restricting healthcare costs for the future.

3.5. VERACITY

Veracity refers to truth telling. It involves comprehensive, accurate and objective communication of information between the practitioner and individual. The obligation of veracity is closely linked with fidelity. Fidelity requires an agreement and kept promise. Veracity and fidelity prohibit deceit. These ethical tenets protect trust. Individuals cannot be expected to trust a care provider if they are not provided the truth. Truth telling is at the core of the patient-provider relationship and is required for the establishment of a trusting relationship.

Developing a strong patient-provider relationship may be difficult due to today's practice environment. Productivity demands reduce time spent with each individual and family. Individuals who receive care in large multi-provider practices may see a different provider at each visit. Health care consumers are savvy today as they have more access to health related information knowledge via the internet. This has positive benefits of an educated consumer; however, it may result in individuals demanding expensive tests or treatments the provider does not believe are in the individual's best interest.

Truth telling seems straight forward and desirable. Delivering news of a difficult diagnosis needs to be handled with sensitivity. The APRN must be straightforward in the effort to deliver the unfortunate news. Culture may influence truth telling. In certain cultures and religions, it is not acceptable to plan for end of life. The APRN may also be asked by family members to not tell the truth to an individual with a terminal diagnosis. The APRN may have to speak to an individual without family present in order to have an honest discussion.

There are times when the APRN may be instructed not to tell an individual the truth. An example is when a nurse advises the APRN that she will need to repeat a phlebotomy procedure due to improper labeling of the tubes. The nurse wants to tell the individual that the specimen inadequate and this is the reason for the additional procedure. This is not the truth. The nurse does not intend harm to the individual, and the procedure needs to be performed. What does the APRN do in this situation?

An attending physician may instruct an APRN not to advise an individual about a mass seen on a chest radiograph. Rather, the physician may advise the APRN to tell the individual that an admission is required due to an abnormality seen on the radiograph. The plan is to advise the individual of the mass after further imaging studies are complete. This is not exactly lying, but the truth is withheld until a later time. The APRN may be uncomfortable with the process of withholding the truth.

3.6. CONFIDENTIALITY

Confidentiality protects individual's privileged information and guards a care provider's trustworthiness. Individuals surrender some privacy by divulging privileged information to a health care provider. Confidentiality obligates the provider to not share privileged information without permission from the individual. Trust is weakened if the individual fears unauthorized disclosure. This may impede the provider's ability to care for the individual.

Federal guidelines have been enacted to protect individual confidentiality. The Health Insurance Portability and Accountability Act (HIPAA) is a federal law intended to protect individual privacy by limiting identifiable data and establishing how this information may be used. Information includes anything related to the past, present or future of that individual's physical or mental health where there is an identifiable piece. Since the Health Information Technology for Economic and Clinical Health (HITECH) Act was passed in 2009, the scope of Health Insurance and Portability and Accountability Act's (HIPAA) privacy and security protections has expanded to notifying individuals of privacy breaches (Fisher & Clayton, 2012).

The consequences of violating HIPAA may result in both civil and criminal penalties, including fines and possible jail time. A health care provider may be individually sued for defamation, invasion of privacy or harassment and face personal liability. APRNs must use caution to protect individual confidentiality and avoid HIPAA violations.

Social media is a growing technology with potential for unintentional HIPAA violations. Misconduct on social media websites may raise liability under state or federal regulations focused on preventing individual abuse or exploitation. If the health care provider's conduct violates the policies of the employer, the provider may face employment consequences, including termination. The reputation of the health care organization may be at stake when a HIPAA or other violations occur (NCSBN, 2018).

APRNs now face new challenges in protecting individual confidentiality. The majority of individuals, family, and providers use smart phones in their daily lives. These phones have Internet capability at the touch of the fingertip. An individual in the care of an APRN make seek to post information on a social media site during the visit. The individual may wish to photograph a procedure being performed by the APRN. The individual being an autonomous human may choose to do this. The APRN must avoid posting any personal identifying information on any social media website. This includes, but is not limited to names, dates of birth, and photographs which may pose risk of identification.

When consulting a specialist, the APRN may wish to share information with the other provider. Sharing information with another provider involved in the care of individual is not a violation of privacy. The APRN must use a secure or encrypted method to share information with another provider involved in a case. APRNs need to use caution when sharing information with other providers to avoid HIPAA and institutional violations.

3.7. PATERNALISM

Paternalism permits health care professionals to act on behalf of humans if an individual is not able to choose or act for him or herself. Paternalism, when utilized in conjunction with autonomy and veracity, allows the practitioner to assist the individual in care related decisions. The provider must act in the fiduciary relationship, placing the needs of the individual above their own personal needs, and the needs of others. This may prove challenging when there are opposing views on the particular treatment of an individual or family.

Paternalistic decisions may occur in the emergency or surgical setting. The APRN in anesthesia may make a decision to provide additional pain relief during a surgical procedure based on vital sign changes. The individual under anesthesia care is unable to verbalize the need for additional pain relief, but the provider will make that decision based on objective findings.

If any of these seven ethical tenets—autonomy, beneficence, nonmalfeasance, justice, veracity, and paternalism—are challenged, a provider will face an ethical dilemma. Understanding these tenets will guide the provider to resolve the dilemma. This may still prove difficult and result in moral uncertainty and distress.

3.8. MORAL UNCERTAINTY, DILEMMAS, DISTRESS, FATIGUE—JUSTICE

Moral certainty is achieved with a very high level of certainty for an action. Moral uncertainty lacks certainty or probability, and makes action questionable. When the resolution is not transparent, it is difficult for the health care provider to act. There may be a sense of constraint from the institution which does not allow the nurse the sense of ability to act (Fourie, 2016).

Moral distress has been defined as the negative feeling associated with a sense of responsibility and a sense of powerlessness (Landry, 2017). Dealing with moral distress is one of the hazards of a career in health care. Moral distress arises when a person or nurse believes they know the right thing to do, but are unable to act due to institutional or other outside constraints (Fourie, 2017). This results in negative self-directed emotions in response to one's perceived involvement in morally undesirable situation (Campbell, Ulrich & Grady, 2016).

Moral distress influences the well-being of nurses, quality of care, and workplace attrition rates (Kelly, 1998; Corley et al., 2001; Corley, 2002; Hamric & Blackhall 2007; Hamric, Borchers, & Epstein, 2012; Whitehead et al. 2015). Moral distress differs from other types of work place dissatisfaction in that it causes individuals to feel morally compromised in some way.

Nurses are challenged to maintain professionalism and responsibility in their everyday practice. Nurses commonly encounter clinical situations that contain ethical conflicts. Examples include administering futile care to an end of life individual against their expressed wishes because the family insists. A nurse may be involved in administering CPR to an elderly individual with terminal cancer whose family has just rescinded the do not resuscitate order. Unresolved conflicts may cause feelings of frustration and powerlessness, especially when nurses are faced with circumstances associated with moral uncertainty or distress.

The discomfort associated with moral distress can be associated with compassion fatigue. Compassion fatigue was identified in association with burnout and is known as secondary traumatic stress disorder (Coetzee & Klopper, 2010). If compassion fatigue is not addressed in the early stages, nurses' ability to continue to deliver optimal care may be compromised. A lack of resources, inadequate positive feedback, and the nurse's response to personal distress can place nurses at risk for compassion fatigue. Addressing the factors which place nurses at risk for compassion fatigue can result in improved workplace retention of caring nurses (Coetzee & Laschinger, 2017).

APRNs face similar challenges in their practice. Additional education in biomedical ethics provided in doctoral level education assists these providers in resolving complex situations and potentially minimizes job dissatisfaction. APRNs, due to the nature of their practices, have more autonomy than nurses. Nurses by scope of practice often work based on the orders of a physician or face employment loss or punishment by an institution for the act of insubordination. APRNs educate individuals, families, and engage in the practice of shared decision making to help to resolve ethical conflicts in their practice. The APRN may consult the institution's bioethics team when a distressing conflict arises.

Justice is the principle of fair and equal treatment for all in research and practice. Due reward and honor are shared by all members of a provider or research team. In research, justice also includes equitable distribution of benefits and burdens of research. Justice represents treating people without prejudice. The APRN must apply the principle of justice to any role in which they act: researcher, educator, clinician, and scholar.

In the role of the researcher, the APRN applies ethical guidelines to authorship. Authorship is defined as having substantial participation in the conception and design of the research study or intervention, or in the analysis and interpretation of data or results. Authorship must include substantial participation in the drafting or editing of the manuscript. The author provides final approval of the version of the manuscript to be published. The author has the ability to explain and defend the study or intervention in scholarly settings (International Committee of Medical Journal Editors (ICMJE, 2017)).

The APRN participating in research will likely be a member of a team. In these cases, the order of authorship is determined by the output from each of the contributing authors. The researcher who makes the largest contribution is entitled to appear as the lead author, or may choose to assume any other position of his or her choice. The lead author should generate the original concept of the work, perform the actual research study, and be identified as the Primary Investigator. The lead author analyzes and interprets the data, and the writing of all or most of the manuscript. In cases where two or more authors equally meet the above requirements, the authors should resolve the dilemma in a collegial manner. The designation of lead author should be assigned to the person who either played the more significant role in the implementation of the research study or wrote the largest portion of the manuscript text (ICMJE, 2017).

Most institutions will have set guidelines for the ethical conduct of research and this will be discussed in another chapter in this book. The purpose of these guidelines is to avoid research misconduct. Research misconduct is defined as deliberate fabrication, falsification, or pla-giarism in reporting research results (APA, 2012). It does not include honest error or differences of opinion. The APRN engaged in research wants to avoid research misconduct as this may result in sanctions from employers, professional associations, and by agencies funding research. The APRN should consult the institutional guidelines to be certain to engage in ethical research.

3.9. INFORMED CONSENT—SURROGACY

Health care providers aim to obtain informed consent from individu-als who can make well informed decisions about care. (AMA, accessed 2018) Impairments to reasoning and judgment may make it impossible for an individual to give informed consent. Intellectual or emotional im-maturity, high levels of stress, mental retardation, severe mental illness, intoxication, severe sleep deprivation, Alzheimer's disease, or uncon-sciousness are examples of conditions in which an individual may not be able to provide informed consent. Providers must find other accept-able sources including family members, surrogates, or legal guardians to provide consent in the aforementioned cases.

Individuals may not fully understand the meaning of a procedure or treatment as described by a provider. Informed consent requires a clear appreciation and understanding of the facts, implications, and future consequences of an action. To give informed consent, the individual must have adequate reasoning faculties and have all relevant facts be-fore consent can be given.

The APRN must consider the notion of competency when seeking consent. Questioning if an individual competent to provide consent is necessary. What is competence? A legal definition of competence is provided in another chapter of this text.

The state of an individual's competency can vary based on health status. Healthcare providers must be aware that individuals may be competent to perform a task at one point in time and not be competent at a later time. In some cases, the APRN must evaluate an individual's capacity to make a decision if the individual experiences periods of confusion requiring admission to the hospital. The APRN would need to assess the individual's orientation to person, place, and time when determining capacity for decision making. The APRN may have to re-turn at a later time to reassess the individual's condition and ability to make decisions, if the initial evaluation revealed a level of confusion. Any discussion requires documentation.

In other cases, an individual may have the capacity for judgment except in the reference to their health state. An example would be an individual who has become accustomed to using opioids to treat chronic pain. Because of the effects of these medications on cognition, this individual may lack the capacity to consider other options. The APRN must always completely and accurately document the individual's state when discussing options for care.

Laws regarding competence were created to protect property rather than individuals (Beauchamp & Childress, 2013, p. 114). Unfortunately, the law does not aid the APRN, as laws regarding competence are not well suited for medical decision making. As competence may vary depending on context, it is not appropriate to globally judge competence. An individual may not have the capacity to make a decision while suffering through an acute migraine headache or a transient ischemic attack, but this does not mean the individual is globally incompetent. The APRN must document any discussion with individuals and note if they are pain free and oriented at the time of the discussion.

A lack of informed consent makes it legally impossible to act. When an individual is unable to give informed consent, another person may be authorized to give consent on his behalf. In the case of minors, parents or legal guardians may give consent. Caregivers for the mentally ill may give consent. In cases of individuals who are critically injured or unconscious, physicians and other members of the healthcare team will administer life-saving treatment. They will act with implied, emergent consent.

If an unconscious or incapacitated individual cannot express consent, the law assumes that the individual consented to treatment for the emergency situation. Implied legal consent is based on two principles: (1) Duty to obtain informed consent is excused if death or irreparable harm may result if the physician delays providing treatment. (2) The law presumes that a reasonable, competent, lucid adult would consent to lifesaving treatment (Canterberry v Spence, 1972).

Courts differ on the definition of a "true emergency." Courts generally will allow the doctrine to protect physicians who act in good faith in caring for an individual with a perceived emergency condition (Thomson v Sun City Community Hospital, 1984). The law works on the assumption of reasonable behavior. It assumes a reasonable individual would want medical care in the event of an emergency (Moore, Moffet, Fider, & Moore, 2014).

Laws support the right of a physician to act in an emergency without expressed consent. It is clear there is protection for physicians' decisions in an emergency situation. Nurses are judged based on doing what another prudent nurse would do in that situation. APRNs are held to similar standards.

In circumstances where an individual is unable to provide consent, a surrogate may be appointed to act on the behalf of an individual. The surrogate has the power to act on behalf of the individual, as long as there is reason to believe that the surrogate is making decisions based on the individual's wishes, values, or interests. Whenever possible, the APRN must keep in mind that all individuals have a right to decide and their choices must be considered even when a surrogate has been assigned. The APRN must assess that the surrogate is indeed acting in the individual's best interest and is respecting the individual's autonomy.

Surrogate decision makers must uphold three standards. The substituted judgment standard requires the surrogate decision maker to make the decision the incompetent individual would have made if competent (Beauchamp & Childress, 2013, p. 69). The pure autonomy standard respects prior autonomous judgments regardless of the existence of a formal advance directive (Beauchamp & Childress, 2013, p. 227-8). Without written advance directives, a surrogate decision maker may make decisions based on their own values and selectively consider events from the individual's life which may not be relevant to the decision at hand.

The final standard is the "best interest" standard, which holds that a surrogate decision maker must weigh options and maximize benefit through a comparative assessment of options—while discounting inherent risks or cost (Beauchamp & Childress, 2013, p. 228). The best interest standard is open to interpretation and is dependent upon who is making the decision. Parents may choose to volunteer a child to donate an organ for a sibling, although the child refuses. The best interest of the individual may override the desire of the donor. The prudent APRN would consider an ethics committee evaluation in such a case.

If there is no advance directive that designates a proxy, the individual's family should become the surrogate decision maker (AMA, 2018). Although the term family is not exact, it includes persons with whom the individual is closely associated. Typically the individual's closest family member is the first choice as surrogate. Family may include partners, spouses, and very close friends.

In cases where there is no one closely associated with the individual, but there are persons who both care about the individual and have sufficient relevant knowledge of the individual, such persons may be appropriate surrogates. APRNs must familiarize themselves with specific state and institutional rules and regulations regarding surrogates. The APRN must be sensitive to possible multiple conflicting views of family members in these circumstances. In the case of a comatose married woman, her husband became her surrogate. However, conflict arose when the individual's mother wanted care withdrawn. The individual's mother petitioned the courts and lost. In this situation, the husband's status as closest family member won out.

3.10. WITHDRAWING AND WITHHOLDING TREATMENT

End of life decisions are viewed as complex and instilled with uncertainty. Each person experiences health decision-making uniquely. In the context of end of life situations, both individuals and their families are challenged with complex decision-making. These situations involve questioning, and uncertainty intersects with a struggle to do the right thing. Families and care providers also struggle with the possibilities of failing to do the right thing according to the expectations of self and others (Milton, 2010).

Withholding and withdrawal of life support is a process through which various medical interventions are either not given to individuals or removed from them with the expectation that the individuals will die from their underlying illnesses. The withholding and withdrawal of life support is legally justified primarily by the principles of informed consent and informed refusal, both of which have strong roots in the common law. The principles hold that treatment may not be initiated without the approval of individuals or their surrogates except in emergency situations, and that individuals or surrogates may refuse any or all therapies.

End of life decisions are often made using a shared decision-making model. Shared decision making is a collaborative process involving care providers, individuals or surrogates the opportunity to engage in health care decision making incorporating best evidence with the individual's values, goals, and preferences (Kon, Davidson, Morrison, Danis & White, 2017). Using this model, clinicians attempt to clarify an individual's values and reach consensus about treatment plans consistent with individual preferences. Critically ill individuals are impaired in their decision making ability, leaving family members and other surrogates to make end-of-life decisions, in accordance with a substituted judgment standard. Health care providers often make decisions for individuals who lack families or other surrogates and have no advance directives, based on a best interest standard.

What may seem the right thing to do to one individual may seem cruel and unjustified to another. Individuals and families may elect to withhold feeding and hydration, and allow death to occur "naturally." However, as the individual is dying, a family member may question if they are causing death by not feeding or hydrating the individual. The goal of non-maleficence is at the forefront when questions arise. It may be reasonable for the family to provide a dying individual a small amount of water as this is not likely to neither cause harm nor change the outcome. Providing pain relief may be acceptable for the same reason.

Just as some health care providers may have mixed motives in caring for dying individuals, some family members may want to ease their loved ones' pain while possibly hastening death. Family members may disagree on the chosen approach and may try to alter the plan by having the individual treated emergently in an acute care facility. They may be challenged to respect the individual's autonomy and decision to withhold treatment. APRNs may provide education and support to individuals and family members when the decision to withhold further treatment is made in an attempt to ensure the individual is spared additional, unwanted medical intervention.

APRNs are often key members of a palliative care team. Palliative care improves the quality of life for individuals and families dealing with life threatening illness through the prevention or treatment of suffering. This includes assessment and management of pain and other physical, psychosocial and spiritual problems in terminally ill individuals (WHO, accessed 2018). The withholding and withdrawal of life support and the administration of palliative care usually involve a multidisciplinary approach, and all involved parties, including the APRN, should participate in planning how such care is realized. The APRN may work to achieve the goal of palliative care, which is to provide comfort. Measures that do not relieve suffering but merely hasten death should be avoided.

End of life care includes difficult decisions. Dying in America is often complicated by discordant treatment teams, insufficient treatment of discomfort, transitions of care settings, and care responsibilities assumed by family members (IOM, 2015). To minimize conflict, the goal of palliative care and the means of achieving that goal should be clearly spelled out in the health record.

Documentation reflects the goal of palliative care to avoid ethical and legal conflict. Opportunity exists for APRNs to assist in the process of shared decision making regarding end of life planning, withholding, and withdrawing of treatment. APRNs in community settings can assist the process by engaging in meaningful discussion with individuals and families long before they are critically ill. According to the IOM, now the National Academy of Medicine (2015), conversations for advance directives do not occur because neither family members nor providers start the dialogue. Both are waiting for the other to initiate the conversation. The APRN works with individuals and families to clarify end of life desires in advance, utilizing clearly written advance directives which could minimize the need for surrogates.

3.11. ORDINARY vs. EXTRAORDINARY TREATMENT

Individuals may be eligible for medical treatment, regardless of whether the treatment is viewed as extraordinary or ordinary. The term ordinary is not equivalent to usual or customary. Ordinary care implies any treatment modality which offers reasonable hope of benefit, and can be used without excessive expense, pain or other inconvenience for the individual (Beauchamp & Childress, 2013, p. 162).

Extraordinary care, if used, would not offer a reasonable hope of benefit. Any treatment which is excessively expensive, excessively painful, or is inconvenient may be considered extraordinary (Beauchamp & Childress, 2013, p. 162). Employing this definition of care would imply that any treatment which offers no reasonable hope or benefit should be avoided, as this would be considered harmful to the individual.

The notion of ordinary and extraordinary care is replaced with the concept of optional management. The following example illustrates this distinction. Treating pneumonia in an elderly community residing female is usual and prudent care. In the case of an 88 year old female with advanced Alzheimer's, COPD, and alcoholism, the family and primary care provider agreed to forego treating this individual's acute pneumonia. Instead, this individual was provided comfort measures in her home where she died within 48 hours of diagnosis.

Opting not to treat the individual's pneumonia seems reasonable utilizing a shared decision making model. Treating the individual's pneumonia could ultimately have prolonged her life; however, the question of benefit should be examined. Treatment in this case would require an inpatient admission, as the individual was not lucid. She would have required ventilator support and invasive management in an intensive care setting. This would make the treatment of pneumonia in this case extraordinary care as it would be expensive, painful, and inconvenient. The APRN well versed in shared decision making can assist individuals and families in choosing the best options for care.

Health care providers may make sound moral judgments by examining the type of treatment to be used. Consideration must be given to the degree of complexity or risk, the cost and availability of the treatment.

Payment should not influence treatment decisions of the moral provider. By comparing the risks of a particular treatment with the potential for benefit, and accounting for individual's base line health status and the current acuity of the situation, prudent decisions regarding care can be made.

When deciding to employ an extraordinary treatment, a health care provider must consider the individual's desires, condition, the likelihood of survival and the cost. Employing a costly and limitedly available therapy may be appropriate if there is significant long term benefit. The availability of organs for transplantation can be scarce. This modality is therefore not readily available to all individuals. Teams are typically involved in the decision making for who should obtain this limited resource. APRNs may be members of these teams.

APRNs encourage individuals to accept those treatments which they believe are reasonable and beneficial, while considering the burdens of a particular treatment. This will vary from person to person. Ultimately the APRN respects it is the individual's responsibility to accept or decline treatments. The APRN exercises best judgment in cases in which an individual's motives may be unclear.

3.12. MEDICAL NUTRITION

Medical nutrition refers to nutritional procedures including assessment and interventions in the treatment of an illness, injury or disease condition. A specially tailored diet is planned based upon the individual's medical, psychosocial history, physical examination, and dietary history. Medical nutrition may reduce the risk of developing complications in conditions such as diabetes, or it may ameliorate the effects of conditions such as hyperlipidemia. Many medical conditions may either develop or worsen due to improper or lack of nutrition.

Invasive interventions such as feeding tubes may be employed to improve an individual's nutritional status when an individual is unable to eat or swallow. The use of feeding tubes in nursing home residents with advanced dementia is a well-known example. In this individual population, the nutritional need is evident. However, providing forced nutrition will not reverse the individual's dementia and the disease will progress.

Nurses play a vital role in providing information and guiding family members through difficult nutrition decisions. Investigators found that nurses believe family members would benefit from guidance in decisions regarding the placement of feeding tubes (Lopez, Amella, Mitchell, & Strumpf, 2010). However, their findings indicate that nurses were reluctant to become involved in these difficult decisions. For nurses to guide family members about the use of feeding tubes, they require education about the rationale for doing so utilizing evidence-based research. APRNs are key members of the health care team able to support the education of individuals, staff nurses and families to reach decisions which are beneficial and optimize quality of life.

Feeding tubes have associated risks and complications, including obstruction and site infection. They require daily maintenance. The demands of this therapy may be more than a family can provide and this in turn may infringe upon the individual and family's quality of life. APRNs must weigh the benefits of nutritional therapy with the associated risks when considering this option for an individual. APRNs may provide recommendations for nasal gastric feeding tube placement on an as needed basis as opposed to a more invasive procedure.

When an individual requires more nutritional support, the APRN can request a consultation with a gastroenterologist for placement of a percutaneous feeding tube. The APRN engages in the process of shared decision making with the family and other members of the health care team. The APRN should support the individual's wishes in the process of determining what the best nutritional therapy is for the individual.

3.13. MEDICAL FUTILITY

Futile medical care exists when there is no hope for improvement in an incapacitating condition. Futile care fails to offer benefit (Jecker, 2014). Quantitative futility is defined as existing when the possibility a treatment will benefit a patient is exceedingly poor. Qualitative futility refers to the quality of benefit of a treatment will be exceedingly poor. Both types of futility indicate the benefit will not have a positive effect on the individual.

Futile care has no possibility of achieving a good outcome and serves only to prolong life. There is no known physical or spiritual benefit derived from such care. Futile care may prolong grieving and give false hope. Caregivers may see themselves as forced to act against the best interests of their individual in cases of futile medical treatment.

In a setting of limited resources, futile care involves the expenditure of resources that could be used by other individuals who have a likelihood of achieving a positive outcome. The utilitarian will argue that a just society should spend and ration its resources sensibly in order to save as many lives as possible. A grim prognosis does not justify an end to care, but a truly futile prognosis requires further consideration by the APRN and members of the healthcare team.

For example, Baby K was born anencephalic with only the brainstem having developed during pregnancy (Ascension Health, 2012). The baby's mother had been notified of her condition following ultrasound and had been advised to terminate the pregnancy by her obstetrician and neonatologist. The mother chose to carry the child to term because of her religious beliefs. The mother and the hospital in which she delivered had opposing views on care for this child.

The hospital physicians strongly advised a Do Not Resuscitate (DNR) order for the child, which the mother refused. Baby K remained on ventilator support for six weeks while a search for another hospital was done. No other facility would accept Baby K. Finally, the child was transferred to a long term care nursing facility after being weaned from a ventilator, but the baby returned to the hospital many times for respiratory problems. Many critics of this case insist that the medical expenses used to keep Baby K on life support for over two years could have been better spent on awareness and prevention efforts of her condition (Ascension Health, 2012).

Some argue that futile clinical care should be a market commodity able to be purchased (Appeal, 2009). If the purchaser of the clinical services has the necessary funds, and as long as other individuals are not being denied access to clinical resources as a result, it may be reasonable to utilize this commodity. In this scenario, Baby K would be able to receive ICU care until funding vanished.

The issues of equity often arise in treatment of end-stage cancer (Khatcheressian, Harrington, Lyckholm, & Smith, 2008). Researchers report lack of provider-individual communication regarding prognosis, goals of therapy, and benefits of aggressive symptom management contribute to the delivery of futile chemotherapy. APRNs engage in open communications to avoid subjecting individuals to futile care.

The purchasing of care is an option in need of examination. If the goal of nursing practice is to do no harm and to benefit an individual, is futile care providing the individual benefit? If the individual or family has the resources to provide the necessary care to keep an individual alive and not tax the system at large, is it reasonable to allow for this type of care?

When caring for an infant who survives an anoxic brain injury and requires home ventilator support, this question is a difficult one. These children require expensive, daily multidisciplinary therapies, including speech therapy, physical therapy, occupational therapy, and nursing care. They require care from primary pediatric services, as well as subspecialty services, such as pulmonary medicine. The parents require education and support in caring for a technology dependent child. As these children grow, they will continue to require services and durable medical equipment.

Resuscitating infants who suffer anoxic brain injuries at birth may result in lifelong care. It is a difficult decision for health care providers and parents to allow a neonate to die without intervention. The parents may choose to have every intervention done to save their infant even after being given a poor prognosis. It may be satisfying to the parent to have the baby in their care regardless of the outcome. Truly informed consent is necessary in these circumstances because of the high level of emotions involved.

APRNs communicate openly with parents in these challenging situations. The APRN thoroughly explains the process of resuscitation and that successful resuscitation does not negate brain injury. The dilemma is who is obtaining benefit from care in this situation—the parent or the child. Ethics committees in the setting of limited resources may determine if some individuals are beyond medical hope and if care would be futile.

3.14. ETHICS COMMITTEES

Ethics committees typically include members from diverse backgrounds who support health care institutions with three major functions: providing ethics consultation, developing and/or revising select policies pertaining to clinical ethics, and facilitating education about topical issues in clinical ethics (University of Washington Department of Bioethics & Humanities, 2013). These committees may assist with interpreting advance directives, withholding and withdrawing life-sustaining treatments, informed consent, and decisions surrounding organ procurement.

Ethics committee members may represent major clinical services and other stakeholders in health care delivery such as clinicians from medicine, surgery, psychiatry, nursing, social work, a chaplain, and a community representative. APRNs may serve as committee members. These committees often include a quality improvement manager, an educator employed by the facility, a lawyer, and at least one individual with advanced training in ethics. The individual with advanced training in ethics may come from philosophy, law, medicine, theology, or anthropology.

A clinician faced with an ethical dilemma requests an ethics consultation when two conditions are met: there is an ethical problem in the care of an individual, and the resolution does not occur after bringing this to the attention of the team responsible for the care of the individual (University of Washington Department of Bioethics & Humanities, 2013). A true ethical dilemma occurs because there is a conflict between principles of autonomy, beneficence, and justice, or between principles and outcomes.

Clinical ethics consultations are interventions by trained members of a bioethics advisory committee to help resolve an ethical dilemma or answer an ethical question that arises in the course of individual care. The consultation is purely advisory. Bioethics committee members and consultants have no authority to make individual care decisions. Individuals and their insurers are typically not charged for ethics consultations.

The process of an ethics consultation consists of several steps. Consultants review medical records and interview the individual, physicians, nurses, family members, surrogate decision makers, and other relevant parties. The consultants provide an analysis of the ethical issue and suggest means to resolve it. This may include a face-to-face meeting with all parties. The case may be presented to a full bioethics advisory committee meeting and discussed. Follow-up is often performed.

The most common issues prompting clinical ethics consultations are conflicts between the medical and nursing staffs over the best care of the individual. Other reasons may include a conflict between the medical-nursing staff and the family over an individual's plan of care. Evidence that the medical staff is not following the wishes of the individual or surrogate results in conflict. Evidence that the family or surrogate decision maker is making a decision that is not in the individual's best interest can also result in an ethical dilemma.

3.15. CASE STUDIES

The APRN may face multiple ethical challenges while engaging in clinical practice. The following scenarios are examples of situations that may arise.

3.15.1. Case Study #1

A nineteen year old female individual presents to the urgent care center with her mother and with a 10 day history of right lower quadrant pain. Both are feeling frustrated due to lack of a diagnosis. The individual was seen 10 days ago in an emergency department and discharged being told she had a hernia which would require evaluation in an ambulatory setting. She then saw her family physician three days later and was referred to a surgeon who would be seeing her in two weeks. She presents this evening due to continuation of the pain and her mother's pressuring her to "find out what is wrong." The individual denies any loss of appetite, nausea, vomiting or diarrhea. She reports dysuria with frequency. She denies that movement or lifting increases her pain. She also denies any bulges to her abdominal wall, just a small "bump" to the right lower abdominal region that is not painful. It is difficult to obtain a history directly from the individual because her mother continually interrupts and answers the questions for the individual.

On further questioning, the individual admits to a vaginal discharge, burning with urination, and sexual activity without barrier protection. She had a boyfriend for the past year with whom she recently ended the relationship. She is uncertain as to whether he had other sexual partners. She reports that he had been her only partner. Her last gynecologic visit was one year ago. She denies a history of previous sexually transmitted infections (STI). Her last menstrual period was two weeks prior and was normal.

After examination, the individual was diagnosed with a sexually transmitted disease. She did not wish to share this information with her mother. The individual's mother pressured the provider for answers and a diagnosis. The provider was challenged to maintain the individual's confidentiality. What ethical principle would guide this provider's decision making? How should she handle the missed diagnosis by the family physician? Are there legal ramifications? What if the individual loses fertility because of the delay in diagnosis? If the mother of the individual was paying for the individual's medical bills, would that change what information she should be given?

3.15.2. Case Study #2

A 78 year old male individual was admitted to the hospital with a brain injury after a fall. He has a history of diabetes mellitus, hypertension, anemia and dementia. He presented with areas of ecchymosis to his forehead. His computerized tomography (CT) scan showed hemorrhagic contusions of the bilateral frontal lobes, left temporal lobe, and small subdural hematomas on the frontal lobes. During his hospitalization he was oriented to person, place, and time and dates for a portion of his stay. The nursing staff reports the individual suffers from occasional confusion, mild short term memory loss, and intermittent agitation. At times he was aggressive to the nursing staff and often refused medications, including insulin and antihypertensive prescription drugs. The APRN managing this individual's care is faced with a dilemma. Can this individual with a documented brain injury and history of dementia refuse his medical therapy? Can he be forced to take his medications? How should the practitioner proceed? Is an ethics committee consult necessary?

3.15.3. Case Study #3

An 82 year old female is admitted from the nursing home for an acute exacerbation of heart failure (HF) and hypernatremia. The individual suffers from advanced Alzheimer's dementia. The individual required diuresis with intravenous furosemide (Lasix) and over the next four days, the HF symptoms and sodium levels improved. Two days later, the sodium levels decreased and a nephrology consultation was obtained. The individual was started on tolvaptan (Samsca) to treat the hypernatremia. This improved the sodium levels, but the individual became hypokalemic, requiring treatment for the elevated potassium. The individual then experienced an episode of syncope resulting in a fall, from which she recovered. The following day, she had an episode of staring off into space which was suspected to be a seizure. The individual was evaluated for a cerebral vascular accident (CVA) and no acute bleeding was identified. The individual continued to experience a complicated hospitalization and worsening of her dementia.

How does the APRN approach an elderly frail individual with multiple complex conditions? Was admission for the HF and resulting complications worth the risk of worsening the individual's dementia? How could this situation be avoided? When is palliative care appropriate for this individual?

3.15.4. Case Study #4

A thirteen year old female comes to the office with her mother for an annual physical examination. During the exam, when she is alone with the practitioner, the individual advises the APRN that she has been sexually active for the past year. The APRN completes the examination and during the follow-up office time, recommends the vaccination for human papilloma virus (HPV). The individual's mother refuses this vaccination as she states her daughter is not sexually active. The individual's mother is concerned that by vaccinating her daughter, she is encouraging early sexual debut. The individual is not vaccinated on this visit and the APRN recommends a follow up visit in two weeks. At the next visit, the individual arrives without her mother and she requests the HPV vaccination. How does the APRN advise this individual? What ethical principles are guiding the APRN's decision to vaccinate this individual? Are there legal issues involved? Does the provider have a duty to tell the individual's mother? Is the provider obligated to counsel the individual to tell her mother?

3.16. REFERENCES

AMA (American Medical Association) (accessed 2018) Informed Consent. Retrieved from https://www.ama-assn.org/delivering-care/informed-consent

AMA (American Medical Association) (2018). Medical Ethics and End of Life: What every patient should know. Retrieved from https://wire.ama-assn.org/delivering-care/medical-ethics-and-end-life-what-every-patient-should-know

APA (American Psychological Association) (2012). Research Misconduct. Retrieved from: http://www.apa.org/research/responsible/misconduct/index.aspx

Ascension Health (2012). Baby K. Retrieved from http://www.ascensionhealth.org/index.php?option=com_content&view=article&id=237&Itemid=173

Beauchamp, T.L. & Childress, J.F. (2013). *Principles of Biomedical Ethics* (7th ed). New York: Oxford University Press.

Campbell, S.M., Ulrich, C.M. & Grady, C. (2016) A broader understanding of moral distress. *The American Journal of Bioethics* 16(12), 2-9.

Canterberry v Spence, 464 F2d 772 (DC Cir), cert denied 409 US 1064 (1972).

Coetzee, S.K. & Klopper, H.C. (2010). Compassion fatigue within nursing: a concept analysis. Nursing & Health Sciences 12(2), 235-243.

Coetzee, S.K. & Laschinger, H. (2017). Toward a comprehensive, theoretical model of compassion fatigue: An integrative literature review, *Nursing & Health Sciences* 20 (1), 4-15.

Corley, M.C. (2002). Nurse moral distress: A proposed theory and research agenda. Nursing Ethics 9: 636–50.

Fisher, J. & Clayton, M. (2012). Who gives a tweet: Assessing individuals' interest in the use of social media for healthcare. *Worldviews on Evidence Based Nursing* 9, 100–108.

Fourie C. (2016). The ethical significance of moral distress: inequality and nurses' constraint-distress. *American Journal of Bioethics* 16(12), 23-25.

Fourie C. (2017). Who Is Experiencing What Kind of Moral Distress? Distinctions for Moving from a Narrow to a Broad Definition of Moral Distress. *AMA Journal of Ethics* 19(6), 578-584.

Hamric, A.B. (2014). A case study of moral distress. *Journal of Hospice & Palliative Care Nursing* 16(8), 457–63.

Hamric, A.B., & Blackhall, L.J. (2007). Nurse-physician perspectives on the care of dying patients in intensive care units: Collaboration, moral distress, and ethical climate. *Critical Care Medicine* 35(2), 422–29.

Hamric, A.B., Borchers, C.T., & Epstein, E.G. (2012). Development and testing of an instrument to measure moral distress in healthcare professionals. *American Journal of Bioethics* 3(2), 1–9.

ICMJE (International Committee of Medical Editors) (2017). *Recommendations for the Conduct, Reporting, Editing, and Publication of Scholarly work in Medical Journals.* Retrieved from http://www.icmje.org/recommendations/

Jecker, N.S. (2014). Medical Futility. Ethics in Medicine University of Washington School of Medicine. Retrieved from https://depts.washington.edu/bioethx/topics/futil.html

Kelly, B. (1998). Preserving moral integrity: A follow-up study with new graduate nurses. *Journal of Advanced Nursing* 28, 1134–45.

Kon, A.A., Davidson, J.E., Morrison, W., Danis, M. & White, D.B. (2017). Shared Decision Making in Intensive Care Units: An American College of Critical Care Medicine and American Thoracic Society Policy Statement. *Critical Care Medicine* 44(1), 188-201.

Landry, C. (2017). Not knowing the "right thing to do:" Moral distress and tolerating uncertainty in medicine. *Clinical Ethics* 12, 37-44.

Lopez, R.P., Amella, E.J., Mitchell, S.L. & Strumpf, N.E. (2010). Nurses' perspectives on feeding decisions for nursing home residents with advanced dementia. *Journal of Clinical Nursing* 19 (5–6), 632–8.

Milton C.L. (2010). Failing to do the right thing: nurse practice and the family experience. *Nursing Science Quarterly*, 23(3), 206–8.

Moore, G.P., Moffett, P.M., Fider, C. & Moore, M.J. (2014). What Emergency Physicians Should Know About Informed Consent: Legal Scenarios, Cases, and Caveats. *Academic Emergency Medicine* 21, 921-7.

IOM (Institute of Medicine now the National Academy of Medicine) (2015). *Dying in America: Improving Quality and Honoring Individual Preferences near the End of Life.* Washington DC: The National Academies Press. https://doi.org/10.17226/18748

NCSBN (National Council of State Boards of Nursing) (2018). A Nurse's Guide to the Use of Social Media. Retrieved fromhttps://www.ncsbn.org/NCSBN_SocialMedia.pdf

TJC (The Joint Commission) (2010). *Advancing Effective Communication, Cultural Competence, and Patient-and Family-Centered Care: A Roadmap for Hospitals.* Oakbrook Terrace, IL.

Thomson v Sun City Community Hospital, 668 P2d 605 (1984).

University of Washington Department of Bioethics and Humanities. (2013). Ethics Committees and Ethics Consultation. Retrieved from http://depts.washington.edu/bioethx/topics/ethics.html

Whitehead, P.B., Herbertson, R.K., Hamric, A.B., Epstein, E.G. & Fisher, J.M. (2015). Moral distress among healthcare professionals: Report of an institution-wide survey. *Journal of Nursing Scholarship* 47(2),117–25.

WHO (World Health Organization) (accessed 2018).WHO Definition of Palliative Care. Retrieved from http://www.who.int/cancer/palliative/definition/en/.

CHAPTER 4

Ethical Considerations in the Care of Vulnerable Adult Populations

JOAN VALAS

4.1. INTRODUCTION

Nurses are held to "high standards of compassion and respect for all—especially those most vulnerable" (Taylor 2010, p. 3) and recognize that the injustice of unequal health care is the result of many factors. The vulnerable may be frail, homeless, and disenfranchised. The term vulnerable populations implies that they are a disadvantaged group of the population that requiring special considerations and protection. The Federal guidance (covered in the Code of Federal Regulations, Title 45 Part 46—Protection of Human Subjects) includes children, pregnant women, mentally disabled persons, or economically or educationally disadvantaged persons as vulnerable. The list can also include unauthorized residents, incompetent patients, prisoners, and the Armed Forces (Code of Federal Regulations, 2019; WHO, 2019; WMA, 2019).

As they are often not "visible"—which can result in further inequalities or disparities of health—these persons enter our health care systems with more acute illnesses that might have been prevented if adequate preventive care had been available. Shi and Stevens (2010) have put forth five reasons to focus national attention on vulnerable populations: they have greater health needs; their numbers are increasing; vulnerability is a social issue resolved through social means; it is intertwined with the nation's health; and there is a growing emphasis on the equality of health, particularly among racial and ethnic minorities. Recognition of those that are vulnerable and at risk is an essential primary preventive measure for the practice of advanced practice nursing.

4.2. VULNERABLE POPULATIONS

The following vignette is an example of the problems facing the nurse practitioner dealing with vulnerable populations.

An elderly female was brought in to the hospital by EMS and was admitted because of an altered mental status. Until recently, she had been able to care for herself and lived alone, according to her neighbors. She is unable to communicate her health history and it is unclear if she has any family members to contact. Her health care needs must be considered as well as the ethical concerns for her care.

Aday (2001) reminds us that the "origins and remedies" arise from the bonded human community and as such all humans have the potential to be vulnerable (p. 1). Humans share the universal condition of vulnerability as well as that of human strength (Nyamathi & Koniak-Griffin & Greengold, 2007 p. xiv). However, most research and policies concerning vulnerable populations focus on subpopulations (Aday, 2001) such as ethnic and racial minorities, women and children, the elderly, the poor, the chronically and mentally ill, disabled, imprisoned, the homeless, and substance abusers. These groups are at risk for poor physical, psychological and social health (Aday 1994; 2001) and have an increased risk to adverse health outcomes, as evidenced by increased morbidity and mortality (Flaskerud &Winslow, 1998; Flaskerud et al., 2002; IOM, 2002).

It is important to distinguish between the terms "vulnerable populations" and "at-risk individuals", as they are often used interchangeably and grouped collectively. Categorizations and use of standardized lists used to describe vulnerable groups should not be used exclusively to describe these populations. Moreover, "a focus on misery, poverty, and crisis alone, [may] contribute to the objectification of a population" (Susser & Patterson, 2001) and only serve to marginalize people in need, creating barriers to care and service. DeBruin (2001) suggests that vulnerability "ought not to be considered as a characteristic of groups . . . rather certain traits may render certain persons vulnerable in certain situations". Often included in these categories are the specific groups detailed above in federal regulations; however, it may be necessary to cast a broader net to ensure inclusion to those who need care the most in consideration of ethics and the concept of health disparities. Nurse practitioners should not limit their understanding of vulnerable populations to a list or a category, but rather look more widely and assess their patients more fully for their individual vulnerabilities.

Gutherie (2005) has noted that there has been a growing need to understand the relationship between health disparities and vulnerable populations among racial and ethnic minorities in the United States. Health disparities may be defined as inequalities of health status as well as the provision, access and quality of care. Health inequalities are particularly apparent when comparing vulnerable populations to non-vulnerable populations (Nyamthi, Koniak-Griffin & Greengold, 2007). Disparity of health care, a core representation of social injustice, has raised national attention on vulnerable groups (Nyamthi, Koniak-Griffin, & Greengold, 2007, p. 6). As a result of a Congress-commissioned study, the Institute of Medicine's (IOM) report entitled Unequal Treatment (2002) concluded that racial and ethnic minorities are less likely to receive needed health services, creating disparities of health and making them more vulnerable and at risk for poor health outcomes. In this report, the IOM also looked at other factors that contributed to these health disparities, such as cultural and linguistic barriers, costs, care delivery sites, health care provider prejudice and stereotyping against racial and ethnic minorities.

Nurse practitioners should consider all of these factors and not limit assessments of their patients to medical needs alone. Nurse practitioners can help to "close the gap in community health" in working with diverse vulnerable populations, not only by having an understanding and first-hand knowledge of the communities (The Future of Nursing, 2010) where they work, but also in recognizing the vulnerability of those who live in these communities. The IOM Future of Nursing (2010) report recommended that nurses be able to critique the ethical aspects of health policy in terms of vulnerable populations (p. 518).

There is no checklist of questions in order to assess for vulnerability just as there is no checklist to assess the culture of our clients; however, the nurse should consider further inquiry and assessment into their clients' economic status and geographic location, health, age, functional or developmental status, and identification of communication barriers and be cognizant of obscure vulnerability associated with race, ethnicity, and gender. Furthermore, assessments and inquiry of vulnerability and culture of clients, populations and communities served by the nurse practitioner in practice or PhD nurse conducting research have many similarities that are helpful to understand.

Cultural competence has "emerged as the mantra of contemporary practice", with an abundance of books and journal articles describing "formulas and instructions for students, educators, and clinicians" on how to become culturally competent which despite nationwide leadership and experts in nursing, medicine, professional organizations and certifying organization, "routine incorporation in patient treatment plans has not been widely achieved " (Dreher, Shapiro & Assesselin, 2016, p. 3) The discussion of guidelines and conceptual models of vulnerability offered below aim to clarify this assessment and its ethical implications on practice and research.

4.3. ETHICAL GUIDELINES AND REGULATIONS FOR THE PROTECTION OF HUMAN SUBJECTS IN RESEARCH

It is important for nurse practitioners to be familiar with federal regulations and ethical guidelines for the protection of human subjects' research. After the World War II War Crime Trials, the Nuremberg Code was established in 1947 as a set of standards to assure research was carried out in an ethical manner. The Office of Human Research and Protection (OHRP) operationally sits within the Office of the Deputy Director for Human Research (DDIR), the National Institutes of Health (NIH) which is part of the U.S. Public Health Service within the Department of Health and Human Services (DHHS). OHPR has published a variety of policy and regulatory guidance materials to assist the research community in conducting ethical research that is in compliance with DHHS regulations. A full historical description of the development of the federal regulations for human subject research is found elsewhere in this book. The ethical guidelines as they relate to vulnerable populations are described here. The National Commission for the Protection of Human Subjects of Biomedical and Behavioral Research was created on July 12, 1974 by the National Research Act (Pub. L. 93-348). The Commission identified the basic ethical principles and developed guidelines that would underlie the conduct of biomedical and behavioral research involving human subjects. The Belmont Report—Ethical Principles and Guidelines for the Protection of Human Subjects (1979) summarize these basic ethical principles. The three basic principles— respect of persons, beneficence and justice—as well as autonomy have relevance to the ethics of research involving human subjects and serve as an analytical framework to guide research. Respect for persons implies that individuals are autonomous agents and that persons without autonomy have the right to protections. Beneficence is the obligation of the practitioner to do no harm and to maximize possible benefits and minimize harm to their subjects and patients. Justice implies fair and equal distribution of benefits and burdens among people, meaning that each person has an equal share. While they are important in their application to research, The Belmont Report does not always provide clear resolutions to the ethical dilemmas faced in research (NIH, 2004).

Research involving vulnerable populations is covered in the Code of Federal Regulations, Title 45 Part 46—Protection of Human Subjects (aka The Common Rule)(Code of Federal Regulations, 2019). This regulation requires that institutional review boards (IRB) take into account the purpose of the research and mandates that research pay particular attention to the special needs and problems of vulnerable populations. This regulation lists children, prisoners, pregnant women, mentally disabled persons, and economically or educationally disadvantaged persons as vulnerable groups. The Common Rule has recently been updated (see Chapter 2 for specifics).

Nurse practitioners involved in research and care of vulnerable populations must consider the special needs of their patients who fall into these vulnerable groups, keeping in mind that inequalities and disparities of health are part of what makes them so vulnerable. The concept of vulnerability is complex and the literature from numerous disciplines is replete with attempts to describe the effects on health care and health outcomes. Several conceptual models exist which describe the relationships among factors associated with vulnerability.

4.4. CONCEPTUAL MODELS OF VULNERABLE POPULATIONS

Conceptual models and frameworks for studying the vulnerable examine why they are more at risk for poor health and experience inferior health care. While several theoretical frameworks have guided vulnerable populations studies (social cognitive theory, theory of reasoned action and health beliefs model), they are not specific to address these risks and experiences (Nyamathi, Koniak-Griffin and Greengold, 2007). Traditional ethical principles focus on the individual and do not cover the wider population.

4.4.1. Aday: Model of Vulnerability

The underlying concept of Lu Ann Aday's conceptual model is risk (1994). Risk assumes that everyone has an equal chance of an adverse health related event. However, certain individuals and groups have more risks than others and these are described as vulnerable populations. They have greater multifaceted health needs that may be debilitating or life threatening and require more extensive health services (Aday, 1994, p. 490). The origins of poor health traditionally focus on the individual; highlighting autonomy and personal responsibility for health. These include age, race, ethnicity and gender. However, a community or societal and environmental or macro perspective of health needs focuses on risks that exist "as a function of the availability of opportunities and resources for maximizing health" (Aday, 1994, p. 490). There is a relationship between the individual and this community perspective. According to this model, vulnerability can be predicted by social status, social capital and human capital. Social status incorporates a person's age, sex, race and ethnicity. Social capital status incorporates an individual's family structure, social networks, marital status, and voluntary organizations. Human capital includes schools attended, jobs held, income and housing of the individual. The availability of these resources has a direct impact on the health outcomes of those who are vulnerable. Ultimately, it appears that "vulnerability reflects the interactions of many factors over which individuals have little control" (Nyamathi, Koniak-Griffin, & Greengold, 2007, p. 7).

4.4.2. Flaskerud and Winslow's Vulnerable Populations Conceptual Model (VPCM)

The VPCM was built upon the work of Aday and others. This model proposes that links exist between resource availability, risk, and health status of vulnerable populations. These resources are similar to Aday's and are described as human capital, social connection and environmental resources. Relative risks are factored into this model and are either behavioral or biological in nature. In this model an increased exposure to risk and limited access to resources results in poorer health status and increased morbidity and mortality. This model was "designed for clinical practice, research and policy interventions aimed at impacting links" between resource limitations and the effect on risk and health outcomes (Nyamathi, Koniak-Griffin, & Greengold, 2007, p. 7).

4.4.3. Shi and Stevens—Vulnerability Model

Shi and Stevens' model is comprehensive, multi-level, and emphasizes both the individual and the community and environmental or ecological risk factors associated with vulnerability. This model highlights a broad range of risk factors that together lead to poor health and health outcomes. Individuals' risk factors are not determined by their individual characteristics alone. This comprehensive model "more accurately reflects realities and avoids . . . blaming the victims" (Shi & Stevens 2010, p. 17). Access to health services, poor quality of care and health status as well as marginalization are reflective of these risk factors. Predisposing risk factors include demographics, personal and cultural belief systems, social structure and social status (i.e., race, ethnicity, gender). Socioeconomic status, human capital and other factors including health insurance and access to care may also influence risk vulnerability. Individual risk factors are categorized as predisposing, enabling, or need, and may influence the community and ecological risk factors that interact with each other and cumulatively influence vulnerability. Predisposing risk factors include individual risk factors of age, race, ethnicity, culture and gender. At the community or ecological level, geographical setting, physical environment and sociocultural norms of the community are factors. Enabling factors socially and materially enhance individual risk factors and include income, education, health insurance coverage and community factors such as the availability of jobs, school and health services. Need risk factors are the existing health problems of the individual, including mental health issues, disabilities and disease rates. The community's risk factors include communicable disease rates and illicit drug availability.

4.4.4. Kachingwe-Huff Model of Culturally Proficient and Ethical Practice

Health care providers should provide proficient care with the necessary cultural knowledge, understand the ethical implications of working with culturally diverse vulnerable populations, and understand that ethical dilemmas may occur as a result of a dichotomy between cultural beliefs/practices of the patient and the health care provider (Kachingwe & Huff, 2015). The Kachingwe-Huff Model of Culturally Proficient and Ethical Practice contends that cultural care can be fostered by incorporating these five components: cultural awareness, cultural knowledge, interpersonal communication skills, cultural collaboration and cultural experiences (Kachingwe & Huff, 2015, pp. 46–47). Most people, including health care providers, innately view others from an ethnocentric perspective leading to distorted perceptions of their patients' health behaviors (Campinha-Bacote & Padgett, 1995; Dowd, Giger & Davidhizar, 1998; Huff & Kline, 2007; Kachingwe & Huff, 2015). Clearly, this is to be avoided in order to provide culturally and ethically proficient care. The five components of this model provide a framework for health care practitioners "to solve ethical problems, issues and dilemmas that may be encountered during a transcultural client-practitioner relationship" (Kachingwe & Huff, 2015).

In consideration of any conceptual model that assists in understanding vulnerability, an advanced practice registered nurse must have cultural knowledge of the clients, populations and communities they serve when applying ethical principles to practice and research. Cultural knowledge requires an understanding and respect of the diversity of cultural groups and incorporating its importance "in an unbiased manner to meet the client's needs" (Kachingwe & Huff, 2015), which is addressed in the ANA code of Ethics (2015).

Provision Eight of the ANA Code of Ethics states that as nurses provide health care to culturally diverse populations and "to create a moral milieu that is sensitive to diverse cultural values and practices" (ANA, 2015, p. 32). The respect for other life styles and values of persons from diverse cultures requires that healthcare providers look introspectively and exam their own values and beliefs. APRNs must also understand and reflect upon their own personal beliefs and values, as there are instances where their values may conflict with their clients. In situations of unresolved conflicts between client and provider beliefs, they may be best handled by referring the case to the institution's ethics committee. However, an understanding of one's own personal beliefs and values, cultural knowledge and ethical principles should be used as a guide to APRN practice in similar situations, particularly involving immigrant populations. When conflicts between the culture of patients and those of the provider exist, the nurse practitioner is best served by bringing in other practitioners for consultation or bringing the issue before the institutional ethics boards to resolve the ethical dilemmas of these conflicts.

4.5. ETHICAL CONSIDERATIONS IN CARE AND RESEARCH OF ILLEGAL ALIENS, INCOMPETENT PATIENTS, PRISONERS, AND THE ARMED FORCES

4.5.1. Unauthorized Residents: Illegal Immigrants

Those born outside of the United States represent an ever growing portion of the U.S. populations. In 2016 more than 13.5% of the U.S. populations (approximately 43.7 million) were foreign born individuals living in the United States according to a report from the Pew Research Center (2018). Of this 43.7 million, 13% are from Europe and Canada, 27% are from South and East Asia, 25% are from other Latino countries and 26% are from Mexico (Radford & Budiman, 2018). Foreign born are defined by the Congressional Budget Office (CBO, 2019) as a person born outside of the United States. Foreign-born or immigrants may have legal permanent status because of a family-sponsored application; they may be refugees or asylum seekers. These residents are issued a "green card" which serves as identification of their legal status. Foreign-born individuals can also hold legal temporary status as a visitor with or without a visa, which grants them a time-limited stay. According to the Pew Research Center (Radford & Budiman, 2018) about one in four immigrants are unauthorized or undocumented to live in the U.S. accounting for 11.0 million or 24.5 percent of the 43.7 million. Of the 43.7 million 33.8 are lawful immigrants. Naturalized citizens account for 19.8 million or 44.1% of that population and lawful permanent residents account for 11.9 million or 26.6% (Radford & Budiman, 2018). In 2016, 66.1% of the foreign born were in the workforce. Of all foreign born, those earning less than $20,000.00 per year accounted for 33.1%, those earning $20,000.00 to $49,000.00 accounted for 39.3% and those earning more than $50,000.00 accounted for 28.9% of that population. Among this population 19.7% were living in poverty and 20.4% had no health insurance (Radford & Budiman, 2018). Many U.S. employers do not provide health care insurance to their low-income employees and past and present federal regulations do not provide Medicaid coverage to unauthorized residents.

Persons without authorized residency or legal citizenship are referred to by many terms in the United States and other countries that have large immigrant populations. In the U.S., the politically correct terminology is highly contested (Dwyer, 2004). Some of the terms used are: unauthorized residents, illegal immigrants, undocumented immigrants and illegal aliens. Whatever the term used, it does not change the fact that these persons have health care needs. In 1965, the U.S. Immigration and Nationality Act eliminated quotas of national origin, allowing only close relatives, refugees and persons of certain professions and skill sets, yet illegal immigration remains a highly contested social and politically polarizing issue. Despite laws and rules against it, immigrants are working and living in every country (Dwyer, 2004). An even more contested and contentious issue is whether these illegal immigrants are entitled to publically-funded health care services. Immigrants, whether legal or illegal, are at greater risk for poor health outcomes (Dwyer, 2004) and are therefore considered vulnerable. Illegal immigration occurs for many reasons, including the escape of war and prosecution, poverty, employment opportunities, and the chance of a better life for themselves and their families. Immigrants in the U.S. often do the jobs that Americans choose not to, and "have the worst jobs and work in the worst conditions" (Dwyer, 2004, p. 35). Certain factors put immigrants at greater risk for poor health outcomes regardless of their legal status. Those factors are not solely related to poor working conditions or language differences but are rather shaped by historical, social, cultural, political and economic factors, known as the social determinants of health. Understanding cultural differences has always been a central focus for the profession of nursing and is addressed through education, which develops cultural competency. Often under-emphasized in cultural competence education are other social factors that may contribute to immigrant vulnerability. It is also important to recognize how the status of being foreign-born or an unauthorized resident impacts the social determinants of health.

There is no one definition of culture and the foreign-born are a diverse group of ethnicities and races. Culture is often confused with race or ethnicity. Culture can be defined as the "integrated patterns of human behavior including thoughts, communications, actions, beliefs, values, and institutions of racial, ethnic, religious, or social groups" (Kleinman, 1978, 1988). It denotes a" historically transmitted pattern of meanings embodied in symbols, a system of inherited conceptions expressed in symbolic forms by means of which men communicate, perpetuate, and develop their knowledge about and attitudes toward life . . ." (Geertz, 1973, p. 89). It is important for nurse practitioners to understand the forces of history, power and political economy in constructing the boundaries of these categories (Schulz and Mullings, 2006) as social determinants of health. It is this powerless state that may make the foreign-born more vulnerable. Health care providers must provide culturally proficient or competent care, understand the ethical implications of working with culturally diverse vulnerable populations, and understand that ethical dilemmas may occur as a result of a dichotomy between cultural beliefs/practices of the patient and the health care provider (Kachingwe & Huff, 2015).

The number of undocumented immigrants in the United States is growing, and the foreign-born and undocumented immigrants have lower rates of public or private insurance (Carrasquillo, Carasquillo & Shea, 2000; Goldman, Smith & Sood, 2005). The foreign born are more likely to live in poverty, are less educated and less likely to have health care insurance, although this varies by the country of origin and immigration status (Truman et al., 2009, p. S278; U.S. Census, 2010) and their unauthorized resident status does not preclude them from purchasing insurance in certain states (Goldman, Smith & Sood, 2005).

U.S. public policy has made those with unauthorized illegal status ineligible for publicly funded health care services in most cases. The 1996 Personal Responsibility and Work Opportunity Reconciliation Act (PRWORA, 1996)(H.R.3734, 1996) made most legal immigrants ineligible for Medicaid during the first five years of their residency. Undocumented persons were already ineligible prior to this act with certain exceptions. Federal Medicaid funds are administered by individual states and are required by PRWORA to enact laws which establish eligibility. Federal funds under Section 1011, Federal Reimbursement of Emergency Health Services Furnished to Undocumented Aliens, are available, however, for payments to eligible providers for emergency health services provided to the undocumented related to hospital inpatient, outpatient and ambulance services (Centers for Medicare and Medicaid Services, 2019). These funds provided $250 billion to all 50 states until 2008. Some states still have funds available and others have exhausted their funds.

Under the Patient Protection and Affordable Care Act (Pub. Law No. 111-148) and the Reconciliation bill (Health Care and Education Act of 2010, Pub. Law No. No. 111-152) known as the Affordable Care Act (ACA) for health reform, passed in 2010, undocumented immigrants are unable to purchase coverage or be eligible for tax credits and will receive no assistance from the federal government (available at Center for Immigration Studies http://www.cis.org). This law will provide access to affordable health care coverage to legal immigrants, refugees and asylum seekers. This does not include those who have been granted protections under the Deferred Action for Childhood Arrivals program (DACA) The status of DACA remains unresolved as of January 2019. However some states such as California undocumented immigrants may be eligible through certain program (Covered California, 2019). Undocumented immigrants will continue to receive Medicaid benefits only for emergency health services under the Emergency Medical Treatment and Active Labor Act (ETMALA) (Berlinger & Raghavan, 2013).

Children and pregnant women have had access to public health care services through federal money given to the states to administrate through what is known as the Children's Health Plan (CHIP). Many states require similar eligibility of legal immigrant status, refugees, and those seeking asylum. CHIP was created by the 1997 Balanced Budget Act to allocate 20 billion dollars over ten years to help states cover low-income children in families ineligible for Medicaid but unable to purchase private insurance. Conditions of this act were restricted in 2007 by President George W. Bush. It was amended by President Barack Obama in 2009 to remove the restrictions. In 2010, the Affordable Care Act (ACA) extended these funds to states with the establishment of state based exchanges (SBE) and starting January 2014 thereby providing more options to patients (Centers for Medicare & Medicaid Service, 2019). As of January 2019 the fate of the ACA is unknown.

As undocumented immigrants are known to have poorer health outcomes, are often socio-economically disadvantaged, and have lower rates of public and private insurance, what ethical responsibility does society have to provide health care services for undocumented immigrants? Dwyer argues that two different answers are elicited from two polarized factions—one he calls "nationalists" and the other "humanists" (Dwyer, 2004, p. 34). Nationalists take the position that society does not have any obligation, basing this perspective on the legal rules and formal citizenship, while humanists state that society does have an obligation (Dwyer, 2004, p. 34). Humanists argue that health is a basic human right. The World Health Organization (WHO) attests that every country in the world now has a human rights treaty that addresses health as a human right and which describes health-related rights and the rights related to conditions necessary for health (WHO, 2019).

4.5.1.1. Social Determinants of Health: The Implications for Ethical Practice

Nurse practitioners working in a variety of settings, including community clinics, public health and emergency rooms, are quite likely to encounter undocumented immigrants. NPs can help and support them overcome barriers of the health care system by providing not only health care services but also providing nonjudgmental ethical and compassionate care. Immigrants often face stigma and marginalization (Derose, Escarce, & Lurie, 2007) from the community at large and even from health care providers because of cultural differences and language barriers, making them reluctant to seek out health care services. Political debates and arguments about immigrants as economic burdens or threats to national safety occur in public spaces through newspapers, television and other media. Undocumented immigrants are not immune to the discourse and therefore do not routinely seek out health care services and only enter the health care system due to an emergency or trauma. Because only emergency medical services are available and they are without access to primary and preventive health care services, they remain vulnerable at discharge. While the Affordable Health Care Act (2010) currently makes health care accessible to many who were previously uninsured, it did not make provisions for the undocumented.

Until political differences are resolved and policies in place to address the problems of immigration, the health of undocumented immigrants remains at risk. This does not eliminate the dilemma and ethical responsibility for nurse practitioners to care for patients in need. Nurse practitioners and researchers work in ever increasingly diverse communities; many of which may be undocumented immigrants. Dwyer states that the selection of patients should be on medical need alone and never on factors of residency, immigration status, or the ability to pay (2004). He also related that the "phenomena of illegal immigration" and adequate health care for them reflects the "complexity of moral thought" (p. 34). These are some of the complexities faced by health care providers working with immigrant populations. Ethical dilemmas arise for nurse practitioners when they allow the immigration status and economic status of clients to enter into their provision of care in any scenario. Similar situations can arise for nurse researchers if their research participants may not have legal residency in the United States. While federal regulations address fair access to and treatment of immigrants in research studies, they do not address their legal status. In such cases in which undocumented immigrants are enrolled in research studies, the nurse researcher must take care to inform them how any information obtained in the study would be used. They must also take care as a researcher to use pseudonyms in order to protect patient anonymity as much as possible.

Undocumented immigrants tend to underreport infectious diseases and go without routine health examinations, immunizations and screenings. Immigrant women are often victims of sexual abuse that goes unreported. Compassionate care includes linking these patients to other supportive services through the healthcare provider's own established community networks, including community social organizations, churches or schools that provide additional health services, and social and legal services for undocumented immigrants. Understanding the implications of the social, economic, and political barriers faced by undocumented immigrants is as important as understanding the cultural traditions and language in providing compassionate care.

To know that someone comes from a particular ethnicity is to know very little about that person as ethnicity "is only one marker of identity" (Turner, 2005, p. 479). Ethnic background, language, gender, socioeconomic status, education, personal and family histories and other factors all contribute to how our patients understand and experience health and illness. Immigrants, legal or illegal, come from varied ethnic backgrounds that are socially, historically and geographically based. Social customs and traditions may or may not determine their health care decisions if they have been separated from their country of origin and have become acculturated into their new homes. Ethnic groups with differing socioeconomic levels may have different perspectives (Turner, 2005, p. 479). How patients experience health from their local perspective is more important than evaluating them or judging them based on ethnicity or their legal status. Arthur Kleinman recommends listening to the narratives of patients or conducting mini-ethnographies to learn about their local and personal perspectives of health and illness (Kleinman, 1978; 1988).

4.5.2. Prisoners

There were 6,613,500 adult prisoners under correctional supervision in (U.S. Department of Justice, 2018). The United States prison population accounts for one quarter of the world's prison population, with an increasing number of racial minorities, women and children. Prisons are often overcrowded and have limited access to health care programs and services despite prisoners' constitutional right to humane medical care (Gostin, 2007). Providing health care and participating in research with prisoners are of concern for the advanced practice nurse working with them. Due to their restricted autonomy, low socioeconomic status, poorer educational background and poor health, prisoners are extremely vulnerable. These factors alone do not allow prisoners to "meaningfully choose" (Gostin, 2007, p. 738) if they wish to participate in medical research. They also are unable to choose their own health care providers and services when needed.

4.5.2.1. Federal Regulations Related to Research of Prisoners

The Nuremburg code (1947) was the first code of conduct for scientific human research recognized internationally. It was written in response to Nazi experiments on prisoners during World War II. It emphasized the "voluntariness" of the subject and stressed that unnecessary physical or mental suffering must be prevented.

Despite these regulations, unethical research involving prisoners continued through the 1970s. A wide variety of research was conducted on prisoners by the U.S. Army, several major pharmaceutical companies and other consumer products sponsors up until the early 1970s (Gostin, 2007). The research includes drugs, diet drinks, detergents, and chemical warfare agents. These declined in the mid-seventies with the formation of the National Commission for the Protection of Human Subjects of Biomedical and Behavioral Research. As late as 1974, prisoner coercion was revealed in the Philadelphia Prison System in the Holmesburg Prison with the research of dangerous hallucinogenic, carcinogenic and radioactive chemicals (Urbina, 2006).

The National Research Act was enacted by the National Commission for the Protection of Human Subjects of Biomedical and Behavioral Research (NCPHSBBR) in 1974 (NCPHSBBR,1979). The act created the federal regulatory framework to protect human research subjects for all federal and funded research. Vulnerable populations protections specific to pregnant women was added in 1975; prisoners in 1978 and children in 1983.

In 1976, a report was published by the National Commission for the Protection of Human Subjects of Biomedical and Behavioral Research for research of prisoners called the Report and Recommendations: Research Involving Prisoners. This report promulgated a federal regulation enacted in 1978 as 45 CFR Part 46 Subpart C, enforced under the U.S Department of Health and Human Services, Office for Health Service Protection and known as the Common Rule, which addressed additional protections for prisoners involved in research including the requirement of informed consent. Updated in 2018, the categories for exempt research was revised and expanded establishing new exempt categories In regard to prisoners Subpart C permits secondary research in a new Category 8. Category 8 allows for secondary analysis of data provided broad consent was secured and documented. The secondary analysis is allowed for prisoners' information or biospecimens provided that the research is not examining the prisoners as a subpopulation (Citi Program 2018).

In 2006, the Institute of Medicine (IOM), under the direction of the U.S. Department of Health and Human Services (DHHS), considered "the need for developing a new ethical framework for prisoner research and to identify regulatory safeguards" (Gostin, 2007, p. 738). Byrne (2005) notes a cultural tension that inherently exists between the prison environment and that of health services research. The restrictive nature of the prison as "custody-control-care" clashes with the "open inquiry environment" of health services research, and so present challenges for the researcher (Byrne, 2005, p. 223). Similar challenges exist for advanced practice nurses working within prison health care systems.

4.5.2.2. Standards for Health Services in Prisons

Health service standards in correctional settings set the bar "to ensure the most basic human rights for prisoners, including access to health care" (Stern, Greifinger & Mellow, 2010, p. 2103). These sets of standards have been developed by the American Public Health Association (APHA 2003), the National Commission on Correctional Health Care (NCCHC, 2008) and the American Correctional Association (ACA, 2003).

4.5.2.3. Correctional Nursing

Correctional nursing, including advanced practice nursing, has emerged as a specialty to care of imprisoned adults and juveniles. A representative from the American Nurses Association (ANA) sits on the board of the National Commission of Correctional Health Care (NCCHC); the organization committed to improving the health care of prisons, jails and juvenile correctional facilities. The NCCHC has offered a voluntary accreditation program based on its standards since the 1970s. Separate standards give guidance to jails, prisons, juvenile detention centers, mental health and drug abuse services for correctional facilities. It also offers a certification as a Certified Correctional Health Professional for health care professionals involved with all aspects of correctional health care (NCCHC 2012). The 2007 ANA Corrections Nursing: Scope and Standards of Practice was reviewed for revisions in 2011 by the ANA and NCCHC. The 2007 principles serve as the "underpinning for corrections nursing" (Trossman, 2011, p. 13). The review will include careful attention to legal implications of practice and ensure that correctional nurses also adhere to the standards of care and the Code of Ethics for Nurses (Trossman, 2011). Advanced Practice Nurses working the within restrictive environment of the correctional system where ethical challenges exist need to understand the "culture clash" (Byrne, 2005, p. 223) between prisoner control and the caring nature of nursing to best meet the needs of their patients. Byrne offers that the strategies used in her research experience optimized ethical and continued participation of prisoners. She suggests that the researcher must have a general knowledge of the criminal justice system and specific prison systems as well as be compliant with security policies. Byrne also suggests the participatory input of the prisoners under study and "awareness of and repeated dialogue with vested individuals and groups", "constant vigilance" and having clear research goals (2005, p. 226). The nurse practitioner in the correctional system may struggle at times to provide care while maintaining prison security for inmates who are socially and culturally diverse and often socially and economically disenfranchised and disadvantaged, many who have not had access to health care before they were imprisoned. The correctional nurse practitioner must see beyond the prisoners' status to be able to clearly assess and treat their patients. For example, citing a situation where prisoners brought in inebriated were not adequately assessed for hypoglycemia and subsequently died; Trossman relates that assessments can make the difference between life and death and that correctional nurses have an "obligation to be responsive to health concerns and not arbitrarily decide someone does not have a legitimate concern" (2011, p. 13). Seeing the clients and their health care needs as separate from their crime is essential for providing ethical care. Other ethical dilemmas faced are similar to those in other settings; for example, the lack of necessary resources to provide care or not enough staff to provide adequate care for the number and acuity of patients on a hospital unit or in an over-crowded prison.

4.6. ARMED FORCES

4.6.1. Research and the Military

Nurse researchers must recognize that military personnel as par-ticipants in research are more vulnerable due to the restrictive nature of their military status and underlying nature of military obedience to serve and obey as opposed to an informed choice to participate. Military subjects are viewed as vulnerable populations, on and off the battlefield, as they are subordinate members of a hierarchical group. Due to this status, they may be unduly influenced to participate in research for fear of retaliation if they refuse (CIOMS, 2016). When conducting research with the US Military, nurse researchers must also be certain of the abil-ity of soldiers to give informed consent to avoid coercion as they may feel compelled to "obey requests", as they are taught to obey all orders ((McManus, McClinton, Gerhardt & Morris, 2007, p. 301).

4.6.2. Physicians

Bennahum (2006) explored the historical perspective of the role of the physician in warfare and asked if history could tell us something about the ethical dilemmas of the military physician. He believes that war teaches physicians to behave ethically, as in the Hippocratic tradi-tion. He concluded that limiting the damage of war has been the focus of both the soldier and the physician "for as long as war has existed" (p. 355).

4.6.3. Military Nursing

Historically, nursing's role in the military has been in the care for injured and sick soldiers and often within a "dangerous environment under threats of violence" (Fry, Harvey, Hurley & Foley , 2002, p. 373). According to Southby, "clinical ethics for nurses in the military versus those in the private sector, and nurses in one of the military services versus another, do not really differ" but "what is unique is the num-ber of stressful experiences in a compressed period of time" (2003, pp. 674, 676) during wartime. The treatment of prisoners of war is ethically challenging to military health care professionals. In a post September 11 era, the controversy over the ethical treatment of military prisoners and detainees has been well documented in the medical literature (Clark, 2006; Miles, 2004, 2008, 2011; Lee, Conant, Jonsen & Heileg, 2006; Holmes & Perron, 2007). Southby (2003) contends that wartime nursing does add professional strain and moral dilemmas from the exposure to casualties that include fellow military personnel, civilians, and prisoners or detainees. The ethical dilemmas are similar to those of nurse practitioners working in the U.S. prison systems noted above; however, these patients are prisoners of war as opposed to prisoners of the state and the crimes are often related to differences of philosophy and values of opposing nations engaged in war time activities.

Nurse practitioners who make decisions about the wounded during wartime utilize the triage system whose "objective is to utilize medical resources as effectively and efficiently as possible and is "a utilitarian rationale" (Beauchamp & Childress, 2013, p.292), violates "every creed of accepted nursing practice" (Southby, 2003, p. 674). This may cause significant moral distress if the less injured are treated first over more significant or catastrophic injuries as they might be using this triage system. Significant ethical dilemmas arise for nurse practitioners working in the military due to the nature of war and in difficult decisions made during triage of who lives and who dies. The conditions of military nursing during "military crisis deployments" puts nurse practitioners especially at risk for moral distress due to austere and/or life threatening conditions, unexpected nature of deployments despite training for preparedness/readiness, and the removal and separation from traditional support systems (Fry, Harvey, Hurley & Foley, 2002, p. 379). "Despite this, [military nurses] are expected to provide expert nursing care under conditions that are different from those of traditional nursing practice" (Fry, Harvey, Hurley & Foley, 2002, p. 379). Upholding underlying ethical principle and "acting in the best interest of the patient" (Southby, 2003, p. 683) is the same for nurses in the military as it is for any health professional.

4.7. INCOMPETENT PATIENTS

Competence is the ability to perform a task or a range of tasks related to a particular decision to be made by an individual. Competence may vary with time or may be intermittent as well as be complicated by various diseases and their progression (Beauchamp & Childress, 2013, pp. 114-120). The concept of competence in decision-making is closely related to the concept of autonomy. Patients must be competent to understand information given to them by their health care provider to make an autonomous decision.

While it has been noted previously that nurse practitioners should avoid lists to determine vulnerability, competency is something the nurse practitioner should assess in their patients in order to determine vulnerability. Being incompetent is itself an identified vulnerable group as much as the state of being incompetent leads to vulnerability. The Patient Self-Determination Act of 1990 gave patients the moral right to make their own decisions about health care and the right to accept or refuse treatments. This act came about because of several landmark right-to-die-cases and based on state laws related to end of life decisions (Grace, 2018, p. 97) and more formally known as advanced directives or living wills. Laws pertaining to legally accepted advanced directives and living wills vary from state to state and nurse practitioners must be familiar with them in the states in which they practice. What happens in circumstances when patients are determined to be incompetent or lack the capacity to make autonomous decisions about their health, and more specifically, how do we know when they are unable to do so? The Patient Determination Act and state laws exist for those purposes.

4.7.1. The Ethical Principle of Autonomy

Originating from the Greek, "autonomous" means governance of self (αυτος = self; νομος = law) and is used to describe the governance of ancient Greek city-states. The term also refers to individuals as autonomous when they are self-determining and free from control of others in accordance with their own plans (Beauchamp & Childress, 2013, p.101). Respect for an individual's right to autonomously make decisions "runs deep in common morality as principle" (Beauchamp & Childress, 2013, p. 101). The Code of Ethics for Nursing calls for the respect for the human dignity of the autonomous individual. Nurses must respect the individual's autonomy and right to make their own decisions (Fowler, 2015) When patients are incompetent, their autonomy is challenged because they are unable to make their own decisions, which then makes them vulnerable.

4.7.2. Autonomous Choice, Competency and Vulnerability

Is a patient competent to make a decision about his or her own health? Health care determinations about competency may lead to over-riding an individual's decisions (Beauchamp & Childress, 2013, p. 101). In such cases, health professionals may turn to informal or formal means to assist them in making health care decisions for their patients. In certain cases, legal incompetence is declared by a court decision and a surrogate decision-maker is appointed. In other cases, health professionals may turn to family members or others responsible for or appointed to act on behalf of the patient, if the patient lacks the ability/capacity to understand the benefits and risks of a therapy, a procedure, or a research protocol.

4.7.3. Paternalism, Autonomy and Vulnerability

Nurse practitioners must understand their own ethical values and should rely on defined standards of practice and ethical principles in making decisions for patients with or without capacity. Many patients and research subjects "are vulnerable to a range of decisional defects or impairments that render them unable to protect their own interests" (Miller & Wertheimer, 2007). Moreover, ethical codes for research are paternalistic in that they are meant to protect subjects. However, ensuring that the patient or research subjects' voices are still heard and perspective considered during decision-making is equally as important. They must also consider any harm to the patient and others in making decisions.

When one with authority restricts or limits the autonomy of a patient, this is referred to as paternalism. Paternalism refers to a parent acting in the best interest of his child by regulating and carrying out decisions on the child's behalf because he or she is not old enough nor has the capacity to make an autonomous decision. Health care providers may find themselves in situations in which a decision must be made for a patient without capacity to do so as an autonomous person. A health care provider has the knowledge, authority and power to determine the patient's best interests but, unlike "a loving parent" (Beauchamp & Childress, 2009, p. 208), must be certain to avoid paternalistic decisions. In health care, the professional is expected to have "superior training, knowledge and insight and thus in an authoritative position to determine the patient's best interests (Beauchamp & Childress, 2013, p.215).This power of information and knowledge may also limit the patient with capacity or an alternate decision-maker when patients lack capacity to do so for themselves. The health care provider can do this intentionally or unintentionally by limiting information, offering or not offering treatment options or by treating or refusing to treat without regard to the patient's wishes (Yeo, Moorehouse, Khan & Rodney, 2010, p. 165). Nurse practitioners must also be clear about how and under what circumstances someone is capable of making an autonomous decision and what is necessary to assure that an autonomous decision is made (Grace, 2018, p. 20). Health care providers have a duty to act in the best interest of the patient in an emergency or life-threatening case, or in an end-of-life situation when patients do not have the capacity to decide for themselves and their wishes are unknown.

4.7.4. The Health Care Professional as the Gatekeeper: Judging Competence

Decision making capacity is not "an all-or-nothing on-off switch, but a patient's bad decision from the health care professional's perspective is not an indicator of lack of capacity and sign of incompetence" (Mitty, 2007). "Capacity runs along a continuum rather than being all on our all off" (Post & Boltz, 2016, p. 44).

Health care professionals often find themselves as gatekeepers in the determination as to whether a patient has the capacity or competence to make a decision. Competence and capacity are often used interchangeably in health care literature. "Health professionals' judgments of a person's incompetence may lead them to override that person's decision" (Beauchamp & Childress, 2013, p. 114) about decisions of care, but they do not have the legal authority to declare patients as incompetent. Competence may fluctuate over the course of an illness, while under the influence of a prescribed medication or illicit drug or with the progression of an illness such as Alzheimer's disease. "Decision-making capacity is specific to the task or situation that requires a decision (Tunzi, 2001). Tunzi (2001) describes four clinical scenarios that should alert clinicians that further assessment is warranted. The first is a patient with abrupt mental status change which might be due to hypoxia, medications, or acute metabolic, neurological or psychological processes. The second alert for further assessment is when a patient refuses recommended treatment and is unwilling to discuss their reasons. A third alert occurs when a patient consents too quickly to treatments that are invasive or carry high risks. The fourth alert occurs when patients may have a known risk factor for decision-making. These include the vulnerable groups described in this chapter, neurological or psychiatric conditions, education levels, language or cultural barriers, or particular age group, such as children or the elderly. Careful assessment is always warranted because anyone in these described groups should not be automatically assumed to have diminished decision-making capacity.

Wong, Clare, Gunn and Holland (1999) outlined three methods of assessing capacity: by the outcome of the decision, the status or membership of the patient to a specific group and by an assessment of the patient's decision-making skills and abilities as applied to a particular decision. In the first method of assessing capacity, the provider's own views, beliefs and values may prevent the provider from seeing the decision from the patient's perspective and thus consider the patient non-compliant and therefore incompetent. Health care providers should be aware of the diversity of cultural life styles, beliefs and values and which may have an impact on patient health care decisions. The second method groups patients as infants, children, the mentally and cognitively impaired and the institutionalized (both patients and prisoners). Judging capacity based on these classifications is not sufficient. While the autonomy of these classifications may be compromised or denied, some will have the capacity to make a decision. The third approach to assessing capacity is a functional approach in which the patient's decision-making skills as they apply to a particular decision are assessed at a particular relevant time. Health care providers using this approach recognize that there are different kinds of decisions with different levels of complexity. "A doubt about capacity represents a doubt about specific tasks or decisions, and not necessarily about all decisions" (Yeo, Moorehouse, Khan & Rodney, 2010, p. 158).

Nurse practitioners should follow appropriate guidelines, standards and resources for evaluating decision-making capacity. For example, The Hartford Institute for Geriatric Nursing and The Alzheimer's Association have resources for assessing the geriatric patient with dementia (available at www.consultGeriRN.org or www.hign.org).

4.8. CASE STUDIES

4.8.1. Case Study #1

The threat of a deadly pandemic flu and vaccine shortage has brought healthcare providers, public health professionals and local public officials together to discuss strategies for setting up the local flu clinics in the community in which you are working. This is the public health emergency preparedness-planning and response group. Given this threat and shortage, multiple sites will be needed to distribute the vaccine to the public. The plan calls for the opening of clinics throughout the municipality in public schools, churches, and municipal buildings as well as at private practitioner offices and the hospital. In the past, the flu vaccine was given to children, the elderly and those with special medical needs as a priority over other populations. The community in question is a suburb of a large metropolitan area that is ethnically diverse and is believed to have a large number of unauthorized resident/ illegal immigrants, although this cannot be verified by local public officials. The healthcare providers and public health professionals have considered that due to the enormity and seriousness of this pandemic, and in light of the vaccine shortage, that another plan to determine which populations should have priority access to the vaccine will be necessary. Personnel from the local community hospital are concerned about a rush on their emergency room and have suggested that all clinics demand proof of residency as a prerequisite for obtaining the vaccine. Given the threat of this deadly pandemic and vaccine shortage, as a member of this decision-making group, how would you prioritize distribution of the vaccine? What ethical goals and standards should this group consider in the preparation of these flu clinics? What are the ethical dilemmas you might face?

4.8.2. Case Study #2

The pandemic flu has taken its toll on the community. More and more patients are requiring ventilator support. There is a shortage of ventilators in your area and a request for additional equipment has been made to the federal government, as the President has declared the epidemic a national disaster. However, decisions as to how to allocate the ventilators to those who critically need them must be made accordingly. You are working as the advanced practice nurse in the medical ICU and the policy is to use the hospital's triage protocols and the CDC's Ethical Guidelines in Pandemic Influenza (2007) to make these types of decisions. Your team is making rounds on the patients, as there are two intubated patients in the ER that are being manually oxygenated with bag/valve/mask devises until a ventilator becomes available. One of the ICU patients is on a ventilator after suffering a severe stroke and did not have an advanced directive on record prior to coming in to the ER via EMS last night. You know that one of the patients in the ER is a 25 year old immigrant mother of five with no health insurance and the other is a 65 year old local business man accompanied by his wife and adult children. What dilemmas would you and your team face in allocating a ventilator to only one of these patients?

4.8.3. Case Study #3

You are a co-investigator on a study with the physician in your NP practice. Many of the patients in your practice have become participants in this collaborative research study. Part of the study requires an interview with clients after the experimental procedure under study has been completed. You learn from several of these patients for whom English is their second language, that they are not sure why this procedure had been done. You also discover that in some cases the consent was signed after the procedure was done. You show those who did sign their signed consent, but they clearly do not understand what they signed or the procedure. You know the physician has been asking his resident and fellow to enroll these patients. You speak to your co-investigator about what you have learned from interviewing some of the patients. The physician does not seem concerned, saying the procedure was to their [the patient] benefit anyway. How do you proceed and what changes would you make in conducting such future collaborative research studies?

4.9. REFERENCES

Aday, L.A. (1994). Health status of vulnerable populations. *Annual Review of Public Health*, 15(1): 487–509.

Aday, L.A. (2001). *At Risk in America: The Health Care Needs of Vulnerable Populations in the United States* (2nd ed). San Francisco: Josey-Bass.

American Nursing Association. (2015). *ANA Code of Ethics for Nurses with Interpretative Statements*. Retrieved from: https://www.nursingworld.org/practice-policy/nursing-excellence/ethics/code-of-ethics-for-nurses/coe-view-only/

Beauchamp, T.L. & Childress, JF (2013). *Principles of Biomedical Ethics* (7th ed.). New York: Oxford University Press.

Bennahum, D.A. (2006). Historical reflections on the ethics of military medicine. *Cambridge Quarterly of Healthcare Ethics: CQ: The International Journal of Healthcare Ethics Committees*, 15(4), 345-355.

Berlinger, N. & Raghavan, R. (2013). The ethics of advocacy for undocumented patients. *The Hastings Report*, 43(1) 140-17.

Byrne, M.W. (2005). Conducting Research as a Visiting Scientist in a Women's Prison. *Journal of Professional Nursing* 21(4), 223-230.

Carrasquillo, O., Carrasquillo, A.I., and Shea, S. (2000). Health insurance coverage of immigrants living in the United States: Differences by citizenship status and country of origin. *American Journal of Public Health*, 90(6): 917–923.

Centers for Medicare and Medicaid Services, Patient Protection and Affordable Care Act (Pub. Law No. 111-148 Health Care and Education Act of 2010, Pub. Law No. No. 111-152. Retrieved from: https://www.cms.gov/about-cms/aca/affordable-care-act-in-action-at-cms.html

Centers for Medicare & Medicaid Services (accessed 2019). The Center for Consumer Information & Insurance Oversight State-based Exchanges. Retrieved from: https://www.cms.gov/cciio/

Clark, P.A. (2006). Medical ethics at Guantanamo Bay and Abu Ghraib: The problem of dual loyalty. *The Journal of Law, Medicine and Ethics* 34(3): 570–580.

Code of Federal Regulations, Title 45 Part 46 Protection of Human Subjects (accessed 2019). Retrieved from: https://www.hhs.gov/ohrp/regulations/finalized-revision-common-rule/index.html.

The Collaborative Institutional Training Initiative (CITI Program) (accessed 2018). Revised common rule. Retrieved from https://about.citiprogram.org/en/course/revised-common-rule-course/

Committee on the Robert Wood Johnson Foundation Initiative on the Future of Nursing, Institute of Medicine (2011). *The Future of Nursing: Leading Change, Advancing Health*. The National Academies Press.

CBO (Congressional Budget Office) (accessed 2019). Retrieved from https://www.cbo.gov/publication/54915

CIOMS (Council for International Organizations of Medical Sciences) (2016). International Ethical Guidelines for Biomedical Research Involving Human Subjects. Retrieved from: https: //cioms.ch/shop/product/international-ethical-guidelines-for-health-related-research-involving-humans/

Covered California (accessed 2019) Eligibility and Immigration. Retrieved from: https://www.coveredca.com/individuals-and-families/getting-covered/immigrants/.

Debruin, D. (2001). Reflections on vulnerability. *Bioethics Examiner* 5(2): 1–7.

Derose, K.P., Escarce, J.J. & Lurie, N. (2007). Immigrant and health care: sources of vulnerability. *Health Affairs* 26(5): 1258–1268.

Dreher, M, Shapiro, D & Asselin, M. (2016). Healthy Places Healthy People: A Handbook for Culturally Competent Community Nursing Practice. Sigma Theta Tau International Honor Society.

Dowd, S.B., Giger, J.N., & Davidhizar, R. (1998). Use of Giger and Davidhizar's Transcultural Assessment Model by health professions. *International Nursing Review* 45(4): 119–122.

Dwyer, J. (2004). Illegal immigrants, health care, and social responsibility. *The Hastings Center Report* 34(1): 34-41.

Flaskerud, J.H., & Winslow, B.J. (1998). Conceptualizing vulnerable populations health-related research. *Nursing Research* 47 (2): 69–78.

Flaskerud, J.H., Lesser, J., Dixon, E., Anderson, N., Conde, F., Koniak-Griffin, D., et al. (2002). Health disparities among vulnerable populations: Evolution of knowledge over five decades in nursing research publications. *Nursing Research* 51 (2): 74–85.

Fry, S.T., Harvey, R.M., Hurley, A.C. & Foley, B.J. (2002). Development of a model of moral distress in military nursing. *Nurs Ethics* 9 (4): 373-87.

Fowler, M.D.M. (ed.) (2015). *Guide to the Code of Ethics for Nurses: Interpretation and Application: American Nurses Association (2nd ed)*. Silver Spring, Maryland: American Nurses Association.

Geertz, C. (1973). Religion as a cultural system. In: *The Interpretation of Cultures*, pp. 87–125. Basic Books.

Goldman, D.P., Smith, J.P., and Sood, N. (2005). Legal status and health insurance among immigrants. *Health Affairs* 24 (6): 1640–1653.

Gostin, L.O. (2007). Biomedical research involving prisoners. *JAMA* 297 (7): 737–740.

Grace, P.J. (2018). *Nursing Ethics and Professional Responsibility in Advanced Practice*. Boston: Jones and Bartlett Publishers.

Gutherie, G. (2005). Bridging health disparities: Addressing unmet needs of women of color. *Journal of Obstetric, Gynecological, and Neonatal Nursing* 5: 385.

Hartford Institute for Geriatric Nursing (accessed 2019). Retrieved from: https://hign.org/.

Holmes, D. & Perron, A. (2007). Violating ethics: unlawful combatants, national security and health professionals. *Journal of Medical Ethics* 3: 143–145.

H.R.3734—Personal Responsibility and Work Opportunity Reconciliation Act of 1996. (1996). Retrieved from: https://www.congress.gov/bill/104th-congress/house-bill/3734.

H.R.4449—Patient Self Determination Act of 1990. (1990). Retrieved from: https://www.congress.gov/bill/101st-congress/house-bill/4449.

IOM (Institute of Medicine) (2002). *Unequal Treatment: Confronting Racial and Ethnic Disparities in Health Care.* Washington, DC: National Academies Press.

IOM (Institute of Medicine) (2011). *The Future of Nursing: Leading Change, Advancing Health.* Washington, DC: National Academies Press.

Kachingwe, A.F. & Huff, R.M. (2015). The ethics of health promotion intervention in culturally diverse populations, pp. 43–63. In: *Health Promotion in Multicultural Populations: A Handbook for Practitioners and Students* (3rd ed.). RM Huff, MV Kline & DV Peterson (eds.). Thousand Oaks, CA: SAGE Publications.

Kleinman, A. (1978). Culture, illness and care: clinical lesson from anthropological and cross-cultural research. *Annals of Internal Medicine* 88: 251–258.

Kleinman, A. (1988). The I*llness Narratives: Suffering, Healing, and the Human Condition.* New York: Basic Books.

Lee, P.R., Conant, M., Jonsen, A.R. & Heileg, S. (2006). Participation in torture and interrogation: an inexcusable breach of medical ethics. Cambridge Quarterly in Healthcare Ethics 15: 202–203.

McManus, J., McClinton, A., Gerhardt, R., & Morris, M. (2007). Performance of Ethical Military Research is Possible: On and Off the Battlefield. *Science & Engineering Ethics*, 13(3), 297–303.

Miles, S.H. (2004). Abu Ghraib: its legacy for military medicine. *The Lance*t, 364 (9435): 725–729.

Miles, S.H. (2008). Torture: the bioethics perspective. In:, From Birth to Death and Bench to Clinical: The Hastings Center Bioethics Briefing Book for Journalists, Policymakers, and Campaigns, pp. 169–172. M. Crowley (Ed.). Garrison, NY: The Hastings Center.

Miles, S.H. (2011). The new military medical ethics: Legacies of the gulf wars and the war on terror. *Bioethics* 25: 1-7.

Miller, F.G. & Wertheimer, A (2007). Facing up to paternalism in research ethics. *The Hastings Center Report.* 37:3: 24-34.

Mitty, E. (2007). Advanced directives: protecting patient's rights. In: *Geriatric Nursing Protocols for Best Practice.* E. Capezuti, D. Zwicker, M. Mezey, D, Gray-Miceli & T, Fulmer (eds). New York: Springer Publishing Company.

NCPHSBBR (National Commission for the Protection of Human Subjects of Biomedical and Behavioral Research). (1974). National Research Service Award Act of 1974. Retrieved from: https://history.nih.gov/research/downloads/PL93-348.pdf.

NCPHSBBR (National Commission for the Protection of Human Subjects of Biomedical and Behavioral Research). (1979). The Belmont Report: Ethical principles and guidelines for the protection of human subjects of research. Retrieved from: https://www.hhs.gov/ohrp/regulations-and-policy/belmont-report/index.html.

National Commission for the Protection for the Protection of Human Subjects Research. (1976). Report and recommendations: Research involving prisoners. https://videocast.nih.gov/pdf/ohrp_research_involving_prisoners.pdf?.

Nuremberg Code (1947). Retrieved from: https://history.nih.gov/research/downloads/nuremberg.pdf

Nyamathi, A., Koniak-Griffin, D., & Greengold, B.A. (2007). Development of Nursing Theory and Science in Vulnerable Populations. In: Annual Review of Nursing Research: Vulnerable Populations, Vol. 25, pp. 3–26. J.J. Fitzpatrick (ed.). New York: Springer.

Nyamathi, A., & Koniak-Griffin, D. (2007). In: *Annual Review in Nursing Research: Vulnerable Populations*, Vol. 25, pp. xiii–xv. J.J. Fitzpatrick (ed). New York: Springer.

Post, F.P. & Boltz, M. (2016). In: *Evidence-based geriatric nursing protocols for best practice, fifth edition*. Boltz, M., Capezuti, E., Fulmer, T., & Zwicker, D. (Eds.). (2016). Retrieved from https://ebookcentral.proquest.com

Radford, J. & Budiman, A. (nd). Facts on U.S. Immigrants, 2016, Statistical portrait of the foreign-born population in the United States. Pew Research Center, September 14, 2018. Retrieved from http://www.pewhispanic.org/2018/09/14/facts-on-u-s-immigrants/

Schulz, A.J. & Mullings, L. (2006). *Gender, Race, Class, and Health: Intersectional Approaches* (1st ed). San Francisco, CA: Jossey-Bass.

Southby, J.R. (2003). Nursing ethics and the military. In DE Lounsbury (ed), *Military Medical Ethics* (pp. 661-686). Washington, DC. Office of the Surgeon General.

Stern, M.F., Greifinger, R.B. & Mellow, J. (2010). Patient Safety: Moving the Bar in Prison Health Care Standards, *American Journal of Public Health* 100: 11, pp. 2103-2110.

Susser, I., & Patterson, T.C. (2001). *Cultural Diversity in the United States*: A Critical Reader. Oxford, UK: Blackwell Publishers.

Taylor, M.D.M. (2010). *Guide to the Code of Ethics for Nurses*. Silver Spring, Maryland: American Nurses Association.

Trossman, S. (2011) Ensuring standards are standard behind bars: Nurses work to review ANA document, promote corrections nursing practice. *The American Nurse*, November/December 2011, pp. 12–13.

Truman, B.I., Tinker, T., Vaughan, E., Kapella, B.K., Brenden, M., Woznica, C.V., et al. (2009). Pandemic influenza preparedness and response among immigrants and refugees. *Am. J. Public Health* 99(S2): S278–286.

Tunzi, M. (2001). Can the patient decide? Evaluating patient capacity in practice. *American Family Physician* 64(2): 299–306.

Turner, L. (2005). Is local cultural sensitivity sometimes insensitive? *Canadian Family Medicine, 51: 478–479.*

Urbina, I. (2006, 13 August). Panel suggests using inmates in drug trials. New York Times, pp. 1.1.

U.S. Census (2010). Retrieved from: https://www.census.gov/programs-surveys/cps.html

Wong, J.G., Clare, I.C., Gunn, M.J., and Holland, A.J. (1999). Capacity to make health care decisions: its importance in clinical practice. Psychological Medicine 29(2): 437–446.

WHO (World Health Organization) (accessed 2019). What is the Value-Added of Human Rights in Public *Health. Retrieved from http://www.who.int/hhr//hhr_activities_eng.pdf*

WHO (World Health Organization) (accessed 2019). Environmental health in emergencies and disasters: a practical guide, Retrieved from https://www.who.int/environmental_health_emergencies/vulnerable_groups/en/.

WMA (World Medical Association) (2013) Declaration of Helsinki: Ethical principles for medical research involving human subjects. Retrieved from: https://www.wma.net/policies-post/wma-declaration-of-helsinki-ethical-principles-for-medical-research-involving-human-subjects/

Yeo, M., Moorehouse, A., Khan, P., & Rodney, P. (eds). (2010). *Concepts and Cases in Nursing Ethics* (3rd ed). Ontario, Canada: Broadview Press.

CHAPTER 5

Ethical Considerations of Care and Research in Mental Health

PAMELA BJORKLUND

In principle, ethics is only meaningful where people—or groups of people—are self-governing and have the opportunity to make choices free from any coercion. Rarely is this the case in the mental health field.
(Barker, 2011, p. 3)

5.1. INTRODUCTION

Respect for the autonomy of the human being is a cherished principle of biomedical ethics (Beauchamp and Childress, 2012). The principle derives from Enlightenment liberal traditions where the capacity for self-governance defines personhood and establishes human dignity and is, therefore, of supreme value (Radden, 2003). Autonomy assumes the inherent equality and dignity of human beings, who are endowed with reason, conscience, free will, and social circumstances free from duress and coercion (United Nations, 1948). The principle of autonomy undergirds the concept of informed consent in health care ethics, practice, and research, where fully informed and autonomous decision-making has been a cherished if not fully inviolable right since the Nuremberg Code, which established in 1947 the essential right of human beings to voluntary participation in research:

> *This means that the person involved should have legal capacity to give consent; should be so situated as to be able to exercise free power of choice, without the intervention of any element of force, fraud, deceit, duress, overreaching, or other ulterior form of constraint or coercion; and should have sufficient knowledge and comprehension of the elements of the subject matter involved as to enable him to make an understanding and enlightened decision (Nuremberg Code in Shuster, 1997, p. 1436).*

In mental health care, however, some mentally ill persons are coerced into treatment without full and informed consent. Mentally ill persons

171

may lack the capacity for fully autonomous, well-reasoned decisions and thus may be subject to the controlling judgments of disproportionately more powerful persons who act 'in their best interests' and 'for the good of the community.' Such people are not free from any element of force, duress, constraint, or coercion; nor do the connections between their reasons and their decisions insure enlightened choice. This reality defines the core vulnerability of persons with mental illness as well as one of the problems with an impartial, principles- or rights-based ethical framework for mental health practice. Where the mentally ill are concerned, autonomy is neither full nor individual. Often, it is diminished and relational—nested inside a contextual web of care-giving relationships, in particular the therapeutic relationship with the primary mental health care provider.

This chapter explores the unique vulnerability of persons with mental illness; situates an ethical framework for mental health care and research inside the domain of applied, professional ethics; and identifies and describes important ethical issues in mental health care and research. In addition, this chapter locates the source of these ethical issues for psychiatric-mental health nurses in their common, everyday practice routines; identifies the ethical approaches that are most useful to achieving moral understandings in mental health care and research; and provides case studies to illustrate and enlighten the preceding discussions. In all cases, permission was obtained to use ethical narratives and case studies.

5.2. PLACING PSYCHIATRIC-MENTAL HEALTH ETHICS IN CONTEXT

5.2.1. Ethics

Ethics is the scholarly study of morality (Lindemann, 2006). Morality is the subject matter of ethics and is commonly thought of as the right or good way to live, work, treat others, organize social life, and so forth. Ethics sets out to understand, justify, criticize, and correct, if necessary, moral beliefs and the ways of life in which those beliefs are practiced (Lindemann, 2006). Thus, ethics is not so much a 'subject matter' as a 'verb'—a mode of doing in thought and action that serves to understand, justify, criticize, correct, and re-establish moral equilibrium in social practices like mental health care and research (Lindemann, 2006; Walker, 2007). Ethics that pertain to the medical specialty of psychiatry/mental health might be termed psychiatric ethics. Given the nursing profession's commitment to holism, health promotion, and disease prevention—and because psychiatric disorders and mental health problems are not necessarily one and the same—the term psychiatric-mental health ethics is preferred here.

Three recognized branches of ethics include metaethics, normative ethics, and practical ethics (Lindemann, 2006). Metaethics is the study of what constitutes morality and where it originates. Normative ethics is the study of moral theories and concepts. It examines the norms, or standards, that are used to guide and evaluate actions. It proposes to explain what is right, what we ought to do, and how we know what we ought to do. Practical ethics is the study of ethical considerations that arise within specific social practices—for example, business, biomedicine, healthcare research, or advanced practice psychiatric-mental health nursing (Lindemann, 2006).

5.2.2. Professional Ethics

The term professional ethics refers to the practical or applied ethics attached to particular professions. Professions have some common characteristics, including specialized bodies of knowledge; responsibility for developing, disseminating, and using that knowledge; a practice orientation that is used for the good of the population served; and the ability to autonomously set educational and behavioral standards for the profession in order to monitor, regulate, and discipline the conduct of its members (Grace, 2018). In contemporary society, a profession's educational institutions, professional associations, and regulatory (licensing and certifying) bodies all play important roles in educating, monitoring, and regulating its members. Contemporary professions, including medicine and nursing, all formulate explicit codes of conduct that represent the discipline's promises to society (Grace, 2018)—for example, the American Psychiatric Association's (APA) Code of Ethics (APA, 2013) and the American Nursing Association's (ANA) Code of Ethics (ANA, 2015), with which all practitioners of psychiatric-mental health care and research should be familiar.

Boxes 5.1 and 5.2 summarize the essential elements of the APA and ANA professional codes. A profession has the autonomy to periodically revise its own standards, scope, and code of conduct to reflect changes in the profession's goals and society's needs as evidenced, for example, by the ever-changing constitution of the Diagnostic and Statistical Manual of Mental Disorders, now in its 5th edition (DSM-5); by the routine updating of codes; or by the supplanting of one code by another, e.g., the replacement of the Declaration of Hawaii (1977) with the Declaration of Madrid (1996).

Box 5.1 - Summary of APA Code of Ethics

Section 1: A psychiatrist shall:

- Not exploit the patient to gratify own needs
- Not violate the boundaries of the doctor-patient relationship
- Not discriminate on the basis of ethnic origin, race, sex, creed, age, socioeconomic status, or sexual orientation
- Not make public appeals based solely upon emotion or utilize patient testimonials
- Not participate in legally authorized execution

Section 2: A psychiatrist shall:

- Conduct himself/herself with propriety in both professional and personal life
- Avoid sexual contact with current or former patients
- Guard against using the inherent inequality of the treatment relationship to influence patients in ways not directly relevant to treatment goals
- Avoid practicing outside his or her area of professional competence
- Intercede with other psychiatrists who jeopardize patient welfare and their own reputations and practices because of mental illness
- Explicitly establish binding contractual arrangements with patients
- Not charge for missed appointments except when this falls within the terms of the explicit contractual arrangement with the patient
- Not split fees, i.e., provide supervision or administration to other physicians or nonmedical persons for a percentage of their fees or gross income

Section 3: A psychiatrist shall:

- Respect the law
- Not engage in illegal activities that bear upon his or her practice
- May protest social injustice without behaving unethically
- May practice acupuncture if allowed by law and if professionally competent to do so

Section 4: A psychiatrist shall:

- Protect the confidentiality of psychiatric records, including the identification of persons as patients
- Release confidential information only with the authorization of the patient or under proper legal compulsion
- Adequately disguise clinical material used in teaching and writing
- Maintain patient confidentiality in consultations where the patient may not have been present and the consultee was not a physician
- Disclose only relevant information and avoid speculation as fact
- Fully describe to examinees the nature, purpose, and lack of confidentiality of examinations performed for security purposes or to determine legal competence or employment suitability

(continued)

Box 5.1 (continued) - Summary of APA Code of Ethics

Section 4 (continued): A psychiatrist shall:

- Assure minors of appropriate confidentiality while including parents and guardians in the treatment, when appropriate
- Reveal confidential information disclosed by a patient only when clinical judgment determines a high risk of danger to patient or others
- May present a patient to a scientific gathering if the patient has provided full and informed consent and the attendees accept the confidentiality of the presentation
- May dissent within the framework of the law if ordered by a court to reveal patient confidences
- May present a current or former patient to a public gathering or news media only if the patient is competent and offers full and informed consent in writing to the enduring loss of confidentiality
- Advise research participants of the investigation's funding sources
- Not evaluate persons charged with criminal acts prior to access to, or availability of, legal counsel
- Avoid sexual involvement with students, trainees, or supervisees

Section 5: A psychiatrist shall:

- Obtain continuing education
- Make referrals only to competent and qualified members of other professional disciplines
- Spend sufficient time to insure that supervisees or collaborating professionals are providing appropriate care
- Never delegate to nonmedical personnel anything that requires the exercise of professional medical judgment
- Agree to the request of a patient for consultation or to such a request from the family of an incompetent or minor patient

Section 6: A psychiatrist shall:

- Hold the therapeutic relationship with the patient above all other considerations in treatment
- Refuse to provide psychiatric treatment to a person who cannot be diagnosed as having a mental illness amenable to treatment

Section 7: A psychiatrist shall:

- Foster the cooperation of those legitimately concerned with the medical, psychological, social, and legal aspects of mental health and illness
- Serve society by advising and consulting with the executive, legislative, and judiciary branches of government
- Clarify his or her status as individual or representative of an organization
- Avoid cloaking public statements with the authority of the profession (e.g., "Psychiatrists know that . . .")

(continued)

175

Box 5.1 (continued) - Summary of APA Code of Ethics

Section 7 (continued): A psychiatrist shall:

- Never offer a professional opinion on a case unless he or she has conducted an examination and has been granted proper authorization for such a statement
- Permit his or her certification to be used for the involuntary treatment of a person only following his or her personal examination of that person, and only following the finding that the person cannot form a judgment as to what is in his/her own best interests and is likely to harm self or others without such treatment
- Never participate in torture

Section 8: A psychiatrist shall:

- Regard responsibility to the patient as paramount

Section 9: A psychiatrist shall:

- Support access to medical care for all people

APA. (2010). *The principles of medical ethics with annotations especially applicable to psychiatry.* American Psychiatric Association.

Box 5.2 - Summary of ANA Code of Ethics

The nurse:

1. Practices with compassion and respect for the inherent dignity, worth, and uniqueness of every person
2. Has a primary commitment to the patient, whether an individual, family, group, or population
3. Promotes, advocates for, and protects the rights, health, and safety of the patient
4. Has authority, accountability, and responsibility for nursing practice; makes decisions; and takes action consistent with the obligation to promote health and to provide optimal care
5. Owes the same duties to self as to others, including the responsibility to promote health and safety, preserve wholeness of character and integrity, maintain competence, and continue personal and professional growth
6. Through individual and collective effort, establishes, maintains, and improves the ethical environment of the work setting and conditions of employment that are conducive to safe, quality health care
7. In all roles and settings, advances the profession through research and scholarly inquiry, professional standards development, and the generation of both nursing and health policy
8. Collaborates with other health professionals and the public to protect human rights, promote health diplomacy, and reduce health disparities
9. Must articulate nursing values, maintain the integrity of the profession, and integrate principles of social justice into nursing and health policy

Source: ANA. (2015). *Code of ethics for nurses with interpretive statements.* Silver Springs, MD: American Nurses Association.

Box 5.3 identifies the historical bedrock for the APA (2013) and ANA (2015) codes. Of particular importance for psychiatric-mental health ethics and mental health practitioners is the Declaration of Madrid, which establishes the specific standards for psychiatric-mental health care and research that have been adopted by all 130 societies of the World Psychiatric Association (WPA) (Tasman & Mohr, 2011; WPA, 1996). Boxes 5.4 and 5.5 summarize the essential elements of the *Declaration of Madrid.*

Box 5.3 - Historic Ethical Codes in Mental Health Care and Research

Nuremberg Code (1947)

- Established 10 principles for permissible medical research with human participants, especially voluntary informed consent (Roberts & Roberts, 1999)
- Emphasized protection of human participants from undue harms/ risks and unnecessary pain/ suffering
- Most important document in the history of the ethics of medical research (Shuster, 1997)

Declaration of Geneva (1948, amended 1968)

- An oath that abjures the physician from using medical knowledge "contrary to the laws of humanity"
- A response to atrocities committed by physicians in Nazi Germany (World Medical Association, 1948)

Declaration of Helsinki (1964, amended 1975, 1983, 1989, 1996, 2000, 2002, 2004, 2008)

- Distinguished between therapeutic and nontherapeutic research: All study participants must be assured of the best proven diagnostic and therapeutic method of care (Roberts & Roberts, 1999)
  —Therapeutic research (clinical research that combines biomedical research with professional care)
  —Non-therapeutic research (non-clinical biomedical research involving human tissues or data) (World Medical Organization, 1996)

Declaration of Hawaii (1977, amended 1983)

- Functioned to provide ethical guidance specific to the profession
- Laid down 10 general ethical guidelines for psychiatrists world-wide
- Emphasized the aim of psychiatry to promote health, personal autonomy, and growth (World Psychiatric Association, 1978)

(continued)

Box 5.3 (continued) - Historic Ethical Codes in Mental Health Care and Research

Belmont Report (1979)

- Provided ethical foundations for current federal regulations including Subpart A (Common Rule) and Subparts B, C, and D for "vulnerable populations"• Specifies three ethical principles that govern research with human participants

  —Respect for persons

  —Treat participants as autonomous agents; insure full and informed consent

    * Protect those with diminished autonomy

    * Beneficence

    * Insure favorable balance of risks and benefits

  —Justice

    * Insure fair procedures and outcomes in the selection of research participants (National Commission for the Protection of Human Subjects of Biomedical and Behavioral Research, 1979)

Declaration of Madrid (1996, amended 1999, 2002, 2005, 2011)

- Declared specific standards for psychiatric practice world-wide
- Adopted by all 130 societies of the World Psychiatric Association as prerequisite for membership

---

Box 5.4 - Summary of Declaration of Madrid

A psychiatrist must:

- Offer best evidence-based treatment available consistent with ethical principles
- Utilize least freedom-restrictive treatment available
- Seek advice and expertise of others when needed
- Advocate for equitable distribution of healthcare resources
- Keep up with scientific developments in the specialty
- Partner with patients to allow free and informed decisions within relationships of mutual trust and respect
- Safeguard human dignity and legal rights in cases of grave disability or incompetence
- Provide no treatment against the patient's will except in cases of danger to life (patient or third party)

  —Uphold the 'best interests' of the patient as paramount in treatment

(continued)

Box 5.5 - Special Situations in Declaration of Madrid

- Euthanasia
    —Duty is to protect life
    —Mental illness may distort patient decisions
- Torture
    —No participation even when under duress
- Death penalty
    —No participation in competency evaluations for execution
- Selection of sex
    —No participation in decisions to terminate pregnancy for purposes of sex selection
- Organ transplantation
    —Role is to insure informed consent and patient self-determination
    —No use of psychotherapeutic skills to influence patient decisions
- Psychiatrists addressing the media
    —Represent the profession with dignity
    —Uphold the dignity of persons with mental illness
    —Make no pronouncements on presumed psychopathology of any person
    —Present research findings accurately and with awareness of their impact
- Discrimination on ethnic or cultural grounds is never permitted

---

(continued)

Box 5.5 (continued) - Special Situations in Declaration of Madrid

- Genetic research and counseling
  - —Duty to insure full and informed consent of participants
  - —Adequate protection of genetic information against misuse
  - —Referral for genetic testing only to facilities with quality assurance and accessible genetic counseling
  - —Genetic counseling for family planning must respect patients' value systems
- Ethics of psychotherapy in medicine
  - —Practitioners of psychotherapy must have proper training
  - —Approach should be scientific and culturally/ethnically sensitive
  - —Full and informed consent of the patient is required
  - —Power differential in the therapeutic relationship must be recognized
  - —Boundaries must be respected
  - —Confidentiality must be maintained except where mandatory reporting is required (child abuse, elder abuse, danger to third party)
- Conflict of interest in relationship with industry
  - —Avoid accepting gifts
  - —Disclose financial and contractual relationships
- Conflicts arising with third party payers
  - —Principles of good psychiatric practice can conflict with organizational imperatives to maximize profits/minimize costs
  - —Maintain professional independence to apply best practice guidelines
  - —Oppose limits on benefits, parity, or limited access to needed medication
- Boundary violations
  - —Sexual relationships with patients are never permitted
- Protection of the rights of psychiatrists
  - —To live up to the obligations of their profession
  - —To practice at the highest level of excellence
  - —To practice free from abuse by totalitarian regimes or profit-driven economic systems
  - —To practice free from discrimination and the stigma of mental illness
  - —To advocate for patients without media ridicule or professional persecution
- Disclosing the diagnosis of Alzheimer's
  - —Patients have the right to know or not to know
  - —Patients and families should be told as early as possible
  - —Exceptions to disclosure in cases of severe dementia, phobia, severe depression

(continued)

Box 5.5 (continued) - Special Situations in Declaration of Madrid

- Dual responsibilities

  —May arise for insurance or employment purposes or as part of legal proceedings to judge competency, fitness to stand trial, criminal responsibility, or dangerousness to self or others

  —Duty is to disclose to the patient the nature of the assessment as non-therapeutic or potentially damaging

  —Must advocate for separation of records to limit exposure of information only to that which is essential for third-party purposes

Source: World Psychiatric Association (WPA). (1996). Madrid declaration on ethical standards for psychiatric practice. WPA, General Assembly, Madrid.

5.2.3. Nursing Ethics

Nursing ethics is a form of practical, professional, or applied ethics. It is in that sense that the terms nursing ethics and professional responsibility can be considered equivalent concepts (Grace, 2018). However, the term nursing ethics is controversial in that some scholars believe nursing ethics is a unique field with considerations that cannot be fully understood by adapting biomedical ethics—that is, the professional ethics of physicians (Fry, Veatch, & Taylor, 2010). Others insist there is nothing morally unique to nursing: Nursing ethics is just a subcategory of bioethics; the same moral issues emerge in health care settings across professions, and the same ethical principles apply to those issues whether one is a physician, nurse, patient, or administrator (Fry et al., 2010). Similarly, even though different professions do have unique characteristics, some argue that claims for a unique ethics for each profession are unnecessary, and different or specialized ethical demands in the mental health context can be met with a broader sense of what it means to be ethically sensitive in health care (Crowden, 2003). Others argue that impartial principles and broad understandings of healthcare professional ethics cannot account for the unique ethical demands placed on the psychiatric provider—for example, to use the 'personal self' as one's principal therapeutic tool (Radden, 2004; Sadler, 2007). Nor do they recognize the autonomy of the psychiatric patient as relational and the nature of psychiatric treatment as a relationship—more often, as a web of relationships wherein influence is inherent; treatment decisions are continuous, not dichotomous; and the subjectivity of the clinician, who is a fundamental component of the situation as a person, is inescapable (Olsen, 2003).

Here, nursing ethics is differentiated from healthcare ethics broadly to emphasize the roots of nursing ethics in everyday nursing practice as opposed to a transcendent realm of universal, impartial ethical principles. Thus, the term nursing ethics refers not merely to the professional ethics of the nursing discipline. More specifically, it refers to the study of nurses' moral concerns, nurses' moral knowledge, and nurses' moral judgments as they arise, are experienced, and are acted upon in the everyday, routinized, but nevertheless unique context of psychiatric-mental health nursing practice at multiple levels across multiple sites (J. Liaschenko, personal communication, September, 2006).

5.3. ETHICAL CONSIDERATIONS IN MENTAL HEALTH CARE

5.3.1. Vulnerability in Mental Illness

5.3.1.1. Diminished Autonomy/Forced Treatment

The mentally ill are vulnerable on several counts, not least of which is their frequently diminished autonomy and decisional capacity. Mental illness is one of the few forms of illness that is commonly treated by force against the person's expressed wishes (Barker, 2011), including such treatment as seclusion, restraint, involuntary medication, involuntary commitment, and restriction of a patient's rights to such things as visitors, phone calls, personal possessions, and taken-for-granted 'privileges' like the right to leave one's room, watch television, eat in a dining room, or associate with others. Clearly, the model of the autonomous patient or research participant is problematic, if not also unrealistic with respect to patients whose self-control, judgment, insight, reasoning ability, and capacity to effectively recognize and communicate needs and concerns waxes and wanes.

Even psychiatric patients who clearly lack adequate decisional capacity may nevertheless retain their moral agency and can still make self-interested choices which, although irrational, are not necessarily harmful to self or others. Autonomy or the capacity to self-govern is predicated upon agency, that is, one's status as a moral agent—a person with inherent dignity and worth who acts in the world for reasons of his or her own. Respecting the autonomy of psychiatric patients entails upholding their moral agency: "To be 'cured' against one's will and cured of states which we may not regard as disease is to be put on a level with those who have not yet reached the age of reason or those who never will; to be classed with infants, imbeciles, and domestic animals" (C.S. Lewis in Barker, 2011, p. 45).

Thus, a major challenge in mental health care and research is to establish whether or to what extent psychiatric patients possess decisional capacity and are capable of giving or withholding informed consent for either treatment or participation in research. In some cases, competence to give or withhold consent must be formally evaluated and documented, usually by a physician, as specified by law. Judgments of competency are typically made in the context of treatment refusals whereupon risks, benefits, and interests must be weighed in the matter of paternalistic interventions like involuntary commitment, forced medication, or any other serious restriction of patient rights. Such paternalistic interventions require not only that the patient lacks decisional capacity but also that the forced treatment or restrictions are in the patient's 'best interests' (Szmukler & Appelbaum, 2008). While the person's best interests may be difficult to determine, considerations include:

- The past and present wishes and feelings of the person concerned, to the degree they can be ascertained, along with the factors the person would consider if able to do so;
- The need to permit and encourage the person to participate as fully as possible in any decisions made for him or her;
- The views of others in the person's relational network with whom it would be appropriate to consult about the person's wishes, feelings, and best interests; and
- Whether the purpose for which any decision is required can be as effectively achieved in a less restrictive manner (Szmukler & Appelbaum, 2008, p. 241).

While 'the protection of others' may be invoked to rationalize forced treatment or restrictions of rights, a potential for dangerousness to others should not be confused with the person's 'best interests,' which can justify involuntary treatment where decisional capacity is lacking. As an ethical and legal consideration, 'protection of others' may justify involuntary detention and treatment, depending on the credibility, seriousness, and magnitude of the risk to others; but it does not hinge on the individual's lack of decisional capacity. The potential for dangerousness to others may be high while the health interest may be minor, and the individual may be fully competent to make treatment decisions despite community safety concerns (Szmukler & Appelbaum, 2008). In sum, the legal justification for involuntary psychiatric treatment in all 50 U.S. states requires the presence of mental illness, which presumes impaired decisional capacity, along with either the potential for danger-ousness to oneself or others or grave disability, which is an extension of the potential for danger to self by means of inability to care for oneself sufficiently to meet basic conditions necessary for life (Olsen, 2003).

5.3.1.2. Treatment Pressures/Therapeutic Relationships

Psychiatric-mental health patients are also vulnerable because they receive mental health care and treatment in the context of a therapeutic relationship in which influence is inherent and unavoidable. The char-acter, or person of the clinician, including his or her virtues, is ethi-cally significant for patient outcomes. The clinician's skills at building, maintaining, and repairing ruptures in the therapeutic relationship are more significant for therapeutic outcome than the clinician's theoreti-cal orientation or therapy-specific training (Olsen, 2003; Radden & Sadler, 2008; Safran & Muran, 2003). This emotionally charged inter-personal process may be the key to treatment outcome; over the course of approximately 50 years of psychotherapy research, the quality of the therapeutic relationship has turned out to be the most robust indicator of treatment success (Muran & Barber, 2010; Safran & Muran, 2003).

The influence inherent in the therapeutic relationship exists on a spectrum of coercion, or treatment pressures that range from (a) persua-sion, suggestions, and recommendations to (b) interpersonal leverage; (c) inducements, incentives, or offers; (d) threats; and (e) involuntary, or 'forced' treatment (Szmukler & Appelbaum, 2008). Persuasion ap-peals to the patient's reason, respects the patient's autonomy, and is least problematic. Suggestions and recommendations lie at the bound-ary between persuasion and interpersonal leverage, which uses the pa-tient's less powerful position and sometimes emotionally dependent relationship with the clinician to exert pressure in a particular direction (Szmukler & Appelbaum, 2008). Inducements present the patient with goods, services, monetary rewards, or other incentives for cooperation with recommended treatment. Although more extreme and problem-atic, threats approximate inducements in that both involve conditional propositions: If the patient accepts treatment, then the clinician will do X. If the patient does not accept treatment, then the clinician will be 'forced' to do Y. At this point, the term coercion rather than treatment pressure is clearly appropriate (Szmukler & Appelbaum, 2008). Forced treatment, of course, lies at the extreme end of the spectrum and de-prives the patient of all autonomy. While inducements, incentives, and threats are ethically questionable if not morally repugnant, they never-theless are commonly used in the U.S. to leverage psychiatric treatment

(Monahan et al., 2005; Robbins, Petrila, LeMelle & Monahan, 2006; Szmukler & Appelbaum, 2008).

5.3.1.3. Exploitation/Boundaries

Due to such factors as impaired reality-testing, limited insight, poor judgment, and other aspects of their diminished autonomy, the mentally ill are especially vulnerable to exploitation, dependence, abuses of power, and the inherent influence and inequality of the treatment relationship. According to the APA Code of Ethics, the therapeutic relationship is "such a vital factor in effective treatment" that preservation of optimal conditions for development and maintenance of a strong therapeutic alliance takes "precedence over all other [ethical and technical] considerations" (APA, 2013, p. 9; Radden, 2002a). Because each individual clinician has a unique and powerful potential to help or harm the patient, extra care must be taken by the mental health provider to observe the boundaries of the treatment relationship, especially because of the "private, highly personal, and sometimes intensely emotional" nature of the relationship (APA, 2013, p. 3; Radden, 2002a). The intensity of the therapeutic relationship can activate needs and fantasies in both patient and provider "while weakening the objectivity necessary for control" (APA, 2013, p. 4; Radden, 2002a). Such interventions as advice-giving, self-disclosure, and other deliberate or inadvertent boundary crossings exploit the power differential in the therapeutic relationship and further weaken the patient's autonomy if they are not accompanied by a clinically sound, contextually appropriate, and well-documented therapeutic rationale.

So important is the issue of boundaries that much of psychiatric-mental health ethics could be considered discourse on boundary violations. All human relationships have boundaries (Jorgenson, Hirsch, and Wahl, 1997). In personal relationships, boundaries tend to evolve over time as a relationship develops or the parties to it grow and change: "For example, the parent and child renegotiate boundaries as the child moves toward adulthood, and the boundaries in an intimate relationship shift as trust between the parties grows" (Jorgenson et al., 1997, p. 50). Boundaries in professional relationships are more rigid; once set, they typically are not crossed or violated without justification. Boundaries flow from the fiduciary nature of the professional relationship, which exists because the professional possesses knowledge and/or skills that the patient lacks and thus seeks. In accepting the trust and confidence of the patient, the fiduciary, or trustee, agrees to act only in the patient's 'best interests' as collaboratively defined (Jorgenson et al., 1997).

Gutheil and Gabbard (1993) have distinguished between benign boundary crossings and harmful boundary violations in mental health care with respect to time, place and space, money, gifts, physical contact, language, self-disclosure, and patient and therapist roles. They have suggested that boundary crossings are benign, therapeutic variants that advance the treatment in a productive way and do not harm the patient. Some of these boundary crossings could be completely appropriate human responses to unusual events that involved physical contact. For example, "[a] patient stumbled as she was leaving the office and fell to the floor. The therapist helped the patient up and made sure that she was all right" (Gutheil and Gabbard, 1998, p. 410); or, "[a] patient entered her therapist's office and announced that she had just received news that her son had died. The patient reached out to embrace the therapist, and the therapist accepted the embrace as the patient sobbed" (Gutheil & Gabbard, 1998, p. 410). Failing to respond humanely at such times might have a negative impact on the patient, perhaps leading to premature termination of treatment, which would be more harmful to the patient than the inadvertent boundary crossing.

A boundary violation, on the other hand, is obviously harmful, constitutes exploitation of the patient, and is likely to destroy the treatment over time. Unlike a boundary crossing, the therapeutic rationale for a boundary violation is usually not identified, discussed, or documented and may be part of an unexamined, repetitive practice (Gutheil & Gabbard, 1998). The harm may range from wasting the patient's time and money to inflicting severe trauma, including the following examples: the therapist who hugs the patient at the end of each session, the therapist who asks the patient to run errands for him, the therapist who conducts sessions outside the office or discloses his or her own personal problems in a way that burdens the patient, and the therapist who makes overt sexual contact with the patient (Gutheil & Gabbard, 1998).

The "edge of appropriate behavior" that defines a boundary is not always clear in mental health care due to the diversity of psychotherapeutic approaches, the need to individualize treatment with targeted strategies for a wide range of variously functioning people in unique situations, and professional norms which change with historical and social conditions (Gutheil & Gabbard, 1998, p. 410). Freud, for example, analyzed his own daughter, Anna; similarly, he analyzed his friend, Sandor Ferenzi, while walking through the countryside during vacations (Gutheil & Gabbard, 1993). Today, mental health treatment of family, friends, and/or self—outside the office, no less—constitutes a boundary violation for which investigation by the appropriate regulatory agency would be required along with professional sanctions.

The purpose of clear boundaries is to create a safe and predictable environment for both patient and provider, in which the therapeutic alliance can flourish and external boundaries create the possibility of productively crossing psychological boundaries through potentially therapeutic mechanisms, including empathy, interpretation of transference and countertransference, and identification with the therapist (Gutheil & Gabbard, 1998). Boundary crossings have both patient care and risk management dimensions. A boundary crossing has the potential to either enhance or compromise patient care, while knowledge of boundaries is important to effective risk management (Gutheil & Gabbard, 1993). Court decisions suggest a trend toward findings of liability for boundary violations even in the absence of gross therapist misconduct; and fact finders—civil or criminal juries, judges, ethics committees of professional organizations, or state licensing boards—often believe that the presence of even minor boundary crossings is presumptive evidence of, or corroborates allegations of, gross therapist misconduct including sexual misconduct, which usually begins with relatively minor boundary crossings (Gutheil & Gabbard, 1993).

Crossing boundaries for therapeutic purposes is an advanced psychotherapeutic skill, and mental health practitioners should practice within both their professional and personal scope. A boundary crossing may be important for a patient's growth and development, but it is not always easy to know how or when to do this. New practitioners typically find it awkward, unnecessarily rigid, inauthentic, or lacking in empathy to strictly and consistently maintain the boundaries of time, place, money, gifts, physical contact, self-disclosure, and role (Gutheil & Gabbard, 1993). It takes sensitivity, knowledge, experience, technical skill, and risk tolerance to know when crossing a boundary is clinically indicated. However, basic risk management requires clear documentation in the patient record of the indications and clinical rationale for deliberate boundary crossings.

Most clinicians make unintentional self-disclosures. For example, they decorate their offices in ways that reflect who they are. Their manner of speech and dress, their style of greeting patients, and all other verbal and nonverbal communications reveal information to the patient. A clinician self-discloses anytime he or she chooses to comment on any particular aspect of the patient's dialogue. The clinician is telling the patient something about what he or she thinks is important. Patients are generally quite expert at noticing and picking up on these inadvertent self-disclosures, which are not the same as deliberate, conscious choices to reveal something personal about oneself as a therapeutic technique, although both deliberate and inadvertent self-disclosures require discussion with the patient. "The boundary issue is not whether self-disclosure occurs or does not occur. Rather, the key issue is what the therapist self-discloses and whether the therapist burdens the patient with personal problems in a manner that reverses the roles in the dyad" (Gutheil & Gabbard, 1998, p. 412).

The vulnerability of the psychiatric patient to harmful boundary crossings imposes a special burden on the provider. With greater opportunity to exploit and dominate, the provider must adhere to stricter standards of good conduct, or virtuous behavior (Radden, 2002b). Virtue ethics, a character-focused approach to ethics, is a helpful, perhaps necessary, if not entirely sufficient model for understanding ethical concerns in mental health care and research (Radden & Sadler, 2008; Sadler, 2007). Virtues are defined as the personal qualities attributed to a person's character and are identifiable through outward action as well as through more subtle manifestations of the person's inner, mental life (Radden & Sadler, 2008). Virtue is evidenced in practice and requires rehearsal, planning, focus, effort, and discipline. Virtue may be acquired through habituation, taught through educational processes, and utilized in the practitioner's capacity for practical reasoning and practical judgment in resolving ethical conflicts (Radden & Sadler, 2008). Because virtue ethics emphasizes everyday conduct, which is laden with ethical significance (Radden & Sadler, 2008), and everyday practice gives rise to the ethical concerns most salient to nurses (Chambliss, 1996), the virtues are important to nurse professionals. Indeed, the virtuous character traits of integrity, compassion, courage, honesty, and humility, to name a few, are explicitly identified in the ANA Code of Ethics as essential to nursing practice (ANA, 2015; Crigger & Godfrey, 2011; Grace, 2018).

5.3.1.4. 'Personal Self'/Stigma

The ethical significance of the 'personal self' of both the patient and the mental health provider cannot be overstated. The personal self of the clinician is an important instrument in effective treatment (Sadler, 2007). The 'self' is a complex amalgam of knowledge, skills, values, ideals, experiences, affects, character traits, self-representations, and outward behavior. It is the practitioner's most salient and valuable therapeutic tool, essential to the therapeutic alliance, which in turn is the most important factor for successful mental health outcomes. The personal self, a commonsense concept with ethical and psychiatric significance, is characterized by agency, the ability to act in the world for reasons of one's own; identity, which distinguishes the self from all else; trajectory, movement along a course that stretches forward into the future; history, awareness of a past belonging uniquely to oneself; and perspective, a standpoint from which to view and experience the world (Sadler, 2007). The personal self is owned; it is 'mine.' However, treatment requires the patient not only to share intimate aspects of the personal self but to reform and reconstruct it in a therapeutic project that is unmatched in our culture with the exception, perhaps, of childrearing (Radden, 2002a). It is an endeavor that heightens both the patient's vulnerability and the responsibilities imposed on the practitioner.

For the patient and others, the boundary between self and mental illness is not always clear. What the clinician considers signs and symptoms of illness may be, for the patient, "prized aspects of the personal self" (Sadler, 2007, p. 116). What Sadler (2007) terms self-illness ambiguity, or more descriptively, the "invasion of the personal space by mental illness," contributes to the vulnerability of psychiatric patients (p. 118). They can feel offended, harassed, and intruded upon by the presumptions and ministrations of well-meaning others who may not themselves fully recognize or appreciate the difference between, for example, the 'person with schizophrenia' and 'the schizophrenic' who has become the illness (Sadler, 2007). Distrustful of their own experience, such patients may question their very identity: "Is this me or is this my illness?" Successful treatment depends in part on "making the self-illness ambiguity less ambiguous" as more aspects of the personal self become visible, comprehensible, and manageable (Sadler, 2007, p. 117).

The conflation or fusion of the patient's personal self with his or her mental illness contributes to social stigma, which compounds the vulnerability of psychiatric patients in presenting them with yet another burden to manage. Not only must they struggle with the mental illness, but they must also contend with the shame, humiliation, and mistreatment that attends social stigma (Sadler, 2007). Stigma occurs as a function of attaching a negative, misunderstood, and exaggerated attribute to a social group that results in global devaluation of group members (Goffman, 1963; Halter, 2008). People with the undesirable attribute may be considered to have brought it upon themselves as a matter of moral failure, poor self-control, or lack of willpower (Halter, 2008). In cases of the mentally ill, the special vulnerability of psychiatric patients extends to the societal reaction to mental illness, which feeds back into conceptions of the personal self (Sadler, 2007). As a function of stigma, their psychic pain is often less recognizable than physical pain no matter how debilitating the mental illness may be. Others in society may still find the pain of mental illness unpersuasive, if they see it at all (Sadler, 2007).

The confusion of personal self with mental illness manifests not only in the patient's distrust of personal experience but also in society's pervasive distrust of the psychiatric patient's psychological integrity, capacity for self-control, responsibility for personal conduct, and ability to safely and cooperatively live in community with others (Sadler, 2007). Radden (2002b) best articulated the problem:

> *[S]cience may eventually allow us to identify and explain states of mental disorder with reference to specific biological markers and underlying causes, thus eliminating much of the negativity, mystery and fear presently surrounding them. Yet some of the systemic prejudice and stigma attaching to such states seem likely to remain as long as our cultural values are unchanged, values which include autonomy, rationality, self-control, personal identity and psychological integrity. With roots deep in the Greek origins of Western culture, these values are entrenched, long lived and antithetical to the ravages wrought by mental disorder. Nothing less than the elimination of these states through prevention and cure . . . could entirely end the negativity attaching to them (Radden, 2002b, p. 411).*

The stigma of mental illness may abate as science advances, but the state of psychiatric science to date has certainly not yet made this possible.

5.3.1.5. Dual Relationships/'Dirty Hands'

Dual relationships are constituted by the necessity of working for the benefit of parties other than, or in addition to, the patient. Dual agency exacerbates the vulnerability of the psychiatric patient and creates ethical problems for the mental health practitioner, whose allegiance might be divided between a patient who needs a certain level or kind of care and an agency that needs to cut costs. Gutheil and Simon (2003) recommend that providers follow the conclusions of the Hastings Center (1978) with respect to issues of double agency: Separate functions should reside in different roles, and patients should be fully informed not only of treatment objectives but also of any conflicts within the provider's priorities or between different professionals' agendas. Tasman and Mohr (2011) advise clinicians to completely avoid treatment situations that place them in a conflict between therapeutic responsibility to patients and third parties. Examples of dual relationships include clinicians treating their own relatives and friends, the same therapist employing concurrent family and individual therapy with a given patient, and clinicians testifying as forensic witnesses for current psychotherapy patients.

A major area for ethical concern in mental health care has been generated by the ways in which health care is financed and access to care and its associated costs are controlled. Managed care may achieve its financial goals with practices that promote dual relationships. Managed care organizations (MCO) may place strains on confidentiality, privacy, trust, and other aspects of the therapeutic relationship by their need to control costs and access to care (Radden, 2002b). Mental health practitioners may find it necessary to act as gate keepers, limiting and rationing health care to insure the viability and/or profitability of the organization (Radden, 2002b). Specific issues of concern include restrictions on the number of clinicians listed on provider panels for a given community, increasing numbers of MCO personnel with access to confidential treatment records, transfer of authority for treatment decisions from providers to less knowledgeable treatment reviewers, refusal to pay for integrated treatment, and insistence on split treatment models in which the patient obtains psychotherapy from a social worker or psychologist and only brief, infrequent medication management visits with a psychiatrist or psychiatric nurse practitioner (Tasman & Mohr, 2011). Such restrictive practices fragment patient care, limit the capacity of medical providers to insure high quality care, and create an ethical bind in which "medical responsibility is not accompanied by a commensurate degree of authority to direct the treatment process" (Tasman & Mohr, 2011, p. 66).

In the world of managed care, the ethical principle of beneficence tends to give way to an ethic of utility. As a consequence, it is increasingly likely that nurses may be forced to act in ways that may be incompatible with ethical practice. The phenomenon of 'dirty hands' is a moral dilemma marked by the experience of being morally compromised and suffering moral distress by doing what is required (Mohr & Mahon, 1996). In mental health care environments that are increasingly driven by market forces, practitioners may find themselves in circumstances where they must adhere to prescribed clinical decisions that may not be in the best interest of the patient (Mohr & Mahon, 1996). There are inherent difficulties and contradictions in a system that treats health care as a market commodity and not as a social good. The fundamental nature of mental health care is relationship, not market transaction.

5.3.1.6. Diagnosis/Explanatory Models

Managed care's approach to containing costs and controlling access to care rests upon a technical, instrumental view of both human beings and mental health care (Phillips, 2002). The challenge of explaining mental illness may be a result of this approach (Brendel, 2002). Explanatory models in mental health care and research have ethical significance because they demonstrate how human existence is construed and what is of value in making human behavior intelligible. Explanatory models lead the practitioner to treat the human suffering of mental illness in particular ways (Brendel, 2002; 2003). Often, the person with mental illness is reduced only to that which can be observed and identified from the outside (Phillips, 2002). The complexity of an individual life is distilled to a cluster of observable, behavioral signs and symptoms organized around a DSM category to which a treatment algorithm or protocol can then be applied. The bio-psycho-social-ethno-cultural uniqueness of the particular person situated in his or her unique historical context is missing (Phillips, 2002).

Adopted from contemporary biological psychiatry, managed care's construal of human existence relies heavily on technical reason, derived from Aristotle's distinction between techne (technical reasoning) and phronesis (practical reasoning) (Phillips, 2002). From the standpoint of technical rationality, a particular problem is always an instance of a general type (Phillips, 2002). Technical reason uses systematized knowledge of the general type, along with specific rules for knowledge application, to address particular problems as if they actually were the general type—that is, without the variability created by individual patients' lives and histories and/or individual providers' varying levels of skill, training, artistry, and experience (Phillips, 2002). Psychotherapies with instruction manuals, treatment algorithms, and other formulaic solutions derive from this kind of reasoning. Such approaches are helpful but insufficient, given human complexity and the limits of the scientific evidence base. They rely solely on the science of the practice, leaving out the practical wisdom of the experienced practitioner (Phillips, 2002).

Brendel (2002) asserts that science and ethics are equal partners in any project to explain mental illness and that the scope of psychiatric-mental health ethics includes focus on the values and norms that guide explanatory models. Explanatory models for mental health care and research are deeply value-laden, because they must involve the best interests of patients and participants, who are people who generally want to be accurately understood and treated as persons, not as disorders or disease entities reduced to diagnostic labels (Brendel, 2002). Pragmatic philosophers such as William James and John Dewey believed that the essential aim of science ought to be favorable practical outcomes for people in their everyday lives and that any explanatory model of mental illness could only be 'true' to the extent it actually promoted beneficial, real-world results for people with mental illness (Brendel, 2003). Consistent with pragmatism of this type, an explanatory model of mental illness that also promotes ethical patient care is more widely applicable within clinical science, where explanations are coherent and plausible only insofar as they are useful and empirically testable in clinical settings (Brendel, 2002; 2003). An explanatory model of mental illness must not only be evidence-based but must promote the beneficial, practical, ethical outcomes of easing mentally ill patients' pain and suffering while achieving more adaptive real-world functioning consistent with their best interests (Brendel, 2002; 2003).

Brendel (2003) has identified three pragmatic, empirical-ethical principles that can guide the mental health clinician to a more widely applicable, outcomes-oriented approach to clinical explanation and treatment. The first pragmatic principle is methodological pluralism. An explanatory model of mental illness based solely on neuroscience ignores the mounting evidence of complex etiological interactions between genetic predispositions and psychosocial stressors and of the treatment utility of combining psychopharmacological and psychotherapeutic approaches (Brendel, 2002; 2003). Mental health clinicians and researchers are ethically and scientifically disadvantaged if limited to a single, reductive, either biological or psychological model of mental illness that cannot account for the indeterminate, open-ended, corrigible nature of both psychiatric diagnosis and etiologies of psychiatric disorder (Brendel, 2002; 2003).

The second pragmatic principle is full participation of the patient in treatment planning in order to achieve optimum results in achieving a mutually acceptable, positive outcome. From a pragmatic view, truth is "the outcome of a deliberative social process aimed at identifying what works in a given situation" (Brendel, 2003, p. 571). In mental health care, the explanation for the patient's difficulties develops over time as the patient, provider, family, and others collaborate and deliberate about the complex, changing dynamics of the clinical situation (Brendel, 2003).

The third pragmatic principle central to mental health practice is the provisional nature of psychiatric explanation (Brendel, 2003). To provide patients with ethical care, practitioners must formulate cases based on the current evidence-base and do so with an awareness of the pluralistic and provisional nature of psychiatric explanation. In mental health care and research, current explanatory models and concepts are never adequate or final (Brendel, 2003).

5.3.1.7. Confidentiality/Privileged Communication

The sensitive nature of the patient's communications in mental health care heightens the stakes for potential breaches of confidentiality. Confidentiality refers to the therapist's responsibility to not release information obtained in the course of treatment to third parties. This is essential for the development of a safe, trusting, therapeutic relation-ship (Sadock, Sadock & Ruiz, 2015). Privilege refers to the patient's right to prevent disclosure of treatment information in judicial hearings; mental health clinicians must treat their patients' communications as privileged as determined by state statute (Sadock et al., 2015; Tasman & Mohr, 2011). Privileged communication is provided by statute in each state in the U.S.; however, not all states extend the privilege to nurses, psychologists, or other non-physician mental health profession-als (Tasman & Mohr, 2011).

Although courts uphold the duty of confidentiality between patient and therapist, which endures after a patient's death, they recognize a higher duty to protect the public safety. This means breaches of con-fidentiality may be required by law in cases of child abuse, threats of suicide, threats of harm to a third party, and allegations of sexual mis-conduct made against a therapist (Tasman & Mohr, 2011). Other excep-tions to confidentiality include patient requests for release of records to third parties, the duty to warn potential victims of a patient's threats to harm them, emergencies, court-ordered psychiatric evaluations, and malpractice litigation initiated by a patient (Tasman & Mohr, 2011). Members of a treatment team may share information with each other without specific permission from a patient; however, team membership should be clarified.

Means of preserving confidentiality may include having all employ-ees of mental health facilities sign confidentiality agreements and/or at-tend regularly scheduled, continuing education events; obtaining signed authorization from patients before releasing information; explaining the need for confidentiality to parents of children and adolescents; obtain-ing confidentiality agreements from all participants in family and group psychotherapy; avoiding gossip or stray communications with relatives of patients or employees not directly involved in the care of patients; properly disguising case presentations; and, as a clinician, refusing to discuss privileged information with one's own family, friends, students, or co-workers (Tasman & Mohr, 2011).

5.4. ETHICAL CONSIDERATIONS IN MENTAL HEALTH RESEARCH

Clinical care and research are both areas for practice, broadly speak-ing; the ethical considerations of mental health care for people with the particular vulnerabilities identified above are also relevant for mental health research with this subset of policy-designated 'vulnerable participants.' The same historic codes and declarations which form the basis for research ethics policies have guided clinical care and professional practice ethics. Conversely, research ethics principles and policies have derived in part from practice ethics, which is appropriate given that research informs effective practice and in part derives its justification from that supporting role (Spetie & Arnold, 2007).

Contemporary research ethics policies began with the Nuremberg Code as a result of reflection and judgment on the atrocities perpetrated upon concentration camp inmates by Nazi physicians (Rhodes, 2010). Since then, the protection of human participants in biomedical research has been the focus of research ethics policy. Informed consent, based on both the principle of autonomy as an ideal of pure self-determination as well as the principle of respect for the actual autonomy of the real human participant, resides at the core of research protections and constitutes the centerpiece of regulatory attention (Rhodes, 2010). The focus on protection of the participants of human research is justified by the lessons of history, by the results of research in experimental psychology that point to a number of pernicious human tendencies across a wide range of societies (Nussbaum, 2010), and by the fact that research inherently involves relationships of asymmetrical power. Relationships with asymmetrical power roles are common in society. (Juritzen, Grimen, & Heggen, 2011; Foucault, 1980). Research ethics is based on a concept of the asymmetry of power. It views the researcher as powerful and potentially harmful, the participant as less knowledgeable and therefore disadvantaged and potentially disempowered within this unequal relationship, and review boards as necessary to protect the participant by striking a better balance of power (Juritzen et al., 2011).

Few ethicists dispute the necessity of protecting those who are least able to protect themselves. Long after the Nuremberg judgments and the widespread revelation of Nazi research practices, history has documented the necessity of such protections (Juritzen et al., 2011). Existing codes of research ethics did not prevent the research abuses and questionable research practices illustrated by (a) the 1963 revelation of investigators injecting uninformed elderly patients with live cancer cells at the Jewish Chronic Disease Hospital; (b) Henry Beecher's 1966 publication in The New England Journal of Medicine of 22 examples of unethical or questionably ethical U.S. research studies; (c) the 1971 debate in The Lancet of the ethics of feeding live hepatitis virus to mentally disabled children at Willowbrook State School from 1955–1970; (d) the 1972 Associated Press exposé of the 40-year Tuskegee syphilis study that was still running 25 years after a reliable treatment for syphilis had been developed; (e) the 1975 U.S. Army acknowledgment of experiments with hallucinogenic drugs on unaware civilians; or (f) the 1999 death of 18-year old Jesse Gelsinger in a University of Pennsylvania/ Schering-Plough gene therapy trial (Beecher, 1966; Edsall, 1971; Goldby, 1971; Krugman & Shapiro, 1971; Pappworth, 1971; Rhodes, 2010; Stolberg, 1999; Weiss & Weiss, 1999).

Social science research also points to the necessity of protecting those who are least able to protect themselves. Replicated findings in social and experimental psychology show that people cannot be relied upon to do what they know is right under certain social conditions—for example, when they can defer to authority and not be held personally accountable, or when group pressure induces them to violate the clear evidence of their own senses where they are the sole voice of dissent (Nussbaum, 2010; Zimbardo, 2008). Numerous examples from experimental psychology show that reliable, apparently decent citizens can be induced by social situations to dehumanize, stigmatize, inflict pain on other human beings, or otherwise violate conventional norms of moral behavior (Nussbaum, 2010; Zimbardo, 2008). Research investigators are not themselves immune to such social pressures; thus, ongoing vigilance in the area of protection of human participants in research is warranted. People with mental illness may be at risk of further psychological distress and exacerbation of their symptoms when enrolled in a research study, and they may be at risk for exploitation and coercion by researchers, clinicians, and even family members in the manner by which informed consent is obtained (McCauley-Elsom, Gurvich, Lee, Elsom, O'Connor & Kulkarni, 2009). However, many mental health problems and illnesses are episodic in nature or have a fluctuating course, meaning that people's mental state—and thus, their capacity to comprehend information and offer informed consent—vary over time (McCauley-Elsom et al., 2009). Autonomy and decisional capacity vary for some of those with mental illness. A subset of people with a wide range of mental health problems may never experience a loss of decisional capacity or ability to give full and informed consent for research participation, which can lead to claims that the classification of all mental health services users as 'vulnerable' is itself disempowering (Allbutt & Masters, 2010). The Belmont Report supports the notion that people with mental illness should have fair access to opportunities to reap the benefits of research. As a social good, research should extend in fair ways to those whose immense and costly suffering is of concern to society as a whole (National Commission for the Protection of Human Subjects of Biomedical and Behavioral Research, 1979).

Weiss and Weiss (1999) reviewed the history of evolving ethics guidelines for the conduct of psychiatric research, including the 1998 report of the National Bioethics Advisory Commission (NBAC), which took an overall stance of protectiveness and placed emphasis on the role of government regulation in safeguarding those with mental illness against exploitation in psychiatric research. The NBAC (1998) report offered 21 specific recommendations across six categories, including the following highlights: (a) With respect to informed consent and decisional capacity in individuals diagnosed with mental disorders, those who are capable of consent should be allowed to consent or refuse research participation without the involvement of others and without coercion. With or without decisional capacity, all conscious people with mental illness have the right to refuse research participation, and decisional capacity should be formally and independently assessed in potential study participants when the research protocol presents greater than minimal risk (Weiss & Weiss, 1999). (b) Psychiatric research must be classified according to risk, including "minimal risk," "greater than minimal risk with the prospect of direct medical benefit to subjects," and "greater than minimal risk that does not offer the prospect of direct medical benefit to subjects." Within each of these classifications, stringent directives guide IRB review and personal and surrogate informed consent (Weiss & Weiss, 1999). (c) Surrogate decision makers have specific duties and must identify and act on the wishes of the study participant; a 'best interest' standard is insufficient for consent to participate in psychiatric research (Weiss & Weiss, 1999).

According to Weiss and Weiss (1999), the NBAC report, which recommended a moratorium on research with participants with impaired decisional capacity, had significant drawbacks that derived from five principal problems, including (a) insufficient awareness of the subtle, widely varying, and fluctuating clinical features of psychiatric disorders; (b) insufficient recognition of the immense societal impact of mental illness and the pressing need for research to address it; (c) insufficient respect for the autonomy and personhood of people with mental illness; (d) insufficient awareness of the practical dimensions of the scientific context; and (e) insufficient integration of existing ethics data on psychiatric research (Weiss & Weiss, 1999).

Overall, people with mental illness are capable of informed consent but have greater difficulties with consent processes compared to medically ill and healthy populations, because the symptoms of mental illness can adversely affect the information-based, cognitive aspects of consent (Weiss and Weiss, 1999). Subjective factors such as attitudes, values, motivations, and context may affect research enrollment decisions (Weiss & Weiss, 1999). Beyond the issue of informed consent, little is known about the effectiveness of ethical safeguards in protecting human research participants. In mental health research, much more education about ethics is needed in the areas of regulatory requirements, the role of the IRB in psychiatric research, differences between clinical care and clinical research, scientific conduct and misconduct, scientific merit and ethical issues in study design, participant recruitment and selection, symptom-provoking studies, medication-free research, placebo-controlled clinical trials, genetics studies, better protection of participants during research participation, relationships between patient volunteers and members of the research team, conflicts of interest in industry-sponsored research, and psychiatric research with children and pregnant women (Rosenstein, Miller & Rubinow, 2001).

Much of the current controversy surrounding psychiatric research focuses on the ethical problems of (a) employing placebo controls instead of comparing new drugs to existing treatments; (b) discontinuing medications for clinical trials, which provokes symptoms and can complicate a patient's recovery; (c) the predominance of industry-sponsored clinical trials and the push to find new uses—that is, new patients with different psychiatric diagnoses—for 'old' psychotropic drugs that are going off patent protection; (d) protecting privacy and confidentiality in genetics research; and (e) conducting psychopharmacology research with children (Angell, 2005; Kolch, Ludolph, Plener, Fangerau, Vitiello & Fegert, 2010; Rosenstein et al., 2001; Spetie & Arnold, 2007).

The latter is a particularly charged issue. Children and adolescents with psychiatric disorders are doubly vulnerable by virtue of both their mental disorder and the fact of being children with a developmental status that entails normal dependency and limited decisional capacity. Along with the historical reluctance of researchers to expose children and adolescents to unnecessary risk during research trials, their protected status as 'vulnerable' has led to a paucity of data on the effectiveness, safety, and pharmacokinetics of psychotropic drugs in children (Spetie & Arnold, 2007). As a result, and with the rationale of not wanting to keep potentially helpful treatments away from children and adolescents who suffer from severe psychiatric symptoms, clinicians may treat pediatric patients by prescribing psychotropic medications 'off-label'—that is, without an FDA-approved indication and without the benefit of any evidence base. This is disturbing for many reasons. At these young ages, the boundary is often obscure between normal and abnormal behavior, which is better understood in adolescents and adults. At younger ages, it is sometimes normal to see such developmental phenomena as separation anxiety, negativism, hyperactivity, tantrums, imaginary playmates, unmodulated aggression, and heightened reactivity to environmental change (Spetie & Arnold, 2007).

Kolch et al. (2010) reviewed and integrated the findings of 138 publications on the ethical and legal issues entailed by psychopharmacological research in children. The need for research with this population is clear; off-label medication use in minors is soaring. The strict paradigm of excluding mentally ill children from research is changing as society recognizes the need to balance the protection of emotionally disturbed children from research against the widespread use of unsafe, ineffective medication. Clinical trials with children may increase; however, legal, ethical, and practical hurdles exist, including legislative barriers, conflicts of interest, problems with assent and consent, problems with study design and small samples, problems insuring minimal risks and burdens, and problems with global justice (e.g., with respect to limited supplies of extremely expensive pharmacogenetic therapies) (Koch et al., 2010). Practitioners must guard against the pressures of both direct-to-consumer pharmaceutical advertising and large monetary incentives to enroll pediatric clients in clinical trials. They must also remember that, in the case of research, children and adolescents are never able to provide consent until they come of age. Parental involvement and consent, even if ethically problematic, is required. As legally guaranteed, minors do have the right to information about the research project and to decline to assent to participate. If a child declines participation, his or her competence to refuse should be formally evaluated.

5.5. ETHICAL SIGNIFICANCE OF EVERYDAY LIFE IN MENTAL HEALTH CARE

The richness and moral complexity of everyday life in mental health care and research cannot be overestimated. When nurses at any level of practice are asked about their ethical concerns, the responses are typically about their everyday, work lives. Stories comprise the typical format, because narrative and analogy are the forms that moral reasoning takes (Walker, 2007). Nurses spend their professional lives as boundary workers, practicing in the interstitial spaces between multiple professions with their multiple, competing interests (Chambliss, 1996). In the health care organization, for example, nurses work at the boundaries of medicine, nursing administration, occupational therapy, respiratory care, radiology, housekeeping, dietary, admissions, volunteer services, health information management, pharmacy, and many other departments (Chambliss, 1996). In all practice contexts—inpatient or outpatient, basic or advanced, independent or group practice—nurses may find themselves case managing patient care in order to negotiate the goals and tasks of treatment and to mediate agreement between patients, families, referral sources, physicians, and all other team members. This reality shapes their ethical concerns.

A multi-year ethnographic inquiry observed and described how emergency department nurses in several mid- to large-size American medical centers conceptualized and responded to the ethical problems they encountered in their everyday work (Chambliss, 1996). Nurses' moral concerns were not abstract; they were not the bioethics issues that interest many physicians—stem cell research, human enhancement, physician-assisted suicide, and medical futility—except as those issues affected the particular persons subject to their care. While the participants were not psychiatric-mental health nurses, this classic work in medical sociology demonstrated that nurses' conceptions of ethical problems were the result of a complex process of socially negotiating the everyday demands of their "in-between" spatial location. Moreover, Chambliss found that responsibility to meet one's ethical obligations was not an individual attribute enacted within the relatively narrow boundaries of the nurse-patient relationship. Rather, it was created and constrained by the larger social context.

In other words, nurses' understanding of what was responsible for them to do was fundamentally shaped by their social location vis-à-vis patients and by their position as subordinates in healthcare systems (Chambliss, 1996). To illustrate the former, by virtue of their proximity to patients, their location in the 'in-between zone,' and their own sense of professional responsibility to advocate for patients, nurses often pick up the slack when things fall through the cracks and other departments or professions default on responsibilities for important (but often unseen) elements of patient care or agency housekeeping. Nurses may also be deeply constrained by the limits of their professional autonomy to follow hospital or agency policies as well as physician directives (Chambliss, 1996).

Every day, nurses juggle the demands of this in-between spatiality, including the orders or directives of health care providers (both physicians and advanced practice registered nurses), the needs of patients, the demands of families, the rules of the law, the boundaries of their legal scope of practice, the bureaucracy of the workplace, the defaulted responsibilities of other departments or agencies, the dictates of administrators, their expectations for professional autonomy, and their own physical and emotional limits (Chambliss, 1996). These conflicts are some of the ethical problems of nursing and explain why nurses' patient care concerns so often involve systems issues and/or conflicts with physicians or administrators—and are construed (or even trivialized) as something 'other' than ethical problems because they do not meet the threshold for the traditional ethical dilemma of biomedical ethics. The higher nurses advance in the healthcare system, the more intense these kinds of conflicts become (Chambliss, 1996).

For example, as nurses'—especially advanced practice nurses'—status, power, authority, knowledge, competence, and skills have grown, their responsibilities have changed, which challenges medical hegemony and/or dominance in health care organizations. Nurses at all levels of practice, but especially at the higher levels, have come to feel that they must, and have a right to define and answer ethical questions for themselves. In part, 'professionalization' describes a shift from a technical to a moral orientation to one's work (Chambliss, 1996). As power goes up, so do responsibilities—and so do ethical conflicts with those who have competing responsibilities and interests. As the organization of health care work changes, so too do the ethical conflicts, as in the case of the surgical nurse who creates a new protocol that changes the work flow of physicians on the surgical team: "The resulting quarrels are seen as moral conflicts, framed in the formal terms of a moral debate. Such debates . . . only arise when there are speakers to deliver them, and with a voice strong and clear enough to be heard" (Chambliss, 1996, p. 99). This is where advanced practice nurses have a critical role to play in educating, informing, supporting, and facilitating the verbal and behavioral expression of nurses' moral knowledge at basic levels of practice as well.

5.6. MORAL FRAMEWORKS FOR MENTAL HEALTH CARE AND RESEARCH

The profession of nursing applies moral theories and frameworks from moral philosophy to understand nursing practice, including utilitarianism or consequentialism, deontological or principles-based ethics, and virtue ethics. Enlightenment moral philosophy, Kantian ethics in particular, produced the moral theories used most often by bioethics and consequently by nursing. American nursing's code of ethics (ANA, 2015) is based on both a Kantian, deontological ethics of duty and an ethics of virtue, outlining both the duties and moral obligations of nurses and the virtues that make for excellence in nursing practice.

5.6.1. Ethics of Responsibility

A useful, alternative model for healthcare ethics essentially encapsulates and describes the narrative, socially negotiated, interpersonal process observed in practice. Walker's (2007) alternative model of moral inquiry has given rise to an ethics of responsibility, which maintains that morality consists of a system's actual social practices and not moral theories. In an ethics of responsibility, the practices characteristic of morality are the practices that implement commonly shared understandings about how responsibilities are to be divided or deflected within a social system (Walker, 2007). These practices of responsibility are commonly shared understandings about who is obligated to do what for whom and who will get to avoid or even remain unaware of certain kinds of obligations. Our various responsibilities, and what it takes to meet them, so often remain invisible to others. An ethics of responsibility tries to shed light on them so that members of a social system can see more clearly how they are all in it together (Walker, 2007). Thus, in this model, a system's practices of responsibility are identified and examined to get at the content of the organization's shared morality so that members can achieve new moral understandings in a continuous process of revising and recreating the present moral order. So how might an ethics of responsibility work in real life?

The social organization of healthcare systems creates and shapes the ethical problems of its members. When power relationships are stable and unchallenged, few ethical crises emerge (Chambliss, 1996). When professional groups, such as nursing, develop new levels of practice that may challenge the existing social order, then moral agendas tend to come into conflict. Practices of responsibility that flow from particular divisions of labor show us these sorts of problems very clearly. For example, a DNP-prepared APRN working in an emergency department had concerns about the hospital's practice of assigning to nursing the responsibility of ratifying current patient medication regimens with hospital admission orders. A form required that providers, both APRNs and physicians, verify home medication regimens with admission and new medication orders. The APRNs ratified their own orders, while the physicians simply initialed a form prepared by RNs. The signed or initialed form constituted medication orders for admission. The ratification process was extremely time-consuming for the nurses. Moreover, when quality control reports revealed a deficiency in compliance, it was seen as a nursing failure; and the nurses at all levels were asked to be more careful in drawing the attention of physician providers to these requirements.

With respect to this clinical scenario, the sorts of questions an ethics of responsibility might ask include the following: Whose responsibility is it to find a solution to this problem? Do the benefits and burdens of current practice fall proportionately on those to whom the responsibility belongs?

This seems to be a systemic problem that falls by default to nursing for unexamined reasons, but is that where it belongs? If not, where would a more ethical system of care place this kind of responsibility?

5.7. CONCLUSION

5.7.1. Ethical Significance of Proximity/Empathy in Mental Health Care

Moral knowledge is inextricable from social knowledge and from one's social location in the larger community, especially with respect to one's responsibilities to and for other human beings (Walker, 2007). Moral knowledge comes from one's proximity to, connections with, and empathy for other people. This informs conscience, or the 'still, small voice within.' Proximity, or closeness to others, shapes and sustains the responsibilities moral agents understand themselves to have. It tends to shape what we think we owe each other (Walker, 2007). For example, a mother tends to feel the weight of her moral responsibility to her child—to whom she is very close—to a different degree than the stranger's child. A nurse tends to feel the weight of her moral responsibility to the long-term patient—for whom she has cared for many weeks or years—to a different degree than the newly arrived referral. In order to comprehend a clinical situation and respond morally to one's child, the stranger, the long-term patient, or the newly referred patient, one must exercise the capacity for empathy—the capacity to understand what it must be like to stand in another's shoes (Bjorklund, 2016).

Empathy is an important source of ethical knowledge. It may be the mental health clinician's most valuable asset. Mutual empathic responsiveness stimulates moral imagination, moral intuition, moral sensitivity, and the capacity for moral distress. One cannot respond morally to others unless one can also see, struggle with, feel with, and ultimately comprehend what is suffered, experienced, and endured by other sentient beings (Bjorklund, 2016). Morality is anchored in powerful feelings such as love and fear, and it relies on our ability to read each other's emotions and intentions.

Enlightenment philosophers believed that the exercise of reason brings human beings to moral knowledge. Religious leaders believe that moral knowledge derives from divine law or the exercise of faith (Taylor, 1985). What guides a person to moral response is conditioned by empathy, which cannot develop and grow in the human organism without human connection, attachment, proximity, and opportunities for reciprocal recognition and response to the subtleties of human expression (Bjorklund, 2016). Faith and reason do not fully inform moral judgments in either the child or the mentally ill person who may have no strong attachment to a faith tradition and may not yet have the capacity for formal operations or abstract reasoning. The gaps in their systems of logic can be wide. They may understand what parents and the larger community hold to be right and wrong; however, the child, like the person with a serious mental illness, is not yet what philosophers would call 'the fully formed, autonomous moral agent' (Bjorklund, 2016). Yet, both are capable of moral behavior, and mental health providers have a responsibility to facilitate it.

5.8. WEBSITES FOR FURTHER INFORMATION

- **American Psychiatric Association: Principles of Medical Ethics with Annotations Especially Applicable to Psychiatry**
  https://www.psychiatry.org/psychiatrists/practice/ethics
- **American Psychiatric Nurses Association: Position Papers (ECT, Seclusion and Restraint, Workplace Violence, Roles of Psychiatric Mental Health Nurses in Managed Care)**
  https://www.apna.org/i4a/pages/index.cfm?pageid=3335
- **American Psychological Association: Ethical Principles of Psychologists and Code of Conduct**
  https://www.apa.org/ethics/code/index.aspx
- **Geriatric Mental Health Ethics: A Casebook**
  http://www.springerpub.com/samples/9780826103192_chapter.pdf
- **Psychiatry Online: Case Studies in Ethics**
  https://focus.psychiatryonline.org/doi/abs/10.1176/foc.9.2.foc197
- **World Psychiatric Association: Declarations on Ethical Standards**
  http://www.wpanet.org/detail.php?section_id=5&category_id=9&content_id=31

5.9. CASE STUDIES

5.9.1. Case Study #1

The patient was an elderly woman with all mental capabilities intact. She was admitted for a hip replacement. A newly certified nurse anesthetist was told by the patient in the pre-op patient interview that she desired a spinal anesthetic instead of a general anesthetic. There were no contraindications to a spinal, so this was the plan decided by both patient and CRNA.

The anesthesiologist assigned to the case (the chair of the department) also interviewed the patient, and he decided that general anesthesia would be used. The CRNA informed him that the patient desired a spinal anesthetic. The MD replied, "Just give her some Versed; she'll never remember." The CRNA felt very uneasy about this and knew that it was wrong, but was intimidated and didn't want to rock the boat. The CRNA went along with the anesthesiologist's plan and did as was instructed.

Over the subsequent nine years, the CRNA never forgot this patient and her inability to be a patient advocate for fear of retribution. She states that now she has grown in confidence and would not let this happen again without some valid reason to override a patient's wishes.

5.9.1.1. Questions for Discussion

1. To whom did the CRNA owe her fidelity? Is the principle of fidelity sufficient to understand the CRNA's ethical conflict? What else requires ethical consideration?
2. Does analysis of this case from a feminist ethics perspective lead to a different ethical outcome? Could the concept of 'gender' be operating in this scenario? How? Where?

5.9.2. Case Study #2

A female in her late 50's was admitted for evaluation because she was not seeking the necessary treatment for her infected leg ulcers. She was a hoarder living in a house that had been condemned. She had been able to obtain groceries and keep herself fed with a roof over her head, despite the deplorable condition of the building. The Department of Public Health had cleaned out the house several times in order to get rid of cat urine, feces, and strange collections of things like her hair, which lay in bowls all over the house. She underwent outpatient commitment, is now in assisted living, and is very unhappy about not being in her own home. The patient is often medication non-adherent, but when she faces revocation of her provisional discharge, she begins to take them again. At what point does she have a right to live in a 'bizarre' way and be left alone, versus having treatment forced on her? Her health was in

jeopardy, as her leg ulcers were infected and she was facing amputa-
tions if she continued to refuse treatment. She is now miserable because
she is not able to live on her own.

5.9.2.1. Questions for Discussion

1. Is there any point in a patient's care when treatment should/must
   be forced?
2. What are this patient's 'best interests,' and how should they be
   determined?
3. What actions might support the 'diminished autonomy' of this
   patient?

5.9.3. Case Study #3

An ACT team specializes in the care and treatment of young adults
aged 18–24 with serious and persistent mental illness (SPMI). The
teams are composed of social workers from the county health department, the mental health center, and the state; nurses from the mental
health center; a psychiatrist; and an advanced practice registered nurse.
The teams are funded from the Department of Human Services and do
not have adequate funds for supplies or patient needs. The primary goal
of the team is to assist patients in goals related to rehabilitation of their
mental illness in order to avoid hospitalization and keep them living
in the community. Specific goals include maintaining stable housing,
learning to stick to a budget, medication and treatment adherence, effective parenting, sobriety, socialization, better physical health, staying
out of jail, and staying out of the hospital.

The ACT team has found that money can be effective in getting patients to complete tasks. For example, they sometimes pay non-compliant patients $2/day to take their medications in front of the staff, or
the patients are given gift cards to Subway or Target after a week of
medication compliance. The team has also given money ($10–$20) for
patients to get necessary lab work they would not otherwise do and also
have given a patient with extreme hand contractures $20 for each visit
to the physical therapist.

Birth control options are discussed with all female patients. Many
already have children and have declined birth control options in the past
for various reasons. A young woman with schizophrenia came into the
office and said she had run out of money. She asked to borrow $50 from
the team's flex fund. She had borrowed money in the past and not paid
it back. The case managers and the nurse decided not to loan the money

to the patient, but instead offered her $50 to get a Depo Provera injection that day plus an additional incentive of $50 every three months for subsequent injections. She agreed to get the injection in exchange for the money even though she had refused birth control in the past.

5.9.3.1. Questions for Discussion

1. Is it ethical to pay a patient to receive birth control? For any reason?
2. Do these scenarios describe inducement or coercion? What is the difference? Informed consent?

5.9.4. Case Study #4

A clinical nurse specialist (CNS) in an outpatient psychiatric clinic evaluated a patient who presented with several psychiatric complaints and an extensive history of major medical problems, including many surgeries and chronic pain. The patient had previously been receiving treatment from another provider and was also being treated at the pain clinic in the same building.

A patient service assistant (PSA) who worked in the psychiatric clinic happened to be passing by the pain clinic one day and saw the patient and recognized her from the psychiatric clinic. She asked a pain clinic staff person why the patient was receiving treatment there and learned that the patient had chronic pain. The patient was in a wheelchair, which shocked the PSA because she had seen the patient outside the clinic, coaching a youth sports team, clearly not in a wheelchair and not apparently in pain. At a subsequent sports event, the PSA took a video of the patient to prove that the patient was not using a wheelchair, and she brought the video to the pain clinic as evidence. The patient was also observed going to her vehicle, standing up from the wheelchair, and effortlessly putting the wheelchair into her vehicle.

Because of the patient's extensive medical history and unsolicited information relayed by the PSA, the CNS diagnosed the patient with Factitious Disorder and met with the collaborating psychiatrist to discuss treatment options. The psychiatrist concurred with the diagnosis. The PSA's information influenced the providers' diagnosis of the patient; however, the CNS believed that she had a duty to perform the most comprehensive assessment possible, including collateral information from others, to arrive at the best diagnosis and treatment plan for the patient. This breach of confidentiality had the potential to benefit the patient if the diagnosis was accurate and treatment was successful.

5.9.4.1. Questions for Discussion

1. Do therapeutic ends ever justify unethical means? Do they justify the ends in this case?
2. Where, when, how was patient confidentiality breached? Was it? Would it be different if the pain clinic was in a different building?
3. Is it legal/ethical to film someone without their permission?
4. Should the patient be told about the breach?

5.9.5. Case Study #5

Many psychiatric medications have not been approved by the FDA for use in children and adolescents. Most of these medications have not gone through clinical trials with children and adolescents.

An adolescent was admitted for a first psychotic episode. At that time, this unit had only one child/adolescent psychiatrist, who was from a foreign country and was a new graduate. He was not yet board certified, and there was a language barrier between him, the patients, the parents, and the staff on the unit. An antipsychotic medication was tried for this adolescent with no significant clearing of the psychosis. The psychiatrist met with the patient for two to three minutes each day, leaving the nursing staff to assess the patient's current condition. The psychiatrist did not meet face to face with the family; all his communications occurred via telephone. After two weeks of this medication trial and no clearing of the psychosis, the psychiatrist decided to perform electroconvulsive therapy (ECT) and communicated this to the family. The psychiatrist did not seek a second opinion with another psychiatrist and did not offer a second medication trial. The psychiatrist left the signing of the informed consent and explanation of the procedure to the nursing staff. When the family arrived, they did not know any details of the procedure or the risks. They agreed to the procedure based on the recommendation of the psychiatrist.

The ECT occurred over the course of a few weeks concurrently with a second medication trial that the psychiatrist decided to begin with the ECT. To complicate matters , the adolescent later admitted that he had been 'huffing' and using 'mushrooms' prior to his hospital admission, which the parents did not know. The patient got better over time, but it is unknown whether the psychosis cleared in response to the ECT, the new medication, or the time away from street drugs.

When asked about the rationale for ECT, the psychiatrist later reported that he felt pressured by the insurance company to get the patient discharged quickly. In addition, the language and cultural differences of the physician, the lack of informed consent obtained by the physician, the lack of a second opinion (which is required for ECT), and only one medication trial before ECT was obtained all present issues.

5.9.5.1. Questions for Discussion

1. Although it commonly occurs, is it ethical to give psychotropic medications to children and adolescents that are not FDA-approved for use with children?
2. What could or should a nurse have done with ethical concerns about the practices of the psychiatrist and the care of this adolescent?
3. As a subordinate in the healthcare hierarchy, and constrained by 'doctor's orders', what are the boundaries of a nurse's role and responsibilities in this scenario?

Identify the psychiatric-mental health ethics issues that are illustrated by this case.

5.9.6. Case Study #6

A psych/mental health department was downsized. Over 50% of the staff was cut. As part of this process, case managers also had to shrink their caseloads. From nearly 600 patients, more than 300 patients were cut. The decisions about which patients would no longer receive services were delegated to two nurse practitioners still remaining on the service. All of the patients had a primary physician and a geriatric nurse practitioner (GNP) assigned to them. The decision of the two NPs was to not make the cuts themselves. Instead, they spent many days on the phone calling all the assigned GNPs to discuss each patient—all 600 of them. The GNPs determined which patients they were comfortable managing on their own and which ones they were not. When the calls were completed, a caseload fewer than 300 patients remained.

5.9.6.1. Questions for Discussion

1. Were responsibilities and roles appropriately matched in this scenario? Should the moral distress of cutting a large caseload in half have been shared by anyone else? Who? Why?
2. Have the 300 patients who lost case management services been treated fairly and justly?
3. What ethical issues, or legal ones, arise from making medical decisions based on finances?

5.10. REFERENCES

Angell, M. (2005). *The Truth About the Drug Companies: How They Deceive Us and What To Do About It*. New York: Random House.

Allbutt, H. & Masters, H. (2010) Ethnography and the ethics of undertaking research in different mental healthcare settings. *Journal of Psychiatric and Mental Health Nursing* 17: 210–215.

American Nurses Association. (2015). *Code of Ethics for Nurses with Interpretive Statements*. Silver Springs, MD: American Nurses Association.

American Psychiatric Association. (2013). *The Principles of Medical Ethics With Annotations Especially Applicable to Psychiatry*. Arlington, VA: American Psychiatric Association.

Barker, P. (2011). *Mental Health Ethics: The Human Context*. London: Routledge.

Beauchamp, T.L. & Childress, J.F. (2013). *Principles of Biomedical Ethics* (7th ed). New York: Oxford University Press.

Beecher, H.K. (1966). Ethics and clinical research. *The New England Journal of Medicine* 274(24): 1354–1360.

Bjorklund, P. (2016). Gossamer threads: Commentary on the impact of digital technology on the developing brain and the capacity for empathy. *Advances in Nursing Science* 39(1): 71-84.

Brendel, D.H. (2002). The ethics of diagnostic and therapeutic paradigm choice in psychiatry. *Harvard Review of Psychiatry* 20: 47–50.

Brendel, D.H. (2003). Reductionism, eclecticism, and pragmatism in psychiatry: The dialectic of clinical explanation. *Journal of Medicine and Philosophy* 28(5–6): 563–580.

Chambliss, D. (1996). *Beyond Caring: Hospitals, Nurses, and the Social Organization of Ethics*. University of Chicago Press.

Crigger, N. & Godfrey, N. (2011). *The Making of Nurse Professionals*: A Transformational, Ethical Approach. Sudbury, MA: Jones and Bartlett.

Crowden, A. (2003). Ethically sensitive mental health care: Is there a need for a unique ethics for psychiatry? *Australian and New Zealand Journal of Psychiatry* 37: 143–149.

Edsall, G. (1971). Experiments at Willowbrook. *The Lancet* 298(7715): p. 95.

Foucault, M. (1980). *Power/Knowledge: Selected Interviews and Other Writings 1972–1977*. New York: Pantheon Books.

Fry, S.T., Veatch, R.M. & Taylor C. (2010). Case Studies in Nursing Ethics, 4th ed. Burlington, MA: Jones and Bartlett Learning.

Gallup Organization. (2018, December 20). Once Again Nurses Top Gallup Poll as Most Trusted Profession 17 Years Running.
 Available: https://www.nationalnursesunited.org/press/once-again-nurses-top-gallup-poll-most-trusted-profession-17-years-running

Goffman, E. (1963). *Stigma: Notes on the Management of Spoiled Identity*. Englewood Cliffs, NJ: Prentice-Hall.

Goldby, S. (1971). Experiments at the Willowbrook State School. *The Lancet, 297*(7702): 749.

Grace, P.J. (2018). *Nursing Ethics and Professional Responsibility in Advanced Practice*, 3rd ed. Burlington, MA: Jones and Bartlett Learning.

Gutheil, T.G. and Gabbard, G.O. (1993). The concept of boundaries in clinical practice: Theoretical and risk management dimensions. *American Journal of Psychiatry* 150(2): 188–196.

Gutheil, T.G. & Gabbard, G.O. (1998). Misuses and misunderstandings of boundary theory in clinical and regulatory settings. *American Journal of Psychiatry* 155(3): 409–414.

Gutheil, T.G. and Simon, R.I. (2003). Abandonment of patients in split treatment. *Harvard Review of Psychiatry 11*: 175–179.

Halter, M.J. (2008). Perceived characteristics of psychiatric nurses: Stigma by association. *Archives of Psychiatric Nursing 22*(1): 20–26.

Hastings Center (1978). In the service of the state: The psychiatrist as double agent. *Hasting Center Report*, 8(2): 1–23.

Jorgenson, L.M., Hirsch, A.B., & Wahl, K.M. (1997). Fiduciary duty and boundaries: Acting in the client's best interest. *Behavioral Sciences and the Law* 15: 49–62.

Juritzen, T.I., Grimen, H., and Heggen, K. (2011). Protecting vulnerable research participants: A Foucault-inspired analysis of ethics committees. *Nursing Ethics* 18 (5): 640–650.

Kolch, M., Ludolph, A.G., Plener, P.L., Fangerau, H., Vitiello, B. & Fegert, J.M. (2010). Safeguarding children's rights in psychopharmacological research: Ethical and legal issues. *Current Pharmaceutical Design 16*: 2398–2406.

Krugman, S. and Shapiro, S. (1971). Experiments at the Willowbrook State School. *The Lancet 297*(7706): 966.

Lindeman, H. (2006). *An Invitation to Feminist Ethics*. Boston: McGraw-Hill.

McCauley-Elsom, K., Gurvich, C., Lee, S, Elsom, S., O'Connor, M., and Kulkarni, J (2009). Vulnerable populations and multicentered research. *International Journal of Mental Health Nursing* 18: 108–115.

Mohr, W.K., and Mahon, M.M. (1996). Dirty hands: The underside of marketplace health care. *Advances in Nursing Science* 19 (1): 28–37.

Monahan, J., Redlich, A.D., Swanson, J., Robbins, P.D., Appelbaum, P.S., Petrila, J., McNiel, DE (2005). Use of leverage to improve adherence to psychiatric treatment in the community. *Psychiatric Service 56*: 37–44.

Muran, J.C., and Barber, J.P. (2010). *The Therapeutic Alliance: An Evidence-Based Treatment Guide to Practice*. New York: The Guilford Press.

National Bioethics Advisory Commission. (1998). *Research involving persons with mental disorders that may affect decision making capacity, Volume 1.* Report and Recommendations of the National Bioethics Advisory Commission. Rockville, MD: National Bioethics Advisory Commission.

National Commission for the Protection of Human Subjects of Biomedical and Behavioral Research. (1979). *The Belmont Report: Ethical Principles and Guidelines for the Protection of Human Subjects of Research*. Washington, DC: U.S. Government Printing Office.

Nussbaum, M.C. (2010). *Not For Profit: Why Democracy Needs the Humanities*. Princeton, NJ: Princeton University Press.

Olsen, D.P. (2003). Influence and coercion: Relational and rights-based ethical approaches to forced psychiatric treatment. *Journal of Psychiatric and Mental Health Nursing* 10: 705–712.

Pappworth, M.H. (1971). The Willowbrook experiments. *The Lancet 297* (7710): 1181.

Peter, E. & Liaschenko, J (2004). The perils of proximity: A spatiotemporal analysis of moral distress and moral ambiguity. *Nursing Inquiry 11* (4): 218–225.

Phillips, J. (2002). Managed care's reconstruction of human existence: The triumph of technical reason. *Theoretical Medicine 23*: 339–358.

Radden, J. (2002a). Notes towards a professional ethics for psychiatry. *Australian and New Zealand Journal of Psychiatry*, 36: 52–59.

Radden, J. (2002b). Psychiatric ethics. Bioethics 16(5): 397–411.

Radden, J. (2003). Forced medication, patients' rights and values conflicts. *Psychiatry, Psychology, and Law, 10* (1): 1–11.

Radden, J. (2004). The debate continues: Unique ethics for psychiatry. *Australian and New Zealand Journal of Psychiatry 38*: 115–118.

Radden, J. & Sadler, J.Z. (2008). Character virtues in psychiatric practice. *Harvard Review of Psychiatry 16*(6): 373–380.

Rhodes, R. (2010). Rethinking research ethics. *The American Journal of Bioethics 10* (10): 19–36.

Robbins, P.C., Petrila, J., LeMelle, S., & Monahan, J. (2006). The use of housing as leverage to increase adherence to psychiatric treatment in the community. *Administration and Policy in Mental Health Services 75*: 49–59.

Roberts, L.W. & Roberts, B. (1999). Psychiatric research ethics: An overview of evolving guidelines and current ethical dilemmas in the study of mental illness. *Biological Psychiatry 46*: 1025–1038.

Rosenstein, D.L., Miller, F.G. & Rubinow, D.R.(2001). A curriculum for teaching psychiatric research ethics. *Biological Psychiatry 50*: 802–808.

Sadler, J.Z. (2007). The psychiatric significance of the personal self. *Psychiatry 70*(2): 113–129.

Sadock, B.J., Sadock, V.A., and Ruiz, P. (2015). *Kaplan and Sadock's Synopsis of Psychiatry: Behavioral Sciences/Clinical Psychiatry*, 11th ed. Philadelphia: Wolters Kluwer.

Safran, J.D. and Muran, J.C. (2003). *Negotiating the Therapeutic Alliance: A Relational Treatment Guide*. New York: The Guilford Press.

Shuster, E. (1997). Fifty years later: The significance of the Nuremberg Code. *New England Journal of Medicine 337*(20): 1436–1440.

Smith, D.E. (1990). The statistics on women and mental illness: The relations of ruling they conceal. In: *The Conceptual Practices of Power: A Feminist Sociology of Knowledge*, pp. 108–138. D.E. Smith (Ed.). Boston: Northeastern University Press.

Spetie, L., and Arnold, L.E. (2007). Ethical issues in child psychopharmacology research and practice: Emphasis on preschoolers. *Psychopharmacology 191*: 15–26.

Stolberg, S.G. (1999, November 28). The biotech death of Jesse Gelsinger. *The New York Times Magazine*, 9136–9150.

Szmukler, G. & Appelbaum, P.S. (2008). Treatment pressures, leverage, coercion, and compulsion in mental health care. *Journal of Mental Health 17*(3): 233–244.

Tasman, A. & Mohr, W.K. (2011). *Fundamentals of Psychiatry*. NJ: Wiley-Blackwell.

Taylor, R. (1985). Ethics, Faith, and Reason. Englewood Cliffs, NJ: Prentice-Hall, Inc.

United Nations General Assembly. (1948, December 10). *Universal Declaration of Human Rights*. Available: http://www.ohchr.org/en/udhr/pages/language.aspx?langid=eng

Walker, M.U. (2007). *Moral Understandings: A Feminist Study in Ethics*, 2nd ed. New York: Oxford University Press.

Widiger, T.A. (1998). Invited essay: Sex biases in the diagnosis of personality disorders. *Journal of Personality Disorders 12*(2): 95–118.

World Medication Association (WMA). (1948). Declaration of Geneva. Geneva: WMA, General Assembly. Available: http://www.cirp.org/library/ethics/geneva/

World Medical Organization. (1996). Declaration of Helsinki. British Medical Journal, 313(7070), 1448–1449. Available: http://www.cirp.org/library/ethics/helsinki/

World Psychiatric Association (WPA). (1978). *Declaration of Hawaii. Journal of Medical Ethics 4*: 71–73. Available: http://www.ncbi.nlm.nih.gov/pmc/articles/PMC1154636/pdf/jmedeth00167-0017.pdf

World Psychiatric Association (WPA). (1996). *Madrid Declaration on Ethical Standards for Psychiatric Practice*. Madrid: WPA, General Assembly. Available: http://www.wpanet.org/detail.php?section_id=5&content_id=48

Zimbardo, P. (2008). *The Lucifer Effect: How Good People Turn Evil*. New York: Random House.

CHAPTER 6

Ethical Considerations in the Care of Pediatric Patients

RITA MARIE JOHN

6.1. OVERVIEW

There is a broad range of ethical issues for Advanced Practice Nurses (APRNs) who practice in pediatrics, ranging from limiting care for the very premature newborn to reproductive health issues in adolescents. There are no simple answers to ethical problems that arise in clinical practice. The APRN faces ethical problems in practice whether she works on an inpatient unit and faces distress due to end of life issues and treatment refusal; works in a NICU with critically ill newborns; in ambulatory care with abusive parents; or works with parents who refuse vaccines for their children. Competence in ethics is essential in clinical practice. There are challenges that the APRN must identify, analyze, and manage. It can be difficult to manage the therapeutic alliance with families, to protect patient privacy and confidentiality, and to use professional authority in an appropriate manner. The integration of ethics in the education of the APRN is critical for adequate decision making in pediatric practice (Cummings, 2016). This chapter serves as an introduction to the problems of pediatric ethical issues. It will review pediatric health care decision-making, practice issues, and role conflict unique to pediatrics. In addition, it will discuss the special problems unique to newborn, infant, child, and adolescent healthcare, followed by a brief discussion of pediatric subjects in a research study. The chapter will conclude with several case studies for further discussion.

6.2. HEALTH CARE DECISION MAKING

Pediatric ethical dilemmas are significantly different than adult ethical dilemmas. With an adult, the provider presents all the options to the competent adult who then decides on the course of action based on his/

her best interests. The ethical principle of autonomy allows a person to make decisions freely, without interference. Respect for autonomy is a core concept in modern ethics (Cummings and Mercurio, 2010; Ross, 2015). The competent adult has the right to control any actions affecting his or her body and clinician cannot override that decision. The adult consent must be voluntary, informed and competent (Ross, 2015).

In addition, autonomy allows the patient the right to refuse treatment and dictates that the APRN must respect that decision. A surgeon who performs a procedure without the consent of the competent adult patient commits assault. Thus, an adult's refusal of treatment is accepted. Adult autonomy is based on the adult having adequate capacity to make the decision, but does not allow the adult to demand treatment that is not medically necessary (Cummings and Mercurio, 2010). If the adult is no longer capable of making a decision, a surrogate is expected to act in the best interest of the adult. In pediatrics, the surrogate must also make the best interest decision. In deciding whether the child can make a decision, the degree of autonomy depends on the child's age, maturity, and intellectual capacity. Young children are not truly autonomous whereas most older children and adolescents have some decision-making capacity.

The principle of beneficence requires that the APRN act in the best interest of the patient, including preventing harm, helping those in danger, and protecting others. This means that the APRN will act in the best interest of the child At times, autonomy is in conflict with beneficence. This occurs when the APRN feels that a particular treatment would be in the best interest of the child, but the patient and the family refuse the treatment. Autonomy usually overrides beneficence (Ross, 2015).

Nonmaleficence assures that the APRN will protect the patient and do no harm. This principle is associated with the expression "above all, first do no harm" (Beauchamp and Childress, 2013). For APRNs, this requires that the care rendered be performed with skill, knowledge, and diligence. Nonmaleficence asks for the obtaining of a consultation when there is doubt. Undoubtedly, this principle comes into play during end of life issues, when sustaining life may not be the best alternative. Lack of training to counsel and inform patients about end of life care choices, genetic counseling, and/or devastating diagnosis may be an area where APRNs and others should defer to other professionals in order to protect patients and avoid harm (Okun, 2010).

APRNs should present all benefits, risks, and alternatives to surrogate pediatric decision-makers. APRNs have a moral obligation to make sure that their own biases do not interfere with presenting all possible treatment options. The APRN must consider three important elements to obtain an informed consent. The surrogate and the patient must have all the needed information to consent. The APRN must assess the understanding of the medical information and the capacity that the surrogate and the patient has for decision making, and must make sure that they have agreed to the treatment plan including any intervention (AAP Committee on Bioethics, 2016).

At times, clinician may not present alternative treatments to parents due to the provider's biases; as clinician, they may not believe that certain alternatives are reasonable (Ross and Frader, 2009). The APRN must consider all alternatives and be aware of bias before approaching patients with treatment plans. Withholding information about reasonable options is not acceptable for the APRN as it could lead to an exercise of power that is unacceptable in this diverse society (Ross and Frader, 2009). APRNs must not substitute their personal beliefs without information about treatment options. In pediatrics, it is critically important that clinician educate parents in order to foster fully informed decision making with a process that allows the risks, benefits and alternative interventions to be fully explored so that parents can act in the best interest of the child.

The Internet has changed the way that families interact with clinician (Tan & Goonawardene, 2017). More patients are turning to the Internet as their first choice for health information and when the Internet information does not match the information that the patient receives from their provider, mistrust can develop (Tan & Goonawardene, 2017). Clinicians need to encourage their patients to discuss whatever they have read online to facilitate and open communication. The information that clinician give to parents must be clear and reflect current research to avoid the informed parent deducing that the provider was not up to date or even misled them. The paternalistic model of healthcare is no longer acceptable in clinical practice; even more so since the Internet has made patients informed consumers.

Even if the APRN feels strongly about an issue, she must ensure that she fully informs the parent of all options to assure the parent or guardian can fulfill their moral duties (Mears, 2010; Ross and Frader, 2009). There are several reasons for parental refusal, including: lack of understanding, cultural beliefs, religious beliefs, denial of the health problem, fear of the treatment, lack of resources, fear regarding side effects, and the belief that alternative treatments may have no side effects (Ross, 2011). Thus, the parent needs continued, ongoing conversation before understanding why a particular treatment has been recommended.

The principle of justice is involved in the decision-making process, as it provides that each person should be treated equally. Nondisclosure of critical information for a surrogate is considered a breach of the principle of justice. It also requires that the APRN treats each person equally and not on the basis of the race, socioeconomic class, age, sex, or social class. This is an area of concern for practitioners in neonatology, where the neonate may be at risk for receiving less care than an older child (Janvier, Bauer, and Lantos, 2007). Health differences may also lead to managed-care constraints and may affect how children are treated. An example of this is lack of coverage for birth control by some insurers leading to an increased risk for pregnancy. Family planning is also the subject of a 1991 ruling by the Supreme court that forbid clinician in public funded family planning clinics for referring a patient for an abortion (Davis and Kodish, 2014).

Laws may also interfere with pediatric practice. A Florida law prevents clinicians from asking about guns in the house (Davis & Kodish, 2014). The Florida Supreme Court upheld the law citing that gun ownership is a private issue. This interferes with the moral obligation of the provider to prevent harm to children, which is central to pediatric practice.

6.2.1. Decision Making in Pediatrics

Young children do not participate in decision-making as they lack the capacity to decide on treatment plans. In adolescents, the principle of autonomy is less clear. The reason for children's lack of autonomy is based on their age, developmental disability, or mental illness, whether temporary or permanent. The role of surrogates in pediatrics is held to a much higher standard in the decision making process, especially if the surrogate is not related (Ross, 2009).

In pediatrics, a surrogate decision-maker is usually designated for the child. The American Academy of Pediatrics (AAP) recent statement for surrogates included four standards—The Best Interest Standard, Harm principle, constrained parental authority, and shared family-centered decision-making (AAP Committee on Bioethics, 2016). This surrogate is typically the parent, as it is felt that the parent will act in the child's best interest. The Best Interest Standard is the guiding principle used by decision makers who must make choices for minors or others who lack the ability to make decisions (Kopelman and Kopelman, 2007). The surrogate will maximize benefits while minimizing harm to the child for whom the surrogate views in a holistic manner (AAP Committee on Bioethics, 2016)

The harm principle points to a threshold for harm below which a parental decision cannot be accepted. For example, refusal of a blood transfusion in a young child has life threatening bleeding would not be accepted and the court would rule in favor of treatment despite parental wishes. Constrained parental authority requires the child's basic needs to be met but recognizes that the surrogate's decision making must consider the needs of the family and balance that with the needs of the child. Shared family-centered decision-making points to the need for collaboration between the family and the clinician.

Parental authority is based on several beliefs: that parents know what is best for their child; parents must live with decisions that are made about their child's medical care; parents have the ultimate responsibility for bringing up their child; and that bonds between family members make the parent most likely to make decisions based on the best interest of the child (Cummings and Mercurio, 2010). Parents' decision-making capacity is more limited than patient autonomy. While an adult decides about their own treatment course, parents must base their decisions on what is in the child's best interest and in the family's best interest.

Obtaining pediatric assent for treatments and procedures is a complex process (Dreisinger and Zapolsky, 2018). Neonates, infants, toddlers, and preschoolers lack the ability to make decisions about health care. On the other hand, school age children and adolescents should be included in the decision making process to the degree to which they have the capacity to assent to treatment (AAP Committee on Bioethics, 2016). The guidelines from the AAP Committee on Bioethics ask that the healthcare provider help the patient develop a developmentally appropriate understanding of the child's condition, what to expect from the testing, make an assessment of the child's understanding, and solicit a willingness to the undergo the proposed plan of care (AAP Committee on Bioethics, 2016).

The child's role in the final decision is less clear. An understanding of children's cognitive level helps to clarify why children may not be fully competent to make a decision (AAP Committee on Bioethics, 2016). Piaget described children between two and seven years of age as preoperational. In this stage of development, the child is not able to consider the whole picture and can only see one aspect of an event at a time. The child is egocentric and is unable to generalize from one experience to a similar one. By the time the child reaches seven, he is entered a concrete stage of operations, giving them the ability for limited decision making (AAP Committee on Bioethics 2016). Around age 11, the child is able to begin to think abstractly and to consider long- and short-term consequences of their decisions. This does not mean that the decision-making capacity is fully developed. The prefrontal cortex develops slowly through early adulthood and affects memory, emotional stability, and long-range planning (Michaud, Blum, Benaroyo, Zermatten, & Baltag, 2015). Adolescents have limitations to the quality of their decisions in that they pay more attention to short-term consequences of actions, are influenced by peers; and have a higher tolerance for risk. Complicating this is that ill children tend to regress to earlier stages of development.

The issues around decision-making for pediatric patients are complex. The APRN must consider the ethical principles of autonomy, beneficence, nonmaleficence, and justice, parental authority in addition to the standards for surrogate decision-making. The decision-making must be viewed within a cultural context as a family may view elders as key decision-makers (Mercurio, Adams et al., 2008).

6.2.1.1. Decision Scenarios

Decision-making is easier when both the surrogate and the child agree with the APRN on the course of treatment. Childhood assent requires four key elements (AAP Committee on Bioethics, 2018):

1. The child should be assisted in understanding his or her condition.
2. The child should be told what will happen during proposed treatment.
3. An assessment must be conducted determining what the child understands and what factors are influencing this understanding.
4. A gathered response from the child regarding the proposed treatment.

Parental/surrogate authority is respected in defining the child's best interest and it is best when an adolescent also agrees with the plan to treat. If the parent and child of less than 18 years agree to treat, then the APRN can go ahead with the treatment plan. When there is an agreement to treat, and that agreement is what the APRN believes is correct, there is no problem in the decision making process. These scenarios are not problematic since both the parent and the adolescent agree on the course of treatment.

If the parents' preference is to treat, but the child refuses treatment, then the child's wishes will generally be overturned by the parent's as the child does not have full understanding of the need for treatment. The child's ability to agree to a treatment plan is largely determined by the child's age and maturity (Dreisinger & Zapolsky, 2018) and determined by his/her competency. Depending on the age of the child, the refusal of the child may need to be considered. This may put the APRN in conflict with the parents and other clinicians. However, the key lies in the child's cognitive ability to carefully weigh all the options. If the APRN asks a 4 year-old if he wants his booster shots, he is likely to reject this treatment option. Cognitively, he is unable to weigh the pros and cons of missing vaccines. However, in adolescence, nontreatment decisions should be considered. If the parents' preference is to treat, but the adolescent refuses, the competency of the adolescent must be fully assessed. In this scenario, the APRN should try to educate the adolescent about the need for treatment. Working with families is key to a successful outcome. It is always better to reach a compromise rather than allow the case to go to court. In general, the younger the child, the more likely the child's refusal will not affect outcome of the case.

In a different scenario, the parent or surrogate may disagree with a treatment plan and refuse treatment for a child who is not competent. In this case, the state can intervene if the parent's decision is deemed to be either abusive or neglectful. The APRN must consider the efficacy of the proposed treatment before seeking a court order to override the parent's refusal. Thus, with a young child, if the parents, as the surrogate decision makers, go against a life-saving treatment for the child, the APRN and other health care clinician can seek court intervention. However, if a treatment option's benefit is not as clear, the APRN must weigh the pros and cons of overriding the caretakers' wishes.

When there is a clearly life-saving intervention for a school age child or younger which is refused by the parents, the parent's authority as decision makers usually will be overturned by the court, particularly if the objection is religious (Ross, 2008). The United States Supreme Court has ruled that religion is not a valid legal defense when it is used to harm the child (Mercurio et al., 2008). The AAP does not believe that a religious defense should be used as a reason to deny treatment of a child when there are highly effective treatments available (AAP Committee on Bioethics, 1997). However, as the child grows, it is possible that if both the parents and the adolescent object to the treatment on a religious basis, the court may uphold the refusal. This was the case in November 2007, when Dennis Lindberg, a Jehovah's Witness with leukemia, refused a blood transfusion and was supported by his guardian, who was also a Jehovah's Witness. The Washington State Court upheld the refusal. Within 12 hours, the child died (Black, 2007).

There is a recent trend of supporting adolescent refusal, particularly if the parents are also refusing treatment (Ross, 2008). A "mature minor" is an adolescent who has not yet reached the age of adulthood (18 in the United States), but who is being treated as an adult. This may be difficult for APRNs when they do not believe that the parent is acting in the child's best interest. These are cases where the APRN may feel the need to take the parent to court. Conversely, if the minor's preference is treatment and that minor is an adolescent, the APRN may need to go to court in order to treat the child if the APRN believes that the parent is not acting in the child's best interest. Consultation with other team members along with an ethics team consultation should be considered prior to reporting the case to child protective services. Child protective services will initiate court proceedings, so the individual practitioner does not have to pay for a lawyer. Again, the main consideration is the efficacy of the treatment. When the treatment is highly efficacious, it is more likely that the court will rule in favor of the APRN. However, when the treatment is not as effective, the APRN must carefully consider the best action. Certainly, the best option with a less efficacious treatment is for the APRN to work with the parents or guardian and the adolescent minor in deciding on the treatment plan.

There are, of course, examples in which an adolescent patient adamantly refuses treatment even when it is advised by both his parents and the APRN. The adolescent may refuse treatment and ask for legal counsel to help them receive no further treatment or may even run away. This happened in the case of 16-year-old Billy Best in 1994, when he refused further chemotherapy for Hodgkin's disease after five treatment rounds. He decided to run away and his parents asked him to come back home. In their plea, they promised Billy that he would not have to resume chemotherapy if he came home. Keeping their promise, the family then refused further treatment and the medical team reported them to Child Protective Services. However, the Massachusetts Court ultimately dismissed the case and the family pursued alternative treatment. Billy is still alive today, and is now publishing a book about his life. His doctors believe that the five treatment courses that he received adequately treated his cancer, but the family believes that their alternative treatment is the reason he is alive today (Ross, 2009).

In a similar case, 16-year-old Abraham Cherrix, also diagnosed with Hodgkin's disease, refused a second round of chemotherapy after the disease reappeared in 2006. The child refused treatment and his family traveled to Mexico for an alternative treatment. When they returned, the parents were charged with neglect and an additional treatment of radiation therapy with a complementary and alternative treatment (CAM) was instituted (Simpson, 2007).

The APRN, faced with parental and mature adolescent refusal of treatment, must be aware of current trends allowing families with mature minors to refuse treatment. In February 2007, the State of Virginia passed a law that allowed families with adolescents 14 and over the right to refuse treatment (Simpson, 2007). Decisional authority was previously clearly in the hands of parents; however, recent trends in decision-making with mature adolescents have changed the way these cases are being decided in court. In cases of refusal where the risk of harm is such that it would constitute medical neglect and place the child at risk for harm, reporting to child protective services and going to court may be the only option. An exception to this can be seen in the 2018 case of 17 year-old Cassandra C. who refused a six-month course of chemotherapy for Hodgkin's Lymphoma and the Connecticut court overruled her refusal, citing her age. It is important to recognize that going to court to allow for a particular treatment to occur is usually fatal to the APRN-family relationship (Ladd and Forman, 2010). It is critical to work with these families so that the best possible outcomes can occur. The APRN should consider not terminating care, but to educate and negotiate with the family so the medical care can continue. In some cases, seeking the state's help may be needed.

The APRN may ensure better outcomes if mutually acceptable treatment plans using shared decision-making are utilized. If the APRN and the family cannot come to an acceptable decision, care may be transferred to another provider, but the APRN cannot abandon the patient.

6.3. PRACTICE ISSUES

6.3.1. Access to Care Issues

6.3.1.1. Insurance Issues

Insurance and managed care constraints may be an area of conflict for the APRN. Institutions may only accept one kind of insurance, and at times, the best care for a rare problem may be in a hospital in a neighboring state where a family on a state-funded Medicaid program will require approval to go out of network. Different insurance providers may require different information and knowing what this information is can be difficult (Okun, 2010). It may take considerable effort on the part of the primary care provider to get a nonparticipating provider covered by the insurance provider. In addition, if a particular institution employs the APRN, she may feel an obligation to refer to a provider within the institution even though the APRN believes another provider may be more knowledgeable in a specific area. An example of this is a child with a rare liver disorder. In this case, the participating gastroenterologist does accept the child's insurance, but there is no hepatologist that accepts this child's insurance. The APRN must discuss the issue with the medical director of the insurance company in order to get the child taken care of by the appropriate specialist. This usually takes extra time on the part of the APRN. Meanwhile, this has delayed treatment and is an access to care delay due to managed care constraints. This can lead to moral distress as the APRN cannot provide the same level of care to all the patients she sees. The APRN needs to get involved in policy through involvement with state and national organizations.

6.3.1.2. Unavailable Treatment

APRNs have reported unavailability of treatments that APRNs felt were necessary because of lack of insurance coverage (Butz et al., 1998). In some cases, a pediatric advanced practice nurse may find that there are no clinicians in a particular subspecialty on an insurance panel. For example, there may be no pediatric neurosurgeon on the insurance panel but the child has a bony tumor of the head. In order to obtain these services, the APRN must contact the insurance company and must generate a request with the rationale for the need for a pediatric neurosurgeon. The APRN who is pressed for time needs to decide when she will do the forms needed for the referral while providing care to patients and balancing her own family demands. This is another area of moral distress for the APRN.

6.3.1.3. Prescription Conflicts

It is not uncommon to find that a particular drug is not covered by insurance and the available alternatives do not have the same action and will not work as effectively. To get this medication for the family, the APRN must fill out appeal paperwork, taking it to the next level after the insurance has refused the medication. This is a time consuming process and takes time away from patient care or from the family. Balancing resources can be difficult for the APRN provider who may have several medically fragile children in her practice. However, without insurance to cover the cost of the medication, there will be an additional financial burden for the family, which may lead to lack of compliance with the ideal treatment regime.

In addition, recent legislation in over sixteen states has limited Medicaid services to the poor including restriction on the number of prescriptions per month. Illinois limits the number of prescriptions that a Medicaid recipient can receive to four per month (Galewitz, 2012).

This kind of limitation may cause families to restrict medical care to children, and APRNs may find that they balance the ideal care with the best possible care given the insurance restrictions. Rationing of resources limits each person's right to equal care. Clinicians do not see patients in isolation, but within a larger community, and, therefore, they should consider the larger community needs as they prescribe. The right of equal treatment requires that careful consideration be given to the treatment plan so that community resources are not distributed disproportionately to a few individuals (Camosy, 2011). This can lead to moral distress for the practitioner as she makes treatment decisions.

There are other areas in prescription writing that may cause conflict for the APRN. Families may request a specific antibiotic for treatment of a common pediatric entity such as acute otitis media. While evidence-based guidelines call for the first-line drug to be high dose Amoxicillin, the family may prefer a third generation cephalosporin which comes at a higher cost for both the insurance company and the family. It also may not be the best first line agent. From a public health standpoint, using the stronger medication when it is not needed can lead to bacterial resistance. It is important to spend the time educating families rather than being pressured to do something that is against good medical practice. A family of a young infant may demand medication for the baby's upper respiratory tract infection. As new warnings about the risk of stroke have been issued by the CDC which warn against the use of this medication in young children, the practitioner must follow the ethical dictum of nonmaleficence: "First do no harm." The family must be educated about the proper use of such medications. The APRN must prescribe treatments that provide the evidence based care and not give in to parental demands. This is another situation leading to moral distress for the APRN.

Families may ask clinician to write for a variety of medications just in case they get sick before their insurance coverage is terminated. Documenting the reasons for these prescriptions may present an ethical dilemma for the APRN. Families want to make sure they have enough medication, but prescribing medications for conditions that are not present is against the law and therefore neither ethically nor legally sound practice. The APRN cannot write for medications for conditions that the patient does not have just because the insurance will cover it for one condition, but not for another.

In some instances, one child in a family may be covered under the insurance, but another child may not. Clinician may be asked to write prescriptions for an uninsured child in the insured child's name and to forge diagnoses that the insured child does not have. Although it is difficult to turn needy families down, clinician cannot commit fraud and violate the Health Care Fraud Act. The APRN must offer the parent alternative means of getting the prescription filled (John, 2007). While the APRN must follow the ethical principle of beneficence, the APRN must always follow the law first.

6.3.1.4. Preferential Treatment

Some practices may ask APRNs to give preferential treatment to patients with private insurance by seeing them out of order, putting the private insurance patient or self-pay before the patient with state insurance. This may lead to moral distress for the APRN because the practice is making it difficult to do the right thing. This leads to longer waits for patients with state insurance. Preferential appointment times may be given to families with private insurance or they may be allowed to walk in without appointments, whereas patients with state Medicaid are required to make appointments.

6.3.1.5. Diagnostics

Insurance companies may designate certain practices as premium practices if they practice more cost effective healthcare. In cost-sharing systems in some managed care companies, a practice's remuneration is inherent on the ability to limit health care costs. There is an incentive to reduce health care expenditures. The companies will specially designate practices if they are deemed more cost effective, and they will be reimbursed for their services at a higher rate. This is a dubious ethical practice (Okun, 2010). The APRN should provide care based on evidence rather than on whether or not the reimbursement to the practice will be higher. These are conflicts that are clearly professional constraints on practice. Section 6.5 contains case examples of ethical conflicts described in this chapter.

6.3.2. Conflicts of Pediatric Advanced Practice Nurses

6.3.2.1. Patient Management

One of the major ethical conflicts for pediatric advanced practice nurses stems around autonomy and the disagreements that arise about patient management. An example of this is when the APRN believes that a patient requires inpatient care and a pediatrician or family practitioner colleague disagrees. Some of the moral distress associated with this conflict might be resolved by having the APRN's practice agreement include the involvement of a third party if there is disagreement between the APRN and the medical consult. When these instances occur, the practice agreement would allow for resolution without conflict between the disagreeing members of the health team. Ideally, a discussion about the best course of action for the patient should be a joint decision that includes all clinician and the family.

6.3.2.2. Billing Issues

Most insurers today cover APRN services at 85% of the insurer fee-for-service schedule (physician rate). To avoid getting a reduced rate, a physician may decide to bill under his name and bill at 100% of the usual fee. This is an ethical dilemma for the APRN, but it is also illegal to bill for services under another's name. APRNs must clearly state in writing in her practice agreement that her employer may only bill at the legal rate.

6.3.3. Institutional Problems

6.3.3.1. Practice Conflicts

Practices may offer clinician a bonus if they increase their patient population or shorten the time that they spend with patients. While time is not the only measure of effective care, it is one of many things that enters into the health care encounter. The APRN may wish to see as many patients as possible to increase billable visits, but may experience moral conflict by not providing the length of visit necessary to adequately care for her patients. This can also be a professional and legal issue.

6.3.4. Family and Pediatric Advanced Practice

6.3.4.1. Nurse Relationships

The issues in this area center around maintaining appropriate boundaries with families, caring for children of friends and family members, accepting gifts, romantic relationships with adolescent patients, being intimate with families and children, and nonmonetary payment for services (Ladd and Forman, 2010). It is important to maintain professional relationships and avoid becoming over involved with families.

6.3.5. Using Professional Authority Appropriately

APRNs may be asked by families to write letters to outside agencies to request further services. In some cases, this may require that the APRN document something that is not true or is not clear from the medical record. Examples of this include writing letters for utilities to get reduced rates or better housing, to confirm parental competence, or about conditions for social security long-term disabilities. It can be quite difficult for the APRN not to sympathize with the family. The need to recognize sympathy for the family must be balanced against the need to avoid being unethical and using the APRN's authority inappropriately. The principle of justice must prevail and the APRN must be truthful. While it is important to advocate for the child and the family, the principle of justice demands fairness from the APRN.

6.3.5.1. Independent APRN Practice

With changes in the laws around independent advanced practice, APRN may decide to open up their own practice. The marketing strategies for promoting APRN private practice must not misrepresent their credentials or skills of any members of the practice. A new DNP graduate should be careful that when she represents herself as a doctor of nursing practice that she considers state guidelines around the use of this terminology. It is important not to guarantee any outcome (Jubuwitz, 2011).

6.4. SPECIFIC AGE GROUPS

6.4.1. Neonates and Preterm Infants

The NICU poses a special problem as the outcome of a preterm infant may fall into gray zones. There are times when medical treatment is clearly beneficial and therefore, the baby's right to be treated falls out of parental decision making. If the benefit of the treatment is as clear, parental choice is more likely to be followed, as the outcome is not clear. Clinician may also decide that treatment is futile and harmful to the infant (Lantos, 2018). In some cases, resuscitation is done but when it is clear that the prognosis is poor, treatment is withdrawn. A newer approach to NICU dilemma recommends that in the face of unanticipated situations, clinician work with parents to discern their own values and ethical beliefs. This change in presentation focuses on clarification of ethical values rather than conflict resolution.

6.4.1.1. History

To understand the present ethical dilemmas in neonatal care, it is important to review some cases that have shaped the landscape of ethical issues in neonatology. In 1963, a neonate was born with Down syndrome and duodenal atresia. The family did not want life-saving surgery done as caring for the child in the future would have posed undue financial stress on the rest of the family. After two weeks, the infant died secondary to lack of ability to absorb nutrition. In 1973, in an essay in the New England Journal of Medicine, Duff and Campbell supported the non-treatment decision, saying that the decision to treat neonates belonged in the hands of families.

Subsequent to this case, there was a profoundly compromised newborn in Maine that the family and physician decided not to treat. Other physicians objected and the case went to the Maine Supreme Court who found that human life took precedence and that the child should have all medical procedures done if this could save his life. The infant died after the court-ordered surgery (Paris et al., 2007).

In contrast, in the Stinson case (1983), an 800-gram newborn with a survival rate of less than 5% was kept alive after he was transferred from a community hospital (where the family had requested no resuscitation) to Children's Hospital of Philadelphia (CHOP). At CHOP, the family was told that the baby would be kept alive at all costs unless he was brain dead. The child was kept alive through several illnesses including a brain hemorrhage. Finally, the baby extubated himself and was allowed to die.

In 1982, in Indiana, Baby Doe was born with Down syndrome and tracheoesophageal fistula. The baby was allowed to die without surgical treatment at the request of the obstetrician and the family (Paris, Schreiber and Moreland, 2007; Pless, 1983). The Indiana Supreme Court upheld the parent's decision, but the federal government felt that physicians are obliged to treat every child. The following year, in New York, an infant was born with a meningomyelocele and multiple congenital defects. The family elected no treatment, but a Vermont lawyer, Lawrence Washburn, brought suit against New York for non-treatment of the child. The Department of Health and Human Services was notified about non-treatment and the case was referred to the New York State Child Protective Service, who did not feel that the case involved child neglect. The child died, but the Surgeon General at the time, C. Everett Koop, informed Congress of the need for treatment for these children (Chambers, 1983).

As a result, Congress passed the Baby Doe Amendment or Baby Doe Law in 1984, effective June 1, 1985. It was an addition to the child abuse law, which stated that withholding food, fluid, and medically indicated treatment from disabled children, was a form of child abuse. However, the United States Supreme Court struck down the amendment in 1986 (Paris, 2007). Out of this act, the "Best Interest Standards" were formed and became the ethical basis for deciding treatment decisions for pediatric patients that could not talk for themselves.

By the late 1980s, one third of neonatologists admitted that they provided medical interventions for sick neonates even when they disagreed with the benefit of the treatment (Kopelman, Irons and Kopelman, 1988). The case of Sammy Linares (1989) and baby boy Messenger (1996) furthered the rights of parents to make decisions regarding their children. In both cases, the fathers removed their infant sons from ventilators and were charged with their murders. Both fathers were set free. In the Linares case, the grand jury never returned a homicide indictment (Paris, 2005). Foregoing medical treatment of critically ill newborns by health care professionals and parents needs to be decided in a setting of shared decision making.

Research completed around this same period showed that there was disagreement among practitioners about treatments for newborns with genetic problems and medical issues. Shaw, Randolph and Manard (1977) surveyed 457 pediatricians and pediatric surgeons about whether they would let parents decide whether to operate on a newborn with biliary atresia and Down syndrome. In their study, 51.7% of the pediatricians would let the parents decide, and 38.4% of pediatric surgeons would let the parents decide. In the same study, 16.5% of the pediatricians and 27.9% of the surgeons would try to persuade the parents to let them operate on the child but would not bring them to court if they would not. Todres, Krane, Howell and Shannon (1977) reported on a survey of 230 pediatricians regarding the same issue. Their study reported that 40.2% of physicians would pursue a court order, and 54.2% would not bring the parents to court. In this study, religious beliefs and affiliations of the physicians significantly affected whether they would pursue a court order. The advances in NICU care were viewed by the medical community with joy and the long term outcomes of the fragile NICU infant were understated (Lantos, 2018).

6.4.1.2. Decisions to Treat the Preterm Infant

The infant mortality rate has steadily dropped since 2005 and in 2016, there were 583 infant deaths per 100,000 people in the United States (Child Trends, 2019). Children less than one year are more likely to die than older children. However, the benefit/burden assessment in assessing the viability of the sick neonate considers survival rates along with neurodevelopmental status.

Good ethics begins with good data (Mercurio, 2010). Disability rates were overestimated by 10% to 50% by clinicians including pediatricians, obstetricians, NICU nurses, nurse practitioners, and neonatologist. Bigger differences in disability rates were seen when estimating outcomes in the more preterm infants (Morse et al., 2000; Blanco, Suresh, Howard, Soll, 2005; Powell et al, 2012). The use of decision aids to aid in making decisions is relatively new. More research regarding the use of the decision aids in clinical practice is needed (Guillen & Kirpalani, 2017). Severely preterm outcome estimators are available at the NICHD website: https://www1.nichd.nih.gov/epbo-calculator/Pages/epbo_case.aspx. At this website, the provider must put in the infant's gestational age, birth weight, sex, and whether antenatal steroids were given within 7 days of delivery along with whether it was a singleton birth. For example, a male, singleton birth at 24-weeks' gestation weighing 700 grams and receiving antenatal steroids has a 64% survival rate, with 44% of those infants having no profound neurodevelopmental impairments, but 27% of the 64% having moderate or severe impairments. There is a 73% risk of death or moderate to severe developmental impairment based on this website's patient outcome estimator. An APRN must consider that these statistics will not reflect whether an extremely premature baby received maximum treatment and therefore the rates of death and impairment may be statistically lower. The AAP concluded that treatment decisions for high-risk neonates should consider the physiologic maturity of the infant, the seriousness of the neonate's medical conditions including birth defects, and the probability of death and disability.

The conversation about the infant's status should begin with a self-assessment of your own religious, cultural and racial stereotypes and negative feelings that you may have. Self-preparation helps to create an environment that encourages trust, listening, and a greater understanding of parental feelings, goals and values. The next step is to create an environment that is safe in which the clinician acknowledges the parent's feelings and elicits their goals, values, hopes and feels. The importance of clarification by repeating the clinician's understanding of what the parents have said can help move the conversation toward shared decision making in which the parental wished are clarified (Lantos, 2018)

Recent research confirms that most disagreements regarding the care of the preterm infant occur when parents want more care than clinicians feel is needed rather than parents wanting to refuse care. Parents are also more accepting of disabilities than clinicians are and parents want the truth but feel hope is important (Lantos, 2018). Clinicians need to be careful to present facts in a way that offers hope to families. The clinicians in the NICU need to be aware of choice architecture and must be present the child's situation in a way that facilitates parent's understanding of the infant's medical condition. By helping clarify the parent's values, goals and priorities, the clinician facilitates and empowers the parents to make meaningful decisions.

In a study by Kempf et al. (2009), 95 high-risk mothers were counseled about fetal risk in advance of delivering their child. The study results demonstrated that palliative comfort care only was desired by 100% of parents when the child was delivered at 22 weeks; but by 24 weeks, only 38% desired palliative comfort care only; and by 26 weeks, none of the parents wanted palliative comfort care only. The results of counseling about morbidity and mortality outcomes of premature infants less than 26 weeks resulted in a substantial proportion of parents desiring comfort care. The importance of discussing outcomes of extremely premature infants prior to delivery in high-risk mothers helped families make difficult decisions. The decision to treat preterm infants born at the borderline of viability will vary from medical centers to medical center. The decision of whether they will treat a baby over 22 weeks but less than 24 weeks will vary around the country. Some centers are reporting a 30% to 50% success rate in infants born at 22 weeks and rates as high as 70% for infants born at 23 weeks (Lantos, 2018). The use of artificial placentas has not reached human trial but this will surely change the landscape of NICU.

The parental decision to treat or not treat preterm infants in the gray zone lead to moral distress in the staff in the NICU. The decision making in an NICU is particular complex as a result of technological advances. The thoughtful and therapeutic use of shared decision making will allow for the APRN to support families as they make decisions about their preterm infant.

6.4.1.3. Allocation of Resources

Some ethicists feel that preterm infants do not receive full treatment because there is less value put on the life of a newborn (Janvier et al., 2007). The argument here is that people would fully treat a 2 month old with sepsis, but would let a 24-week gestation newborn die because he only had a 50% chance of survival without sequelae. The question around newborn resuscitation and care is that fetuses are not viewed as living by some and therefore in the initial minutes following birth, may be seen as less of person (Janvier et al,, 2007). According to Janvier et al. (2007), the newborn is placed in a special moral category, resulting from the transition from fetus to person. Decisions to treat newborns differently from other age persons suggest that newborn's lives are less valued (Janvier et al. 2007), or that the law makes definitive cut off dates. NICU treatment for preterm and critically ill newborn infants is scrutinized more than adult intensive care units.

The decision to put a neonate on ECMO or other expensive therapeutic measures can be difficult and should be decided based on just resource allocation (Kirsch & Munson, 2018). The authors point out that in consideration of the use of the therapeutic measures such as echo that it must be a bridge to another modality such as a transplant, a bridge to recovery, a bridge to a long-term device, or a bridge to a final decision (Kirsch & Munson, 2018). Resource allocation must be fair in appointment and access and must protect a vulnerable child from exploitation or exclusion of the benefit. In addition, potential for harm or undue benefit must be considered (Kirsch & Munson, 2018). The allocation of a limited resource such as echo becomes problematic when there are multiple infants with the need for echo but only two machines. The allocation of limited resources can be decided based on the following: lottery, social worth, overall population health, helping the sickest patient or societal benefit (Kirsch & Munson, 2018).

6.4.1.4. Maternal-Fetal Conflict

When a mother is pregnant, she has full power of decision-making regarding her obstetrical treatment at the time of delivery, which may be at odds with the best choices for the baby. The principles of respect for patient autonomy, beneficence, nonmaleficence, and justice guide decisions, whereas feminist theory and the ethics of care help frame the answer. A woman who refuses to have a cesarean delivery when faced with a large fetus with heart rate abnormalities should be educated about the consequences of such a decision, but the autonomous pregnant woman has the right to refuse treatment. The American College of Obstetrics and Gynecology states that with regard to maternal decision making capacities, they would not support going to court to force a cesarean section to protect the fetus (American College of Obstetricians and Gynecologists, 2016). The guideline support the use of open communication using the RESPECT model. The acronym stands for rapport, empathy, support, partnership, explanation, cultural competence, and trust (American College of Obstetricians and Gynecologists, 2016). Guidelines should be in place within hospitals and birthing centers to resolve conflicts, and shared decision-making should be used when there is a conflict. The APRN/nurse midwife may be involved in the care of the infant and may be called on to educate the mother about the care of these infants and the possible outcomes. Communication using the RESPECT model is the key to ethical decision-making, with intervention by the courts rarely needed (American College of Obstetricians and Gynecologists, 2016).

6.4.1.5. Newborn Screening

In the early 1960s, phenylketonuria (PKU) testing of infants was introduced and by 1967, the test was mandatory in 37 states (El-Hattab, Almannai, & Sutton, 2018). The expansion of newborn screening to congenital hypothyroidism took place in 1973, and by the mid-1980s, several other metabolic conditions were added to newborn screening panels. In the late 1980s, it became clear that early introduction of penicillin prophylaxis prevented death in patients with sickle cell disease. Therefore, screening for sickle cell disease was added to the panel. In the early 1990s, tandem mass spectrometry was developed and its use in newborn screening increased the number of conditions tested. The use of tandem mass spectrometry technology led to expansion of the newborn screening program. These new tests also raised questions about the necessity of screening for conditions that could not be effectively treated (El-Hattab, Almannai, & Sutton, 2018). New genetic testing including a targeted gene panel or whole exome sequencing were considered as new ways to screen newborns but due to high cost, prolonged turnaround, and the uncertainty of variants with unknown clinical significance, these methods are not viable at this time (El-Hattab, Almannai, & Sutton, 2018).

The Advisory Committee on Heritable Disorders in Newborns and Children (ACHDNC) give their recommendations regarding the newborn screening program panels in the United States. Individual states make the final determination and thus screening panels do vary from state to state (El-Hattab, Almannai, & Sutton, 2018). The APRN must consider where a child was born in order to rule out rare conditions in a symptomatic patient. (El-Hattab, Almannai, & Sutton, 2018). The guidelines for testing newborns at birth include that the disease tested for should be an important public health problem, that there is an effective treatment, and that the test is acceptable to the population (Wilson and Junger, 1968). Categories of newborn screening include organic acids, fatty acids, amino acids, hemoglobin disorders, hearing, endocrine disorders, and other diseases such as cystic fibrosis (National Newborn Screening and Genetic Resource Center, 2019). As of July, 2018, the

Health Resources and Services Administration recommended that 35 core conditions be included in the newborn screen with an additional number of 26 conditions that are second tier recommendations (Health Resource and Services Administration, 2018). Different states' newborn screening programs vary, but all screen for the 35 core conditions. New tests continue to be added to the panel based on observational data and expert opinion (Health Resource and Services Administration, 2018).

Today, the Secretary of Health and Human Services' Advisory Committee on Heritable Disorders and Genetic Diseases in Newborns and Children makes recommendations regarding what tests should be included in the newborn panel. More recently, there is a proposal to screen for severe combined immunodeficiency and for congenital cyanotic heart disease, which would bring the core panel to 31 different screening tests. All states have not yet implemented these two new recommendations.

Advocacy groups have played an important role in the addition of tests to the panel. However, some of these groups are tied to industry and some of the diseases now included in some state panels are not a large public health threat. An example of this is Krabbe's disease, which was added to the New York State newborn screening panel despite the fact that the condition only affects 40 infants per year nationwide.A few states like New York also screen for Krabbe, Fabry, Niemann-Pick, adrenoleuko-dystorphy, Gaucher, and Hurler syndrome, the benefit of screening for these disease is not yet proven (El-Hattab, Almannai, & Sutton, 2018)

Conversely, screening for congenital hypothyroidism has prevented developmental disabilities as newborn screening allows this disease to be picked up before there are any physical manifestations of hypothyroidism. If parents refuse newborn screening, they may opt out of early identification of diseases like PKU and hypothyroidism that can be effectively treated in the newborn period. Early treatment of these diseases reduces mortality and morbidity as the diagnosis of the disease before the development of symptoms is critical. Some recommendations of the newborn screening panel are problematic as there are no effective treatments to date.

Newborns are now screened for both cystic fibrosis (CF) and sickle cell disease (SCD). As a result, there is an increase in the number of patients identified as of carrier of the disease. While genetic testing of children is not recommended in order to protect the child's privacy and autonomy, newborn screening is an exception to this rule. There has been considerable debate about the potential benefits and harm. Table 6.1 outlines the pros and cons of carrier state identification. It could be argued that disclosure of sickle cell carrier state is important because of the increased risk of heat stroke associated with the carrier state

(Ross and Clayton, 2009). There is no data about cystic fibrosis carriers having increased risk of any disease. The confirmation of CF carriage requires a burdensome confirmatory process to distinguish between a false positive and truly positive testing (Rosenfeld, Sontag, Ren, 2016).

Parents must be informed that screening tests are being done and that parental permission should be obtained. Most states continue with the newborn screening program as an "opt out" test and therefore no permission is required before the testing is done (El-Hattab, Almannai, & Sutton, 2018). In order for parents to opt out, they must know in advance that a test is being performed and then must proactively opt out of the program if they do not want their baby screened in the nursery. The issue is whether or not the broadening of these tests continues to fulfill the criteria for a public health screening program. Parents should be educated about these tests and active consent should be obtained to fully respect parental autonomy (Ross and Clayton, 2009). If the parent refuses newborn screening, the child may be placed at risk for long-term sequelae such as intellectual disability from untreated PKU or hypothyroidism.

In addition, there are pilot programs to screen for lysosomal storage disorders, fragile X, and Duchene's Muscular dystrophy. Since these disorders may not show up until later in life, there are questions as to whether it is ethical to test newborns for diseases that will not be symptomatic until later. Some of the concerns about newborn screening for the infant include psychological harm, stigmatization, and discrimination from being identified as having a costly disease (El-Hattab, Almannai, & Sutton, 2018)

The introduction of new tests to the newborn screening panel should be carefully studied for long-term effects. There are issues related to parental refusal of newborn screening, as some of these screening tests do screen for very treatable conditions. The present estimate is that 1:500 to 1:1000 births will have a disorder identified by newborn screening with

TABLE 6.1. Pros and Cons of Carrier State Identification.

Pros	Cons
Awareness about Clinical implications of carrier status	Anxiety or distress from learning of an abnormal test
Awareness of future reproductive choices	Misunderstand of genetic implications
Empowered by knowing genetic information	Potential discrimination and stigmatization on the carrier
	Continued worry about the carrier
	Possibility of non-paternity

hearing loss, primary congenital hypothyroidism, cystic fibrosis, sickle cell disease, and medium-chain-acyl-CoA dehydrogenase (MCAD) deficiency being the most common conditions (American College of Obstetrics & Gynecology, 2015). While newborn screening is an opt-out test, the majority of parents do not even realize what is being done and see it as a PKU testing. Parents may be unaware of the broad nature of the testing. While the need for newborn screening and the risk and benefits should be thoroughly explained to the parent, it is rarely done in hospital. The first notification that the child was screened may the notification of an abnormal result from the state newborn screening unit.

6.4.1.6. Vaccine Hesitancy

Hesitancy of accepted medical treatments such as vaccines is a source of concern for all healthcare clinician (Edwards & Hackell, 2016). Childhood immunizations are still a persistent area of concern for parents and clinician. Recent outbreaks of vaccine preventable diseases across the globe are a persistent area of concern with some parts of the United States reporting over 5% of the children are unvaccinated due to personal beliefs exemptions (Edwards et al., 2016). While the overall rate of vaccination is high, there is room for improvement (Hill, Elam-Evans, Yankey, Singleton, & Kang, 2018).

State laws requiring vaccines stem from a 1905 landmark case in which the United States Supreme Court endorsed school immunization requirements and gave states the right to reinforce these laws (Omer et al., 2009). In 1922, the Supreme Court found that school immunization requirements were constitutional (Omer et al., 2009). The trends in state immunization policies have made universal vaccination more difficult (Edwards et al., 2016). Due to changes in molecular immunology, there are an increasing number of vaccines available. In addition, cost-effectiveness analyses are changing policy decisions around immunizations.

Early in the 1900s, vaccination was mandatory and required to protect the public health. Today, the ethical issues around universal vaccination revolve around securing the greatest good for the greatest number of people versus protecting the rights of individuals. In the United States, a parent cannot be forced to vaccinate a child.

If a national mandatory requirement for vaccination of all children despite parental objections existed, society would minimize the effects of deleterious disease consequences, promote societies' duty to protect children, and maximize equal distribution of health programs and their prudent use (Hendrix, Sturm, Zimet, & Meslin, 2016). If the vaccination of children was an elective decision, it would promote the personal liberty to refuse or choose, and would minimize any adverse vaccine events. Today, vaccines are recommended and are not mandatory in the hopes that the Best Interest Standard will prevail, and families will want to protect their children against vaccine preventable diseases.

There are three reasons that parents can elect to exempt their children. There are exemptions for children who have valid medical reasons for not taking the vaccine such as allergies, exemptions for parents whose religious beliefs oppose immunizations, and exemptions for parents who have philosophical beliefs that can be cited when they refuse to immunize their child (Omer et al., 2009). At the present time, philosophical exemptions due to moral, personal or other beliefs are allowed in 17 states. (National Conference of State Legislators, 2019). West Virginia and California have removed both religious and philosophical objections to vaccine refusal but most states allow for religious objections (National Conference of State Legislators, 2019). Parental concerns due to perceived vaccine safety issues have led to increasing numbers of parents refusing or delaying vaccines.

The APRN must be aware of parents' need for correct information about vaccines. Parents need appropriate information about vaccines in order to make informed decisions. Unfortunately, there are a large number of official looking websites that promote vaccine hesitancy and these Internet site need to be countered with appropriate information. The largest portion of parents who changed their minds did so because of information from health care clinician (Edwards et al. 2016). One study reviewed United States newspaper print information from 1995 to 2005 and found that 37% of the articles gave negative information about immunizations (Hussain et al., 2011). Thus, APRNs must be aware of the importance of providing appropriate evidence-based resources for vaccine information.

TABLE 6.2. Types of Parental Reactions to Vaccine

Immunization advocate	Vaccine acceptance with a strong relationship with their health care provider
Go along to get along	These parents lack knowledge but do not question vaccine and would vaccinate their child
Cautious acceptor	Minor concerns are present but will vaccinate with the proper education
Fence-sitter	Significantly concerned about vaccines and have a neutral relationship with their health care provider. They have knowledge about vaccine
Refuser	Refuse vaccines due to concerns about safety, distrust in the medical system, or religious beliefs

(Adapted from Edwards et al., 2016)

A study of vaccine attitudes, concerns and information sources showed that parents of young children felt the most important resource of information about vaccines was the child's doctor or nurse (Kennedy, Basket, and Sheedy, 2011). Due to the dissemination of unreliable information to parents, parents may refuse and want to space out vaccines (Edwards et al, 2016). A list of reliable websites and books are found in Box 6.1. If the family refuses to immunize their child, the APRN should ask the family to sign a release from liability to a malpractice suit if the child was infected with the vaccine preventable disease and had a bad outcome. This is available from the following website-- https://www.aap.org/en-us/Documents/immunization_refusaltovaccinate.pdf

The American Academy of Pediatrics encourages continued involvement with families who refuse vaccines but recognizes that some practices may dismiss patients who refuse to vaccine due to concerns about exposure of the children with vaccine preventable diseases in the waiting room (Edwards et al., 2016). The recommendation is that the policy of children being vaccinated in the practice or be dismissed from the practice needs to be transparent in the practice so that families will understand the philosophy of the practice (Edwards et al., 2016). However, if the APRN wants to terminate the relationship, she must transfer the care of the patient to another provider before she terminates the relationship. She cannot abandon the patient and refuse to care for the child (Gilmour et al., 2011).

From an ethical standpoint, the APRN must assess the level of information that the parent has and explore the beliefs of the parent. The APRN then can educate and give appropriate information including websites and books (See Table 6.3) (Edwards et al., 2016). Parents must have misinformation corrected and the correct information communicated in an effective forum so that informed decisions can be made in the best interest of their children (Edwards et al., 2016).

Some of the reasons that clinicians give to validate their reasons for terminating patient relationships include philosophical differences, and the risks of exposing immunized patients to non-immunized patients with diseases that are vaccine preventable. For example, a child with a cough whose parent has refused immunization against pertussis may be present in the waiting room along with infants who have not yet been fully protected by vaccine. In 2019, Washington State declared a measles epidemic which is also being experienced in NYS (Yan & Goldschmidt, 2019). Vaccination coverage for MMR, DTaP, and varicella vaccine at entrance to kindergarden was close to 95% during the 2016-2017 school year with a median exemption rate of 2%. However, coverage varies within states, and even in states with overall high rates, there can be clusters of low vaccination rates (Seithers et al. 2017).

6.4.2. Child and Adolescent

6.4.2.1. Predictive Genetic Testing

The area of genetic testing has expanded dramatically over the last ten years and today genetic tests can be both diagnostic and predictive. The testing available has increased accuracy and can include a single gene test, multiplex gene panel, whole exome sequences (WES) or whole genome sequencing (WGS). While these advances may help

TABLE 6.3. Websites and Books with Reliable Information about Vaccines.

Websites with Reliable Information about Vaccines
• www.medlineplus.gov—National Library of Medicine
• www.cdc.gov—Centers for Disease Control
• www.nih.gov/icd—National Institute of Health
• www.who.int—World Health Organization
• https://www.aap.org/en-us/advocacy-and-policy/aap-health-initiatives/immunizations/Pages/Immunizations-home.aspx - AAP immunization website
• https://www.chop.edu/centers-programs/vaccine-education-center — Vaccine Education Center at Children's Hospital of Philadelphia website
• www.immunize.org—Immunization Action Coalition Website
• www.vaccinateyourbaby.org—Put out by two websites
• https://www.immunize.ca —The Canadian website encouraging immunizations.
• https://www.caringforkids.cps.ca —Canadian Pediatric society
• www.iom.org—Institute of Medicine
• www.meningitis-angels.org
• www.nfid.org—National foundation for infectious disease
• https://www.niaid.nih.gov/research/vaccines
• www.nmaus.org—National Meningitis Association
• www.pkids.org—Parents of Kids with Infectious Disease
• https://www.texaschildrens.org/departments/immunization-project/vaccine-preventable-disease —Center For Vaccine Awareness and Research, Texas Children Hospital
Books with Reliable Information about Vaccines
• Offit, P.A. (2010) Deadly Choices: How the anti-vaccine movement threatens us all.. New York, NY: IDG Books.
• Fisher, M.C. (2005) Immunizations and Infectious Diseases: An Informed Parent's Guide. Elk Grove Village, IL: American Academy of Pediatrics.

improve the lives of Americans, they also lead to new ethical dilemmas. Personalized information about modifiable risk factors may provide children and adolescents with the information they need to modify their lifestyle in order to avoid disease. However, this generation is the first group of children and adolescents that have the ability to get this information, but how this will affect them is not yet known.

Predictive genetic testing can be divided into categories of diseases that manifest in adults, diseases that manifest in childhood, and testing that identifies carrier information. There is universal consensus in the AAP that predictive testing in children for adult onset disease and testing for carrier status should be delayed. A mature adult must make decisions about genetic testing Genetic testing can affect the psychological well-being of the person if they are at risk for a disease and can lead to stigma as well as discrimination in the workplace. Genetic information can also pose legal, ethical and social risks for family. Genetic information is difficult to interpret and the differences between causation and association may be difficult for parents. (Botkin et al., 2015; Committee on Bioethics, Committee on Genetics, and The American College of Medical Genetics and Genomics, Social, Ethical and Legal Issues Committee, 2013; reaffirmed 2018). The kind of genetic condition and the possibility of preventive treatment determined whether geneticists will provide genetic testing

There are psychosocial, clinical, and reproductive implications to these tests and there is not yet enough research as to the long-term effects of knowing this information. In terms of testing for adult onset condition, clinicians need to discuss with the parents and/or adolescent the reason to do predictive testing. In the face of lack of treatment, clinicians need to encourage predictive testing until adulthood when the decision can be made with a more complete understanding of the implications (Botkin et al., 2015; Committee on Bioethics et al., 2013, reaffirmed 2018).

While more extensive testing is available, ASHG (2015) recommends the use of targeted gene panels or single gene testing to confirm the child's clinical presentation. Limiting the analysis using genome scale sequencing is an acceptable alternative to target the genes of interest. Genome scale sequencing is appropriate when limited genetic testing fails to identify the mutation and may be needed even when targeted gene panels or single gene testing has not been done. There is no indication for genome-scale sequencing in healthy children. The issue around secondary findings based of genome-scale sequencing is also addressed in the latest guidelines and encourages the lack of disclosure of secondary findings unless they have health significance for the child (Botkin et al., 2015; Committee on Bioethics et al., 2013, reaffirmed 2018).

Chromosomal microarray (CMA) is a more common and cheaper test used in children with developmental delays including autism, congenital anomalies, and developmental delays (Botkin, 2015). This testing is also difficult to interpret and may have secondary findings of unknown clinical significance.

Direct to consumer genetic testing originally only tested for paternity and ancestory testing. Today genetic health testing is available online from both US based companies and overseas companies. These companies may offer direct testing for genetic conditions without any counseling by clinicians and genetic counselors. A parent can test their child without any assent. In addition, the quality of this testing may not be as rigorous as a medical center lab.

Preadoption testing is not recommended and it is felt that adoptive parents should have the same access to their child's genetics as the birth parents. Therefore any genetic testing is only done in the face of a childhood onset disease with appropriate clinical presentation.

There are harms of knowing a genetic diagnosis for the child and adolescent that may increase anxiety for the parent and child, increase guilt for the parents, problems with employment and insurance, detection of paternity, changes in how the child is viewed by the parents, and alteration of self-image for the child. For example, in a family with history of retinoblastoma, knowledge of whether a child has the gene for retinoblastoma can allow for surveillance and early detection of the disease, thereby preventing loss of vision. However, if the family refuses the genetic test, the question may be asked: "Are they acting in the child's best interest?"

In the case of Fragile X syndrome, the number of trinucleotide repeats is often associated with the severity of the disease, so knowing the genetic make-up of the child can determine the prognosis. In terms of reproductive issues, parents may avoid having further children in order to prevent having another child with the disease and may make family planning decisions based on the knowledge of their disease Genetic testing can also allow families to make life decisions about retirement based on the information.

Knowledge that a child has a genetic disorder may affect family relationships and the child may be rejected, overindulged, or scapegoated. Vulnerable child syndrome (Green and Solnit, 1964) may result, causing the parents to treat the child as though something is going to happen to the child, and restrict his activity. Unaffected children may be treated differently as a result of the identification of a problem with their sibling.

TABLE 6.4. Important Issues in Genetic Testing in Children and Adolescents.

- Genetic confirmation of a clinical suspicion that will enable appropriate management
- Delay genetic testing with adult onset diseases
- Testing should be discouraged if potential harm outweighs any benefit to the child or adolescent
- If the benefit or harm falls in a gray area, extensive education and counseling based on their ability and maturity should be done.
- Clinician must obtain parental permission along with adolescent's or child's assent
- If the provider feels the test is not in the best interest of a child, the provider needs to advocate on the behalf of the child
- Any research must focus on the genetic testing proposed benefits including the psychosocial impact of the genetic testing results.
- Pharmacogenic testing should be done only if directly benefits the child
- Parents should not do direct to consumer genetic testing

Adapted from Botkin, 2016; Committee on Bioethics et al., 2013, reaffirmed 2018

Ethical issues regarding genetic testing also center on privacy and confidentiality as well as the right to know and the right to not know. A family member who has knowledge of his genetic disease may not choose to disclose the disease if is not likely to result in serious harm to another family member. Genetic testing may affect a child's future ability to get life insurance as the insurers may be able to get this information from the clinical records of the patient (Rothstein, 2018). The insurer's themselves feel that they should have access to this information despite the fact that it may not predict the lifespan of the person.

Testing for certain diseases may be supported by the APRN if there is clear benefit to the child. For example, in hypertrophic cardiomyopathy, drug therapy may be of benefit to the child to prevent sudden death (Botkin et al., 2015). If the APRN is in doubt, she should refer the patient to the geneticist. If the APRN believes that the genetic test may cause more harm than benefit to the child, the APRN must act as an advocate for the child. They can refuse to do the testing as it does not benefit the child.

6.4.2.2. Special Needs Children

Families who care for children with special health care needs (CSHCN) have multiple demands on them that are different from families raising well children. The enormity of the obligations can change the family dynamics—limiting attention to other children, changing employment status of a parent, limiting recreational activities, and making day-to-day decisions. The family is responsible for carrying out complex regimes with little support from outside agencies. This may lead to lack of adherence and trigger a referral to child protective services for medical neglect. The APRN must develop a plan using shared decision-making that meets the needs of the family and the CSHCN. For the seriously ill CSHCN, the APRN should raise the issue about advanced care plans and palliative care before the child is actually dying. Discussion around what should be done for a child with a terminal condition must be discussed before an acute event occurs (Okun, 2010).

For clinicians, one of the issues with special needs children is the extra time required in caring for these children versus caring for a well child, often without appropriate reimbursement (Okun, 2010). While a sense of duty and obligation to patients is part of clinical practice, clinician must be compensated for the time spent caring for these patients as they do take away time for other patients. There is additional paperwork for insurance companies to approve equipment and medication and this additional time is also not compensated.

The APRN must develop expertise in counseling and informing patients about issues around death, sexuality, genetic risk, and prognosis. Discussion around harm versus benefit for a variety of procedures and surgical options must be held to promote beneficence. Families who want treatments that are not proven may be refused by clinician if there is no clear benefit to the child (Okun, 2010). This may lead to difficult communications with families regarding refusal to give unproven treatment. However, good ethics demand refusal of unproven treatments.

6.4.2.3. Nondisclosure of a Diagnosis to a Child or Adolescent

While patient autonomy may be clearer in adult ethical situations, pediatric patients require a significantly different approach due to the importance of family and their necessity to act in the best interest of their child. Disclosure of a disease may carry the burden of stigmatization and discrimination along with cultural and religious concerns for families (Kulkarni et al., 2001).

Culture clearly needs to be considered in disclosures (Dreisinger & Zapolsky, 2018). Outside Western cultures, communication by innuendo rather than direct communication is the norm. Telling a patient a diagnosis directly may be seen as disrespectful and can disrupt family relationships (Kuldarni et al., 2001). In certain cultures, family autonomy is far more important that individual autonomy and reflects the fact that different cultures handle ethical considerations in different ways

(Swota and Hester, 2011). Therefore, when discussing disclosure with families, the APRN must consider the entire life of the patient, including an understanding of the family, community, and culture (Swota and Hester, 2011).

Ethical issues about nondisclosure center on basic concepts in pediatric ethics such as child autonomy, truth telling, beneficent deception, nonmaleficence, confidentiality, cross cultural considerations, and family autonomy. The APRN may meet families who request nondisclosure of any diagnosis to the child due to religious or cultural reasons. Family autonomy must be considered in cross-cultural ways. In Western society, moral dilemmas may require consideration of family autonomy. Most professionals prefer to be truthful with their pediatric patients. Truth telling is closely aligned with the ethical duty of respecting the autonomy of others (Kuldarni et al., 2001).

The military's previous policy of "Don't ask, don't tell" regarding sexual orientation and passed by Congress in 1996 reflects the concept of beneficent deception (Kuldarni et al., 2001). The concept of avoiding telling the truth, if truth can do more harm than good, has lost popularity. In cases where parents do not want an older child or adolescent told of a diagnosis, the diagnosis must be considered. For example, in an adolescent, where HIV is often a sexually transmitted diagnosis, the responsibility to protect the rest of society must be considered. While it can be argued that the strongest argument for nondisclosure is the wishes of the parents, consideration of the public's health also must be considered in a sexually active adolescent. Legal concerns may overshadow these decisions, and in cases where there is a risk to the rest of society, the APRN can get a court injunction based on the principle of beneficence and the Best Interest Standard.

The patient may also feel a loss of trust and significant anger toward the members of the healthcare team who failed to disclose the diagnosis. The APRN may experience guilt, fear, empathy, liability, and anger about failing to be honest with the patient. Nondisclosure may lead to frustration, as the APRN may not be able to talk directly to the patient and get his/her input into medical treatment decisions. Some of the reasons for nondisclosure cited by the parent may be the child's age, the lack of symptoms, and the reduction in self-esteem if the child knew about his disease.

Medical decision-making is problematic when the interests of the child and the interest of the parents are not in concert. The child or adolescent who does not know the diagnosis cannot weigh in on treatment options. In an adolescent who is able to consider treatment options, the nondisclosure takes this right away from the child. A pragmatic right-based justification seems appropriate in the adolescent who is able to make decisions (Kulkarni et al., 2001). In these cases, an ethics consult may be helpful to the APRN and the health care team.

6.4.2.4. Caring for Abused Children

According to legal mandates, the APRN is required to report suspected child abuse. Child abuse may take the form of physical abuse, psychological abuse, sexual abuse, or neglect (Centers for Disease Control, 2018). At times, questioning parents lead the APRN to suspect that the child is being exposed to excessive violence, which also needs to be reported even if the APRN is concerned about the therapeutic relationship with the parent. It is important to remember that the APRN must act in the best interest of the child no matter what the relationship is with the guardian or parent—protecting the child is the focus of the APRN's care.

There are several different ethical situations around child abuse in which the APRN may experience moral distress. Parents may suffer from mental illness, substance abuse, or domestic violence leading to child abuse. A child should ideally be raised in an environment that will foster his growth and development. While this may mean the removal of the child from the natural guardians, all efforts should be made to keep the family together with supports and ongoing treatment. Placement in a foster care may result in multiple homes, multiple school placements, loss of parental and family support and the termination of foster care at 18, leaving the child without adequate life skills for adult life (Council on Foster Care, Adoption, and Kinship care and Committee on Early Childhood, 2012). Placement with foster care may not be the best option for the child in the long run, so it should be used only if the parent's situation is unable to be remediated (Council on Foster Care, Adoption, and Kinship care and Committee on Early Childhood, 2012). The APRN who cares for foster children must monitor their progress and report concerns to child protective services.

APRNs may be involved in child abuse cases in which the child experiences a severe injury as a result of abuse. This can occur in the ED, PICU, or in long term care facilities. In these cases, lifesaving medical treatment may be needed. In some of these children, the perpetrator is not clear and the parent—perhaps one of the perpetrators—may be involved in making decisions. If it is determined that the child is suffering, will not recover, and the quality and extent of life will not be restored, consideration of termination of lifesaving support should be raised with the parents. In cases where the parents might be charged with a crime if the child's life support is terminated, the parent may be more concerned about what is best for them instead of the child (Gladsjo et al., 2004). In these cases, the court will appoint a guardian ad litem, who is an attorney who advocates for the best interests of the child. These attorneys explore the situation based on interviews with the healthcare team, including the APRN and the parents. They issue a report to the judge about the child's situation in order to help the court make a decision. Discontinuing life-sustaining interventions may cause disagreements between the health care provider and families (Fisher, 2011; Gladsjo et al., 2004). Parents may not be able to consider the best interest of child when there is a potential conflict of interest, an insufficient understanding of their child's condition, or parental refusal to acknowledge the seriousness of the child's condition. Difficult decision-making can be helped by a referral to an ethics team to review the decision making process and improve the parent's understanding. This may also help avoid court involvement in these cases.

Covert surveillance is another issue in cases of Factitious Disorder by Proxy, also known as Münchausen syndrome. This disorder occurs when a well-child is subjected to multiple medical procedures to find out what is wrong with the child when, in truth, the parent or guardian is making up a child's symptoms for medical attention. About 10% of the children die as a result of their parent's attempt to falsify their symptoms. Most perpetrators are careful about their deceitful activities and finding them in the act of falsification of symptoms is difficult. This may lead to planting cameras or using hidden mirrors to catch the parent in the act. There are two ethical sides to the use of covert spying. One side believes that the spying will lead to a loss of trust and set up a dishonest relationship between the parent and the provider (Fisher, 2011). The child is used as bait, which some believe is unacceptable and leads to the provider losing sight of their main responsibility of child protection. As the family is unlikely to do this in a hospital setting, this method is difficult to implement. On the other hand, if the parents are confronted openly about the problem and asked to participate in a recovery program, the relationship may be preserved.

APRNs may have negative feelings about guardians who have abused their children. It is important to acknowledge those feelings if the APRN is going to continue to work with the family. If the APRN's feelings cannot be worked through, the care of the family should be transferred.

6.4.2.5. End of Life: Palliative Care

Pediatric palliative care meets the needs of children of all ages who need relief from physical, psychological, social, financial, spiritual suffering and to promote a positive family function and adaption with the goal of improving the child's quality life. Pediatric palliative care also promotes informed decision-making and promotes coordination of care (Section on Hospice and Palliative Medicine, and Hospital care, 2013). There are clear guidelines for pediatric palliative care endorsed by the AAP and the National Hospice Foundation. When a pediatric patient has a serious, life threatening illness, the guidelines for palliative care stress the importance of assessing and documenting the child's views and preferences regarding their medical care and their choices be weighed in the final decision-making (National Consensus Project for Quality Palliative Care, 2018).

There are four values that form the basis of care for children (Mercurio, Forman et al., 2008):

1. Pain and suffering is unacceptable and should be alleviated.
2. Pain and suffering include physical pain but have a psychological, emotional, and spiritual dimension.
3. Each child should be treated with respect.
4. The family of the pediatric patient is the responsibility of the primary care provider.

APRNs, similar to other clinician, may lack formal training in palliative care and may not have the knowledge base to set up high quality programs. Parents lack an understanding of what palliative care and what it could do for their child in an event of a serious illness (Zawistowski, Black, Spruill, & Granowetter, 2018)

The provision of palliative care to children a part of every program that delivers palliative care. Recent guidelines for quality palliative care were endorsed by the AAP and stress the need for comprehensive palliative care (National Consensus Project for Quality Palliative Care, 2018). The APRN working in palliative care must be clear with families that there are many unknowns about palliative care including time of death.

The APRN not directly involved in palliative care team should continue to work with the family to provide optimal treatment. The APRN must also acknowledge that caring for a patient with a rare disease may require continued reassessment to provide optimal comfort care. There are several pediatric palliative care programs available for APRNs who wish to improve their care of terminally ill children. Table 6.5 is a list of curricula that are now available for APRNs and other members of the healthcare team who want additional training in palliative care.

TABLE 6.5. Palliative Care Training.

Association/Name of Curriculum	Website
American Association of Colleges of Nursing ELNEC Core Curriculum	http://www.aacn.nche.edu/elnec/trainings/national#core
Initiative for Pediatric Palliative Care	http://www.ippcweb.org/curriculum.asp
National Hospice and Palliative Care Organization	http://www.nhpco.org/i4a/pages/index.cfm?pageID=5889
Center to Advance Palliative Care	http://www.capc.org/palliative-care-professional-development/clinical-site-visit-directory
American Academy of Hospice and Palliative Care	http://www.aahpm.org/certification/default/resources.html
	This is a physician website but it has good resources for learning more about palliative care.

For the adolescent who is diagnosed with a terminal illness, the issues around decisions are more complex due to determination of decisional capacity. In the case of a dying adolescent who has been through multiple treatment regimes, maturity levels may be remarkable and patients should be granted their preferences on how they want to spend the rest of their life (Ross, Leigh, & Anthony, 2018). Adolescents may deny their impending death and continue to act as though they will survive. Acceptance of this may take time and the APRN must gently communicate the reality of their present illness (Ross, Leigh, & Anthony, 2018). As with adults, adolescents should be allowed to determine the aspects of palliative care intervention which they desire. The adolescent must understand the risks of all the treatment options, understand the medical information, make a voluntary choice, and comprehend the nature of the decision. An adolescent's conception of death should be considered in order to allow him to make end of life decisions (Ross, Leigh, & Anthony, 2018).

A parent may oppose the disclosure of the adolescent's transition to a terminal illness. To avoid any problems, the provider should initiate a conversation about truthfulness about the diagnosis and prognosis with the family from the beginning. This will help reduce anxiety in the adolescent and foster a trusting relationship. Most parents understand the importance of truthfulness and good ethical practice. At times, the parent may not want the child to be told about the transition to palliative care. The APRN must make sure that the parents know that if the child directly asks, the APRN will be truthful. In these cases, having the family talk with a spiritual advisor may be helpful. Again, an ethics consult may be needed in difficult cases.

6.4.3. Adolescents

6.4.3.1. Issues in Reproductive Health

Ethical issues are frequent in adolescent healthcare centered on the right to confidential reproductive healthcare. Over the past thirty years, laws to give adolescent access to reproductive health care without parental consent have enabled adolescents to obtain confidential reproductive health care (Guttmacher, 2019). The reason for expanded adolescent's rights in the past 30 years stems from the knowledge that some teens will not seek health care if their parents are required to be notified. Statutes known as "state minor consent laws" allow adolescents to seek treatment for sexually transmitted diseases, contraception, and reproductive issues without the consent of parents (English, 2007).

6.4.3.1.1. Disclosing Adolescents' Information to Parents/ Guardians

Clinics with public funding may give adolescents access to confidential family planning services, contraception, and pregnancy-related care. Depending on the state, these laws also allow adolescents to consent for treatment for mental health and substance abuse treatments. APRNs may treat adolescents for these issues without the consent of the parent depending on the state law. However, there are states where parent's rights have been infused into the right of adolescents to seek reproductive health care. In the case of abortion, in 11 states as of January 2019, at least one parent must be notified before an abortion can take place but 21 states require that at least one parent consent to a minor's abortion (Guttmacher Institute, 2019). However, the Supreme Court ruled that parents cannot overturn the adolescent's right to an abortion, and in some states, the laws allow a judge to override parental notification if the adolescent can show maturity in health care decision making process.

Adolescents are allowed to consent to a variety of health care services such as sexual and reproductive health care, mental health care, and substance abuse treatment. Despite the advances in minors' rights, not all states allow adolescents to have access to the above services. Recent parental rights notifications now state that state consent laws apply to minors 12 and over or in some cases, only if they are married, pregnant, or already parents in order to consent (Guttmacher Institute, 2019). In some states there is no case law and APRNs may provide medical care if they feel the minor is mature. For example, 26 states and the District of Columbia allow minors to consent for contraceptive services; only 20 states allow only certain categories of minors can consent, and only 4 states have no law (Guttmacher Institute, 2019).

When an adolescent is pregnant, only 32 states allow adolescents to seek prenatal health care without parental permission. There are 13 states where there are no explicit policies regarding providing care to adolescents. In 14 states, the APRN can notify the parent of the adolescent's pregnancy if the APRN feels it is in the best interest of the child (Guttmacher Institute, 2019). In these 13 states, there is no requirement to notify the parent. The APRN must always consider what is in the best interest of the child. Depending on the state law, once the pregnancy ends, these adolescents may be considered minors again even though they are parents. It is the responsibility of the APRN to know state law for adolescents. Some pregnant adolescents seek to become emancipated minors after their pregnancies. An emancipated minor has the right to consent to treatment regardless of the parent's wishes. The adolescent must follow the procedures required to obtain a certificate of emancipation for that state and the APRN must actually see the certificate to provide routine medical care. For homeless adolescents, some states allow treatment without documentation.

The Guttmacher Institute website is an excellent current resource of information regarding adolescent healthcare and state laws. The ethical issues concern the importance of adolescent confidentiality. If the law requires reporting, then the APRN must tell the patient the reason that they will notify parents.

Finally, in caring for adolescents for reproductive issues, parents may find out about the office or emergency room when they receive an insurance statement either via the Internet or by a paper statement. Adolescents must be informed that this may happen and there is no way of preventing the insurance company from issuing an explanation of benefits.

6.4.3.1.2. Sterilization of Minors with Developmental Disabilities

The issues around sterilization of minors with developmental disabilities are controversial due to the long history of abuse of sterilization of women in the United States (Mercurio, Adam et al., 2008). In

1942, the Supreme Court declared human procreation was a fundamental right (Committee on Bioethics, 1999, reaffirmed 2006). This law made the sterilization of any individual more difficult and by the 1970s, there were several regulations that prevented federal programs from sterilizing individuals with developmental disabilities (Mercurio, Adam et al., 2008). The surgical sterilization of the developmentally disabled remains controversial and there are significantly different laws from state to state (AAP Committee on Bioethics, 1999, reaffirmed 2006). The AAP encourages pediatricians to develop relationships with local agencies and legal resources to understand and sort through the complex information around state and federal law (AAPCommittee on Bioethics, 1999).

The argument against sterilization of developmentally disabled minors focuses on respecting the integrity of the body, risks of surgical sterilization, and avoidance of limitations on the child's development and decision-making (Goldman & Quint, 2011). Parents of developmentally disabled children may have hygiene, mood change, pregnancy, and sexual activity concerns. It is argued that sterilization does not change an adolescent's sexual desire and only changes the risk of pregnancy. Parents must understand that sterilization carries risks and the benefit of sterilization must be for clear medical indications. The family with a child with developmental disabilities should consider that sterilization will prevent pregnancy, but it will not prevent sexual abuse or exposure to sexually transmitted diseases. Ethical concerns about sterilization of adolescents with development disabilities focus on the right of the child not to be treated as an object, but as a human being with basic rights (Goldman and Quint, 2011).

The APRN caring for these families should start the discussion about sexuality as the child enters puberty, exploring the concerns of the family and discussing contraception options to prevent pregnancy. Aside from the legal issues, there are religious beliefs that may interfere with presenting the pros and cons to parents. In cases where the APRN cannot give unbiased care because of religious beliefs, transfer of care to another provider is imperative.

6.4.4. Issues Surrounding Social Media

Social media such as Facebook, Twitter, Linkedin, and Internet searches of patients can be way of obtaining information about patients (Jent et al., 2011). Social media is a way of developing and maintaining relationship across distances. However, depending on the privacy setting, significant personal information can be obtained via these sites.

A preliminary study of 302 graduate students showed that 27% of clinicians sought information about their patients via social media sites (SMS) (Lehavot, Barnett and Powers, 2010). By exploring an adolescent's SMS posting, the APRN may find herself in a unique dilemma, as the APRN must decide what to do with the information that is obtained especially if the patient is posting information about self- or other-directed violence. If the APRN fails to act, she may be liable for not acting on the posting information even though she may have believed that the posting was not truthful (Lenhart and Madden, 2012). The adolescent may also believe that an APRN's searches are an invasion of privacy and this can disrupt the therapeutic nature of the relationship (Jent et al., 2011).

Jent et al. (2011) reported a survey of 109 pediatric medical residents, interns, and medical students in South Florida who used medical vignettes to explain that they had visited the SMS of a patient and presented the subjects with options after reading the patient's personal posts. Both faculty and trainees reported that they felt SMS to be public information. However, the trainees were the only ones who reported going on to SMS for information. Although going onto a patient's website may be an ethical violation, this did not appear to influence health provider's decision-making to do so.

Given the exposure of the younger generation to technology and SMS, the APRN must consider ethical guidelines before using SMS in clinical practice and obtain permission before seeking information about patients on their websites. Clinician should not seek information about a patient from an Internet or SMS search. Using social media together with an adolescent, and with the parent permission, may be a more acceptable way of exploring information posted on a SMS with a provider.

6.4.5. Pediatric Subjects in a Research Study

The ethical principles of respect for persons, justice, and beneficence are important in pediatric as well as adult research. The application of these principles in pediatric research must be considered against a child's developmental level, family decision-making, and risk to the child. Institutional Review Boards (IRBs) involved in approving pediatric research protocols view children as a vulnerable population and therefore focus on maximizing safety in pediatric research protocols (Rose, 2017a). Healthy children usually participate in research studies that involve no more than minimal risk unless it offers direct benefit to the child or it offers only minor increase over minimal risk (Rose,

2017a). While the Institute of Medicine has tried to standardize minimal risk, each local IRB will view this differently and there is variability in the risk assessment of each IRB (Rose, 2017a).

Informed consent of both the child and parent is important in pediatric research. When there is more than minimal risk, both parents may be required to sign the consent. Rose's review of research practices in children, points out that pediatric assent, the researcher must make sure that the child has an understanding of health and must have a clear explanation of the tests (Rose, 2017b). The child should agree to the study without any coercion and should understand what participation in the study involves. Pediatric patients can benefit from research and can be involved in study with higher than minimal risk but maximizing pediatric safety in studies is important (Rose, 2017b). Pediatric patients pose unique problems in all aspects of healthcare. The APRN caring for children must consider their special ethical dilemmas and work with families to promote the best outcomes.

6.5. CASE STUDIES

1. The parents of a 32-week gestation age infant girl do not want intervention for the neonate. The child is otherwise well, but has respiratory problems and needs intervention. What is your approach to this problem?
2. A 39-year-old mother was recently diagnosed with breast cancer. She is BRA-2 gene and wants her 16 year-old tested for the gene. The child does not want to be tested. How would you approach this issue? What are the ethical principles in this situation?
3. During a pertussis outbreak, there are five parents in your practice with young infants refusing the DTaP vaccine. What is your approach and why?
4. A mother of an 8 year-old brings the child to your office for a well-child visit. The mother has refused vaccines and today tells you that if you want to give vaccines you will need to negotiate with the child. How do you approach this situation? What are the ethical dilemmas with vaccine refusal?
5. A 13 year-old discloses that she is sexually active with her boyfriend. She is not using birth control but is using condoms consistently by her report. How do you approach this situation? What are the ethical and legal issues with reproductive healthcare for adolescents?

6. A 15 year-old boy has a green penile discharge. He appears in the office without his parents. The clinic staff states he cannot be treated. What are the APRN's responsibilities? How do you approach this situation? How would you educate the staff?
7. A 15-year-old child with muscular dystrophy is developing increasing shortness of breath. He has previously expressed his desire to not have life support. The mother wants the child have a tracheostomy. What is the APRN's response? What ethical dilemma does this cause?
8. A mother of a 19 year-old who is mildly developmentally delayed is concerned about her daughter's interest in boys. What is the APRN's response? Why?

6.6. REFERENCES

American Academy Pediatrics Committee on Bioethics, http://pediatrics.aappublications.org/collection/committee-bioethics.

American Academy Pediatrics Committee on Bioethics. (1997). Religious objections to medical care. Pediatrics, 99: 279–281. doi: 10.1542/peds.99.2.279.

American College of Obstetricians and Gynecologists. (2015). Newborn screening and the role of the obstetrician–gynecologist. Committee Opinion No. 616.. Obstetrics & Gynecology, 125, 256–60. Retrieved from https://www.acog.org/Clinical-Guidance-and-Publications/Committee-Opinions/Committee-on-Genetics/Newborn-Screening-and-the-Role-of-the-Obstetrician-Gynecologist. Accessed February 1, 2019.

American College of Obstetricians and Gynecologists. (2016). Refusal of medically recommended treatment during pregnancy committee Opinion No. 664. Obstetrics & Gynecology, 127, e175–e182. Retrieved from https://www.acog.org/-/media/Committee-Opinions/Committee-on-Ethics/co664.pdf?dmc=1&ts=2019020 6T1354585908.

Beauchamp, T.L. & Childress, J.F. (2013). *Principles of Biomedical Ethics* (7th edition). New York, NY: Oxford Press.

Black, C. (2007, November 29). Boy dies of leukemia after refusing treatment for religious reasons. *Seattle Post-Intelligencer*. Available at http://seattlepi.nwsource.com/local/341458_leukemia29.html.

Blanco, F., Suresh, G., Howard, D. & Soll, R. (2005). Ensuring accurate knowledge of prematurity outcomes for prenatal counseling. *Pediatrics 115*, e478-e487.

Botkin, J.R.; Belmont, J.W.; Berg, J.S.; Berkman, B.E.; Bombard, Y.; Holm, I. Mcinerney, J (2015). Points to consider: Ethical, legal, and psychosocial implications of genetic testing in children and adolescents. *American Journal of Human Genetics 97*(1), 6-21. doi: 10.1016/j.ajhg.2015.05.022.

Camosy, C.C. (2011). Ethics for the pediatrician: Just distribution of health-care resources and the neonatal ICU. *Pediatrics in Review 32*(5): 204–207. doi: 10.1542/pir.32-5-204.

Centers for Disease Control. (2018). Child maltreatment prevention. Retrieved February 3, 2019. Available at https://www.cdc.gov/violenceprevention/childabuseandneglect/index.html.

Child Trend (2019). Infant, child and teen mortality. Retrieved from https://www. childtrends.org/indicators/infant-child-and-teen-mortality.

Committee on Bioethics, Committee on Genetics, and The American College of Medical Genetics and Genomics, Social, Ethical and Legal Issues Committee. (2013; reaffirmed 2018). Ethical and policy issues in genetic testing and screening of children. *Pediatrics 201*, 131, 620-625. DOI: 10.1542/peds.2012-3680.

Committee on Bioethics (2016). Informed consent in decision-making in pediatric practice. *Pediatrics, 138*(2), e20161484. DOI: 10.1542/peds.2016-1484.

Committee on Bioethics. (1997). Religious objections to medical care. *Pediatrics 99*(2): 279–281. doi: 10.1542/peds.99.2.279. Reaffirmed October 2006.

Committee on Bioethics (1999). Sterilization of minors with developmental disabilities. *Pediatrics 104*(2): 337–340.

Council on Foster Care, Adoption, and Kinship care and Committee on Early Childhood (2012), Health care of youth aging out of foster care. *Pediatrics 130*(6), 1170-1173 doi:10.1542/peds.2012-2603.

Cummings, C.L. & Mercurio, M.R. (2010). Ethics for the pediatrician: autonomy, beneficence, and rights. *Pediatrics in Review 31*(6): 252–255. doi: 10.1542/pir.31-6-252.

Cummings, C.L. (2016). Teaching and assessing ethics in the Neonatal ICU. *Seminars in Perinatology 40*, 261-269. http://dx.doi.org/10.1053/j.semperi.2015.12.016.

Davis, D.S. & Kodish, E. (2014). Laws that conflict with the ethics of medicine: What should doctors do? *The Hasting Center Report 44*, 11-14. https://www.jstor.org/stable/44159112.

Dreisinger, N. & Zapolsky, N. (2018). Complexities of consent: Ethics in the pediatric emergency department. *Pediatric Emergency Care 34*(4), 288-290.

Duff, R.S. & Campbell, A.G.M. (1973). Moral and ethical dilemmas in the special care nursery. *New England Journal of Medicine 289*: 890–894. doi: doi:10.1056/NEJM197310252891705.

Edwards, K.M. & Hackell, J(2016). The Committee on Infectious Diseases, & The Committee on Practice and Ambulatory Medicine. (2016). Countering vaccine hesitancy. *Pediatrics 138*(3):e20162146. Retrieved from http://pediatrics.aappublications.org/content/pediatrics/138/3/e20162146.full.pdf. Accessed February 1, 2019.

El-Hattab, A.W.; Almannai, M. & Sutton, V.R. (2018). Newborn screening: History, current status, and future directions. *Pediatric Clinics of North America 65*, 389–405. https://doi.org/10.1016/j.pcl.2017.11.013.

Fisher, M.A. (2011). Ethics for the pediatrician: caring for abused children. *Pediatrics in Review 32*(7): e73-78. doi: 10.1542/pir.32-7-e73.

Gilmour, J.; Harrison, C.; Asadi, L.; Cohen, M.H. & Vohra, S. (2011). Childhood immunization: when physicians and parents disagree. *Pediatrics 128*, Suppl 4: S167–174. doi: 10.1542/peds.2010-2720E.

Guillen, U. & Kirpalani, H. (2017). Ethical implications of the use of decision aids for antenatal counseling at the limits of gestational viability. *Seminars in Fetal & Neonatal Medicine 23*, 25-29. https://doi.org/10.1016/j.siny.2017.10.002.

Gladsjo, J.A.; Breding, J.; Sine, D.; Wells, R.; Kalemkiarian, S.; Oak, J. & Friedlander, S.F. (2004). Termination of life support after severe child abuse: the role of a guardian ad litem. *Pediatrics, 113*(2): e141–145. doi: 10.1542/peds.113.2.e141.

Goldman, E.B. & Quint, E.H. (2011). Arguments against sterilization of developmentally disabled minors. *Journal of Child Neurology 26*(5): 654–656. doi: 10:1177/0883073811402077.

Guttmacher Institute (2019). State policies in brief: An overview of minors consent law. Available at https://www.guttmacher.org/state-policy/explore/overview-minors-consent-law.

Health Resource and Services Administration. (2018). ACHDNC recommended uniform screening panel Retrieved from https://www.hrsa.gov/advisory-committees/heritable-disorders/rusp/index.html Accessed Feb 1, 2019.

Hendrix, K.S.; Sturm, L.A.; Zimet, G.D. & Meslin, E.M. (2016). Ethics and childhood vaccination policy in the United States. *American Journal of Public Health, 106*(2), 273–278. doi: 10.2105/AJPH.2015.302952.

Hill, H.A.; Elam-Evans, L.D.; Yankey, D.; Singleton, J.A. & Kang, Y. (2018) Vaccination coverage among children aged 19–35 months — United States, 2017. *MMWR Morbidity and Mortality Weekly Report 67*, 1123–1128. DOI: http://dx.doi.org/10.15585/mmwr.mm6740a4.

Hussain, H.; Omer, S.B.; Manganello, J.A.; Kromm, E.E.; Carter, T.C.; Kan, L. & Salmon, D.A. (2011). Immunization safety in US print media, 1995–2005. *Pediatrics 127*: S100-S106. doi:10.1542/peds.2010-1722O.

Janvier, A.; Bauer, K.L. & Lantos, J.D. (2007). Are newborns morally different from older children? *Theoretical Medicine and Bioethics 28*: 413–425. doi: 10.1007/s11017-00709052-y.

Jent, J.G.; Eaton, C.K.; Merrick, MT; Englebert, N; Dandes, S; Chaptman, AV & Hershorin, ER (2011). The decision to access patient information from a social media site: what would you do? *Journal of Adolescent Health 49*(4): 414–420. http://dx.doi.org/10.1016/j.adohealth.2011.02.004.

John, R (2007). Beneficence, prescriptions, and the nurse practitioner. *Advance for Nurse Practitioner 15*: 55–57.

Kennedy, A.; Basket, M. & Sheedy, K. (2011). Vaccine attitudes, concerns, and information sources reported by parents of young children: results from the 2009 Health Styles survey. *Pediatrics 127*: S92–S99. doi:10.1542/peds.2010-1722N.

Kirsch, R. & Munson, D. (2018). Ethical and end of life considerations for neonates requiring ECMO support. *Seminars in Perinatology 42*, 129-137. https://doi.org/10.1053/j.semperi.2017.12.009.

Kopelman, L.M.; Irons, T.G. & Kopelman, A.E. (1988). Neonatologists judge the 'Baby doe' regulations. *The New England Journal of Medicine 318*: 677–683. doi:10.1056/NEJM198803173181105.

Kopelman, L. & Kopelman, A. (2007). Using a new analysis of the Best Interest Standard to address cultural disputes: whose data, which values? *Theoretical Medicine and Bioethics 28*: 373–391. doi: 10.1007/s11017-9050-0.

Kulkarni, R.; Scott-Emuakpor, A.B.; Brody, H.; Weil, W.B.; Ragni, M.V. & Gera, R. (2001). Nondisclosure of human immunodeficiency virus and hepatitis C virus coinfection in a patient with hemophilia: medical and ethical considerations. *Journal of Pediatric Hematology and Oncology 23*(3): 153–158.

Ladd, R.E. & Forman, E.N. (2010). Ethics for the pediatrician: pediatrician/patient/parent relationships. *Pediatrics in Review 31*(9): e65-67. doi: 10.1542/pir.31-9-e65.

Lantos, J. (2018). Ethical problems in decision making in the neonatal ICU. *The New England Journal of Medicine. 379*, 1851-60. DOI: 10.1056/NEJMra1801063.

Lenhart, A. & Madden, M. (2007). Social networking site and teens, Pew Internet and American Life Projects. Available at http://www.pewinternet.org/Reports/2007/Social-Networking-Websites-and-Teens.aspx. Accessed July 20, 2012.

Lehavot, K.; Barnett, J.E. & Powers, D. (2010). Psychotherapy, professional relationships, and ethical considerations in the myspace generation. *Professional Psychology: Research and Practice 41*(2): 160–166. doi:10.1037/a0018709.

Mercurio, M.R. (2010). Ethics for the pediatrician: imperiled newborns: limiting treatment. *Pediatrics in Review 31*(2): 72–75. doi: 10.1542/pir.31-2-72.

Mercurio, M.R.; Adam, M.B.; Forman, E.N.; Ladd, R.E.; Ross, L.F. & Silber, T.J. (2008). American Academy of Pediatrics policy statements on bioethics: summaries and commentaries: part 1. *Pediatrics in Review 29*(1): e1-8. doi: 10.1542/pir.29-1-e1.

Mercurio, M.R.; Forman, E.N.; Ladd, R.E.; Maxwell, M.A.; Ross, L.F. & Silber, T.J. (2008). American Academy of Pediatrics policy statements on bioethics: summaries and commentaries: part 3. *Pediatrics in Review 29*(5): e28-34. doi: 10.1542/pir.29-5-e28.

Mercurio, M.R.; Maxwell, M.A.; Mears, B.J.; Ross, L.F. & Silber, T.J. (2008). American Academy of Pediatrics policy statements on bioethics: summaries and commentaries: part 2. *Pediatrics in Review 29*(3): e15-22. doi: 10.1542/pir.29-3-e15.

Michaud, P.A.; Blum, R.W.; Benaroyo, L.; Zermatten, J. & Baltag, V. (2015). Assessing an Adolescent's Capacity for Autonomous Decision-Making in Clinical Care. *Journal of Adolescent Health 57*, e361-e366. http://dx.doi.org/10.1016/j.jadohealth.2015.06.012.

Morse S.B., Haywood J.L., Goldenberg R.L., Bronstein J., Nelson K.G., Carlo W.A. (2000). Estimation of neonatal outcome and perinatal therapy use. Pediatrics, 105, 1046-1050.

National Consensus Project for Quality Palliative Care. Clinical Practice Guidelines for Quality Palliative Care, 4th edition. Richmond, VA: National Coalition for Hospice and Palliative Care; 2018. https://www. nationalcoalitionhpc.org/ncp.

National Conference of State Legislators. (2019). States with religious and philosophical exemptions from school immunization requirements. Available at http://www.ncsl.org/research/health/school-immunization-exemption-state-laws.aspx Retrieved on February 3, 2019.

National Newborn Screening and Genetic Resource Center. (2019). National Newborn Screening Status Report: Updated 11/2/2014. Available at: http://genes-r-us.uthscsa.edu/sites/genes-r-us/files/nbsdisorders.pdf. Retrieved February 5, 2019.

Okun, A. (2010). Ethics for the pediatrician: Children who have special health-care needs: ethical issues. *Pediatrics in Review 31*(12): 514–517. doi: 10.1542/pir.31-12-514.

Omer, S.B.; Salmon, D.A.; Orenstein, W.A.; deHart, M.P. & Halsey, N. (2009). Vaccine refusal, mandatory immunization, and the risks of vaccine-preventable diseases. *New England Journal of Medicine 360*(19): 1981–1988. doi: doi:10.1056/NEJMsa0806477.

Paris, J.J.; Schreiber, M.D. & Moreland, M. (2007). Parental refusal of medical treatment for a newborn. *Theoretical Medicine and Bioethics 28*: 427–442. Doi: 10.1007/s11017-007-9046-9.

Powell, M.R.; Kim, U.O.; Weisgerber, M.C.; Simpson, P.M.; Nugent, M. & Basir, M.A. (2012). Readiness of obstetric professionalsto inform parents regarding potential outcome of premature infants. *Journal of Obstetrics & Gynaecology 32*(4), 326-331. https://doi.org/10.3109/01443615.2012:656743.

Pless, J. (1983). The story of baby doe. *The New England Journal of Medicine 309*: 664.

Rose, C.D. (2017). Ethical Conduct of Research in Children: pediatricians and their IRB (Part 1 of 2). *Pediatrics 139*(5), 39(5):e20163648. DOI: 10.1542/peds.2016-3648.

Rose, C.D. (2017b). Ethical conduct of research in children: pediatricians and their IRB (Part 2 of 2). *Pediatrics 139*(6), e20163650. DOI: 10.1542/peds.2016-3648.

Rosenfeld, M.; Sontag, M.K.; Ren, C.L. (2016). Cystic fibrosis diagnosis and newborn screening. *Pediatric Clinics of North America 63*, 599–615. http://dx.doi.org/10.1016/j.pcl.2016.04.004.

Ross, L.F. (2008). Ethical and policy issues in pediatric genetics. *American Journal of Medical Genetics C Seminars in Medical Genetics, 148C*(1): 1–7. doi: 10.1002/ajmg.c.30162.

Ross, L.F. & Clayton, E.W. (2009). Clinical and ethical considerations in managing carrier detection. *American Journal of Public Health 99*(8): 1348–1349. doi: 10.2105/ajph.2009.161554.

Ross, L.F. & Frader, J. (2009). Hypoplastic left heart syndrome: A paradigm case for examining conscientious objection in pediatric practice. *The Journal of Pediatrics 155*(1): 12–15. doi:10.1016/j.jpeds.2009.03.008.

Ross, L.F. (2015). Theory and practice of Pediatric bioethics. *Perspectives in Biology and Medicine 58*(3), 267-280. DOI: https://doi.org/10.1353/pbm.2016.0008.

Ross, P.; Leigh D. & Anthony, H. (2018). Palliative care in adolescents and young adults with cancer—Why do adolescents need special attention. *The Cancer Journal 24*(6), 336-341 doi: 10.1097/PPO.0000000000000341.

Rothstein, M. (2018). Time to End the Use of Genetic Test: Current in contemporary bioethics. *The Journal of Law, Medicine & Ethics 46* (2018): 794-801. DOI: 10.1177/1073110518804243.

Section on Hospice and Palliative Medicine, and Hospital Care, (2013). Pediatric palliative care and hospice care commitments, guidelines, and recommendations, *Pediatrics 132*(5), 966-972. DOI: 10.1542/peds.2013-2731.

Seither R.; Calhoun K.; Street E.J.; Mellerson, J.; Knighton, C.L.; Tippins, A. & Underwood, J.M. (2017). Vaccination coverage for selected vaccines, exemption rates, and provisional enrollment among children in kindergarten — United States, 2016–17 School Year. *MMWR Morbidity & Mortality Weekly Report 66*, 1073–1080. DOI: http://dx.doi.org/10.15585/mmwr.mm6640a3.

Shaw, A.J.; Randolph, J. & Maynard, B. (1977). Ethical issues in pediatric surgery: a national survey of pediatricians and pediatric surgeons. *Pediatrics 60*: 588–593.

Simpson, E. (2007, March). Kaine signs 'Abraham's law' bill on choice to refuse treatment. *The Virginia Pilot*. Available at http://hamptonroads.com/node/240161.

Tan, S.S. & Goonawardene, N. (2017). Internet Health information seeking and the patient physician relationship: A systematic review. *Journal of Medical Internet Research 19*(1), e9. doi: 10.2196/jmir.5729: 10.2196/jmir.5729.

Todres, I.D.; Krane, D.; Howell, M.C. & Shannon, D.C (1977). Pediatricians' attitudes affecting decision-making in defective newborns. *Pediatrics 60*: 197–202.

Yan, H. & Goldschmidt, D. (2019). Washington measles outbreak climbs while other states grapple with the disease. Retrieved from https://www.cnn.com/2019/02/04/health/washington-measles-outbreak/index.html. Accessed February 6, 2019.

Zawistowski, C.A.; Black, C.; Spruill, T. & Granowetter, L. (2018). Parental Knowledge and Opinions on Palliative Care for Children. *Pediatrics 141*(1).

CHAPTER 7

Ethics and Women's Health

CAROLINE M. HEWITT

Advocates of comprehensive women's reproductive health believe in a woman's decision to have a safe and satisfying sexual life including safe motherhood, access to diagnosis and treatment of sexually transmitted infections, management of reproductive tract malignancies, and protection against gender discrimination, gender inequity and inequality. Women—more specifically, their potential for reproduction—are often at the center of an ethical and political maelstrom. It is therefore important to understand the significance of the ongoing domestic and global debates surrounding women's reproductive rights. This chapter will discuss two prevailing ethical approaches supporting women's right to reproductive health: Feminist Bioethics and Public Health Ethics. Also discussed will be the current United States' legislative climate concerning women's reproductive rights and freedoms. Case studies will be presented at the end of the chapter applying both principles of feminist bioethics and public health ethics within our current health care environment.

7.1. FEMINIST BIOETHICS

Thomas Beauchamp and James Childress developed their influential approach to bioethics based upon the application of four general moral principles particular to ethical problems: autonomy, justice, nonmaleficence and beneficence (Beauchamp & Childress, 2009; Dodds, 2000). Despite Beauchamp and Childress's insistence that all four principles have a role to play in bioethics, some philosophers have argued that autonomy has become "the first among equals" (Beauchamp & Childress, 2009, p. 216). To quote from Beauchamp and Childress, regarding their definition of autonomy:

Autonomy is to be understood as 'personal rule of the self that is free from both controlling interferences by others and from personal limitations that prevent meaningful choice, such as inadequate understanding'. The principle of respect for autonomy requires respecting those choices made by individuals whose decisions are free from external interference or personal limitations (2009, p. 99).

From a feminist perspective, the definition of autonomy provided by Beauchamp and Childress, with its emphasis on informed consent, is narrow and does not fully reflect women's experiences. For Dodds (2000), the notion of informed consent—within the paternalistic society in which we live and given the cultural association between "femininity" and "irrationality"—may actually limit women's autonomy. Feminist bioethics, therefore, is an attempt to reshape the 'conceptual terrain' on which women, and others subject to oppressive social conditions, are expected to make health care decisions; it is a discipline focused on identifying those features of healthcare that exacerbate, or ameliorate, oppression (Dodds, 2000). Feminist philosopher Susan Sherwin argues that feminist bioethics must be understood as an ethics of the oppressed:

"Feminists share a recognition that women are oppressed in our society and understanding that their oppression takes many different forms, compounded often by other forms of oppression based on features such as race, ethnicity, sexual orientation, and economic class. Because feminists believe that oppression is objectionable on both moral and political grounds, most are committed to transforming society in ways that will ensure the elimination of oppression in all its forms." (Sherwin, 1992, p. 48).

7.1.1. Personhood

Control over a woman's reproductive life is an issue of concern in both feminist and public health bioethics. Whether about women's autonomy or welfare of a larger society, reproductive choices like abortion or the use of contraception continue to be debated nationally and internationally. Feminist bioethics is concerned with identifying and ameliorating features of health care which exacerbate oppression. The current United States abortion debate pits the rights of women against the rights of the fetus, also known as autonomy versus the moral rights of the fetus (Gibson, 2004). The essential conflict revolves around the disagreement over the moral status (personhood) of the fetus. According to Gibson (2004), there are three basic positions regarding the moral status of the fetus: conservative, moderate and liberal. The conservative view is that the fetus has a right to life from the moment of conception;

the more moderate view is that the fetus comes into the possession of the right to life at some stage during pregnancy and the liberal view is that the fetus does not, at any stage of gestation, have a right to life. The abortion debate, therefore, is not so much over women's rights, but rather over the moral status of the fetus (Gibson, 2004).

Gibson (2004) goes on to suggest that the argument over fetal moral status rests on the concept of personhood, yet this very concept is essentially contested. As described by the three positions regarding the definition of fetal moral status, there is ongoing debate over the definition of personhood. When disagreement exists over the proper use of a concept or when no exemplar exists—and this concept is fundamental to the abortion debate—then, Gibson argues, this debate is irresolvable (2004).

7.1.2. Moral Absolutists

For those who approach the definition of the concept of personhood from a conservative position (commonly referred to as pro-life or anti-choice), fetal life begins at conception, and there is little ambiguity in the abortion debate. Taking a deontological approach to ethics—that is, an ethics consisting of duty and moral obligation—abortion is wrong. This conservative position is fundamentally deontological in its reliance on a single moral rule: do not kill. This is in opposition to teleological ethics which acknowledges more subtlety in the gradations between right and wrong. In other words, deontological ethics are concerned with determining the rightness or wrongness of actions, while teleological ethics are concerned with determining the goodness or badness of actions (Lake, 1985). In teleological ethics, actions themselves assume their distinctively moral character by virtue of their adherence to the rules. For these moral absolutists, circumstances have no bearing on the morality of abortion, including in cases of endangerment of a mother's life or rape. In all cases, abortion is intrinsically wrong by virtue of its violation of the moral rule against killing for a moral absolutist (Lake, 1985).

7.1.3. Relational Autonomy

The difference between non-feminist and feminist approaches to abortion lie in the relative attention each gives in its analysis of the interests and experiences of women. Feminist analysis regards the effects of unwanted pregnancies on the lives of women individually and collectively as a central element in the moral examination of abortion.

Women must be regarded as full moral agents, responsible for making moral decisions about their own pregnancies (Sherwin, 1992). However, the moral status of the fetus needs to be considered as well. As described by Gibson (2004), this 'relational' conception of moral status views the mother and fetus not as two independent beings whose moral claims have to be balanced against one another, but rather focuses on the relationship between the fetus and mother. The moral status of the fetus is unique because a fetus exists only in relationship with a particular other on whom it is entirely dependent for existence. It is because of this relationship that the fetus is morally significant, as it is out of relationships that our moral obligations arise. However, fetuses do not have an absolute value because they have no existence independent of this relationship. Their value is that not of an individual human being, but of a human relationship. Personhood is understood in terms of social relations; for Sherwin, humans are fundamentally relational beings. The self is relational in that each of us develops as a person through our relationships with others. It is the variety of relationships and roles in which a human being participates in their membership of a community that gives them their value as persons (Sherwin, 1992). For feminists, therefore, personhood is understood in terms of social relationships; personhood is our capacity to participate in a variety of relationships. This feminist definition of autonomy is a re-working, rather than a rejection, of the Kantian ethics. Autonomy is viewed as something that resides in the individual self. But as the self is constituted and re-constituted within a network of relationships, so too is the capacity for autonomy (Gibson, 2004).

7.2. PUBLIC HEALTH ETHICS

Bioethics evolved around key principals of respect for persons—including the autonomy of persons capable of self-determination and protection of those who are incapable—the duty to do good (beneficence) and to do no harm (non-malfeasance) and justice. Public health ethics can be regarded as "macro" beneficence (Dickens and Cook, 2007). Whereas bioethics is concerned with protecting the rights of the individual through informed consent, in public health, consent comes from legislated authority or from governmental mandates to protect populations from harm (Dickens and Cook, 2007).

Utilitarianism is generally the moral theory most often applied to matters of public health. Utilitarianism is the moral theory concerned with the consequences of actions; the good consequence being that which most positively affects the greatest number of people. Utilitarians value well-being and accept only one principle of ethics: the principle of utility, the good to be maximized (Beauchamp and Childress, 2009). Hedonistic Utilitarians, such as Jeremy Bentham and John Stuart Mill, view utility entirely in terms of happiness or pleasure. More recent utilitarian philosophers argue that values other than happiness—knowledge, health, success, and enjoyment, for example—also contribute to well-being. This principle has been translated into the formula of doing the greatest good for the greatest number, and therefore has obvious applicability in public health policy and service (Beauchamp and Childress, 2009).

Utilitarians disagree whether the principle of utility pertains to particular acts in particular circumstances or to general rules that themselves determine which acts are right and wrong (Beauchamp and Childress, 2009). For 'Act' Utilitarians, the consequence of an act must first be considered. That action which results in the greatest good must be the action chosen. 'Rule' Utilitarians, on the other hand, first look to ethical rules which then direct the action to be taken.

7.2.1. Reproductive Health

Global unity concerning the urgency of improving women's reproductive health and rights is reflected in the historic 1994 International Conference on Population and Development (ICPD) held in Cairo, Egypt. Confirmation of the fundamental rights of women and men was later made at the 1995 International Conference on Women in Beijing, China (Townsend, 2007). Both of these conferences recognized that reproductive health failures embodied in unsafe childbearing involve more than just clinical medicine and must also be addressed as public health concerns (Cook & Dickens, 2002).

Generally, reproductive health implies that people are able to have a satisfying and safe sex life, the capacity to reproduce, and the freedom to decide, if, and when, and how often to do so. This concept of reproductive health offers a comprehensive and integrated approach to health needs related to reproduction. It places women at the center of the process, and recognizes, respects and responds to the needs of all women, not only those of mothers. The 1988 World Health Organization (WHO) definition of reproductive health was adopted and expanded at the ICPD and International Conference on Women. It reads:

"Reproductive health is a state of complete physical, mental and social well-being and not merely the absence of disease or infirmity, in all mat-

ters relating to the reproductive system and to its functions and process-
es. Reproductive health therefore implies that people are able to have a
satisfying and safe sex life and that they have the capacity to reproduce
and the freedom to decide if, when and how often to do so. Implicit in this
last condition are the right of men and women to be informed and to have
access to safe, effective, affordable and acceptable methods of family
planning of their choice for regulation of fertility which are not against
the law, and the right of access to appropriate health-care services that
will enable women to go safely through pregnancy and childbirth and
provide couples with the best chance of having a healthy infant." (UN,
1995)

Within this context, reproductive health care is defined as the con-
stellation of methods, techniques and services that contribute to reproductive health and well-being by preventing and solving reproductive
health problems. It also includes sexual health, the purpose of which is
the enhancement of life and personal relations, and not merely counseling care related to reproduction and sexually transmitted diseases
(Cook, Dickens & Fathalia, 2008).

7.2.2. Safe Motherhood

A major burden for females is related to their reproductive function
and reproductive potential. Reproduction is not a disease (Cook, Dickens & Fathalia, 2008). A list of reproductive health indicators is as follows:

* Safe motherhood
* Fertility by choice (contraception, abortion)
* Sexually transmitted infections
* Female genital cutting (circumcision/mutilation)
* Infertility
* Cancers of the Reproductive Tract

The differential incidence of unsafe motherhood has been described
as making the greatest discrepancy in any health statistic between developed and developing countries worldwide (Cook and Dickens,
2002). It is estimated that every year worldwide, about 515,000 women
die of complications of pregnancy and childbirth. Furthermore, at least
7 million women suffer serious health problems after childbirth, and
an additional estimated 50 million women suffer adverse health effects
after childbirth (Cook & Dickens, 2002). To put these figures in context
of developed and developing countries, the risk of pregnancy-related

death for a Canadian woman is 1 in 8,700 compared to that of a woman in Rwanda which is 1 in 6 (Cook & Dickens, 2002). Safe motherhood depends on women's avoidance of untimely and otherwise inappropriate pregnancy.

Unsafe or otherwise unwanted pregnancies may result in unsafe abortions, either because abortion is not legally and safely available or, if legally available, there are no qualified practitioners to provide it; these situations raise obvious ethical concerns. The above-cited 1994 and 1995 watershed conferences both addressed the public health implications of unsafe abortion. The 1994 Cairo ICPD resolved "to strengthen their commitment to women's health to deal with the health impact of unsafe abortion as a major public health concern and to reduce the recourse to abortion through expanded and improved family planning services" (Cook & Dickens, 2002). The 1995 Beijing Conference developed a platform for action which resolved, "unsafe abortions threaten the lives of a large number of women, representing a grave public health problem as it is primarily the poorest and the youngest who take the highest risk" (Cook & Dickens, 2002).

7.3. CASE STUDIES

Two prevailing ethical approaches, feminist bioethics and public health ethics, recognize the centrality of women's experiences. There exist overlap in themes and interests between feminist bioethics and public health ethics, specifically that of the experience of the disenfranchised, which includes feelings of powerlessness and repression. Feminist and reproductive health advocates support and echo each other's concerns and approaches and similar ethical principles are argued from both perspectives. However, for purposes of academic purity, the following case studies will be presented from a feminist bioethical approach separately from public health (utilitarian) approaches.

7.3.1. Personhood and Partial Molar Pregnancy

Catherine, a 36 year old biochemist, and devout Roman Catholic, was thrilled to learn she was pregnant with her second child. She and her husband had been trying to get pregnant for the last six months. However, the couple was devastated to learn at the initial prenatal visit and sonogram, that this pregnancy was considered a "partial molar" and the viability of the fetus uncertain. Incidence of spontaneous abortion is high, and the likelihood of the birth of a viable fetus is very low. Partial molar pregnancies increase the risks of maternal preeclampsia, hypertension, hyperemesis and hyperthyroidism (Chiang and Berek, 2010). Catherine is faced with an ethical dilemma: who has a greater moral status, mother or fetus? Should Catherine proceed with an abortion or proceed with the pregnancy despite the risks to her own health and the very low likelihood of a viable infant? Catherine believes fully with the conservative view of personhood; that is, Catherine believes that life begins at the moment of conception. Even faced with the low likelihood that this fetus will be viable, for Catherine, conception has occurred and life exists; therefore, to do anything to interfere with this pregnancy is tantamount to murder. Catherine views herself as a faithful Catholic who will do all in her power to follow the teachings of the Church. For Catherine, to follow the rules of the Church is more important than any circumstances which may interfere with this moral absolutism, even the potential for her own mortality.

Catherine's husband, Bob, however, does not share Catherine's moral absolutism. Bob is a feminist. Bob believes that personhood can only be understood in terms of social relationships. Since Catherine's fetus is only a fetus, and therefore unable to engage in any relationship other than the one with Catherine, and Catherine is an adult fully capable in engaging in many complex relationships, Catherine, therefore, holds a greater moral status than her fetus. Like Catherine, Bob understands the low likelihood that the pregnancy will ultimately progress to a viable infant, and he too understands the health risks for Catherine should she continue with the pregnancy. Bob reasons that Catherine holds a greater moral status than the fetus and therefore it is Catherine's right to exercise her own autonomy, and within a feminist bioethical framework, it is ethical for Catherine to choose to terminate her pregnancy. Bob further reasons that because Catherine is a full moral agent, responsible for making moral decisions about her own pregnancy, should she decide to continue with the pregnancy, based upon her own moral reasoning, then that is her own right.

What ethical principles are involved? How would you as a provider help them with a decision? What are your legal and ethical responsibilities to the patient? The fetus? The father?

7.3.2. Utility in Family Planning

Maria is a nurse practitioner working in a county health department's family planning clinic. She has just walked into an exam room to be greeted by a very nervous 16 year old female who wants contraception. The client reports being sexually active for six months with one partner and is using condoms inconsistently for contraception. Maria has an ethical dilemma: should she perform her "typical" new patient gyne-cologic exam (which includes a pelvic exam, pap smear and collection of cervical cultures for screening of sexually transmitted diseases) or follow the updated practice guidelines which negate the need to per-form the above mentioned test in the traditional manner? Needing some context through which to think through this dilemma, Maria decides to apply the moral theory of Utilitarianism to help guide her practice.

Utilitarians themselves disagree whether the principal of utility per-tains to particular acts in particular circumstances or to general rules that themselves determine which acts are right and wrong (Beauchamp & Childress, 2009). For Act Utilitarians, the consequence of an act must first be considered. That action which results in the greatest good must therefore be the action chosen. Rule utilitarians, on the other hand, first look to ethical rules which then direct the action to be taken. Maria needs to consider each type of utilitarianism within the context of her dilemma. Would following one or the other type of utilitarianism lead to a different outcome or a similar outcome?

7.3.3. Act Utilitarianism

"What would be the consequence of not performing the traditional exam", asks Maria, "which action would lead to the greatest happi-ness or well-being for the greatest number"? The most obvious and most directly experienced happiness would be enjoyed by the client. Maria imagines the client would be relieved she did not have to endure this uncomfortable, invasive and extremely embarrassing examination. Another positive outcome would be economic. From a bioethical utili-tarian perspective, not performing the exam would more efficiently al-locate limited healthcare resources: time and supplies. By not having to perform the exam, Maria would be spending less time with this client visit and thus have more time to attend to the 10 clients waiting to be seen. In terms of other resources, by not using the liquid-based pap now, it would be available for another client, for whom the pap test is indicated (according to national guidelines). The cost to the state labo-ratory would also be less. This is one less test to be run and interpreted both by the technician and pathologist. Lastly, supplies required to per-form the pap would not be used; neither disposable speculum supplies nor the staff time and energy required to clean and sterilize the equip-ment would be required.

In addition to the two positive consequences of following the updat-ed practice guidelines, Maria can also think of a negative consequence of this action. The remote possibility exists, reasons Maria, that this adolescent client could have an asymptomatic gynecologic neoplasm, which by virtue of not performing the full gynecologic exam, could be missed. This would be an undesirable consequence of not performing the traditional exam.

7.3.4. Rule Utilitarianism

Opposed to Act Utilitarianism, which is concerned with the consequence of actions, Rule Utilitarianism is concerned with rules as guidance for actions. The action of following the rule, opposed to the consequence of the action, is the motivation for Rule Utilitarianism. For Maria, the most obvious rule, in this context, is to do no harm. The principle of nonmaleficence is commonly used as the guiding principle in biomedical ethics (Beauchamp & Childress, 2009). Using the same process she used in examining her actions, Maria attempts to reason through which approach—to perform the exam or not to perform the exam—would cause the least harm. Maria is unsure if she should only consider potential harm for the client, or if she should consider potential harm to herself, as well. She reasoned that within the context of the rule of utility, if harm came to herself, the clinician, then she would be unavailable to care for other people in need, and thus would not be following rule utilitarianism.

In regards to what harm could be done to Maria if she were not to perform the exam, the harm would be financial. Most health insurance reimbursement rates to clinicians are based on time spent with the client as well as number of body systems examined. If no pelvic exam was performed, then Maria would bill the client's insurance company a lower fee. Less money would be coming into the clinic and less money paid to the clinician. "If do not perform the lengthier and more complex exam, I make less money and therefore will not be able to afford to continue to work in a public clinic and provide care to this underserved population," reasons Maria.

"Do no harm", thinks Maria, "what if I miss one of those asymptomatic gynecologic cancers? Although it is such a remote possibility, I still have to acknowledge the existence of that very small risk. It certainly would be harmful to the client if I were to miss a cancer."

Maria considered two potentially harmful outcomes for not performing the exam, and she now considers how not performing the exam would "do no harm" to the client. By not performing the exam, Maria would be avoiding inflicting discomfort (perhaps even pain), and embarrassment (perhaps trauma) on this individual. Before considering her arguments both through Act and Rule Utilitarianism, Maria wants to review the strength of the evidence which informed these "new national guidelines".

7.3.5. Implications for Practice

Maria has thought long and hard about how to best care for this client. Using utilitarianism as a guide, Maria has considered the consequence of her decision not to perform a pelvic exam. She has also considered what least harm will befall herself and the client if she were to follow the principal of nonmaleficence. Maria has also considered the current clinical evidence and national guidelines pertaining to adolescent reproductive health care.

In reviewing her arguments, Maria recalls how she thought of two positive consequences, in term of happiness for the greatest number, if she were to not perform the exam; the client would be happy and fewer health resources, including her own time, would be used. Maria does continue to worry about the very small risk that she may miss an asymptomatic gynecologic cancer. If she were to follow the principal of nonmaleficence, Maria imagines the greatest benefit to the client, in term of no harm, from not performing the exam. She does acknowledge the decrease in revenue by providing a shorter, less extensive visit, but she did not take a job in a public health clinic to get rich. Worrying about reimbursement when providing care at a clinic in which the majority of clients have no health insurance at all seems to be wrong, thinks Maria.

The risk of missing a gynecologic cancer would most certainly be doing harm. This thought haunts Maria. However, the risk of an adolescent presenting with an asymptomatic gynecologic cancer is extremely unlikely; studies looking at gynecologic cancers classify "young" as less than 50 years (Grimes & Wallach, 1997). Also, considers Maria, the public health system is based upon allocation of limited resources to those at greatest risk. "I need to be more concerned about this client getting pregnant than I do having a rare vulvar cancer, and therefore I need to do everything in my power to provide evidence based, nonjudgmental care and education and ensure she will return to follow-up visits. Whether I follow Act or Rule Utilitarianism, both approaches seem to bring me to the same conclusion: I will follow the current evidenced-based practice and not perform the traditional pap."

Maria explains to the client that she did not need to perform a pelvic exam, but spends the time educating the client about contraception, STD prevention and safer sex practices. She collects a urine sample for screening of chlamydia and gonorrhea and a pregnancy test since the client reported inconsistent condom use. Maria prescribes oral contraceptive pills. The client is very pleased with the time and consideration she receives; she feels Maria really listened and feels secure she was prescribed the very best contraception for her.

7.3.6. Utility in Infertility

Issues relating to reproduction are often ethically fraught. Matters relating to assisted reproduction are medically complicated, financially expensive and present several ethical dilemmas. Assisted reproduction invites concerns of custom, culture, religion and personal freedom and when complex and expensive technologies are added to the mix, the ethical dilemma become even more complicated.

This third case study presents a reproductive choice scenario and discusses it from a Utility bioethical approach. Francis is a 43 year old single mother of a 14 year old daughter, and who is seeking fertility treatments to conceive a second child. She has saved enough money from her job as a manager at the local supermarket to pay for the donor sperm. The first two IVF cycles, covered by her health insurance, have been unsuccessful. Francis desires a third IVF cycle that her insurance will not cover. Francis' physician, a reproductive endocrinologist, supports her choice to seek another cycle.

Francis understands that the likelihood of a successful IVF conception is very low, and it has been explained to her both the maternal and fetal risks of pregnancy at her advanced maternal age: hypertension, preeclampsia, gestational diabetes, and preterm birth. Despite these medical risks, and the low likelihood of success, Francis is determined not to give up her dream "of having another child". Francis borrows money from her sister to pay for another IVF cycle.

From a mainstream autonomy perspective, it is Francis' decision alone to reproduce or not. However, from a Utilitarian approach (Act Utiliarianism), the possible consequences of her action (to proceed with another IVF cycle) must be considered. Is continuing with another IVF cycle a 'good action', one which most positively affects the greatest number of people? For Francis, the best consequence will be that she will have a healthy, term infant which will provide fulfillment of her desire to have another child. A 'bad' consequence may be as follows: a twin gestation causing numerous health problems for Francis and/or hypertension and gestational diabetes which might result in Francis' hospitalization for several weeks. If Francis were to develop uncontrollable preeclampsia and subsequently deliver 30 week infant twins, the infant twins would have to remain in the Neonatal Intensive Care Unit (NICU) for ten weeks (while Francis remained in the hospital with complications secondary to a pregnancy- related deep vein thrombosis).

The potential 'bad' consequences would not be experienced by Francis and infants alone. Francis' 14 year old daughter would be required to stay with an elderly uncle while her mother was in the hospital, and might become increasingly despondent during her mother's absence. Francis' health insurance has an inpatient limit and most of her own hospital care and her infants' would not be covered and therefore Francis would be responsible for majority of the costs. What costs Francis would not be able to pay would have to be covered by the hospital itself, which is a publicly funded hospital. Thus the ultimate burden would be paid by the taxpayers. Francis would still be indebt to her sister.

As described in this case, the potential 'bad' consequences are numerous and affect many individuals and communities in addition to Francis. There is no one available to help Francis fully understand the potential consequences of her decision to proceed with another IVF cycle: Francis' physician has an ethically conflicting financial interest should she proceed with another IVF cycle. Francis cannot imagine the complexity of potential pregnancy-related health problems she may experience and Francis does not know that her health insurance plan has an inpatient limit.

Francis desires another child even though the potential consequences of her action to conceive another child through IVF are numerous and harmful. Francis does not fully understand these potential consequences and moves forward with another IVF cycle.

7.4. UNANALYZED CASES

1. Anastasia is a 23 year old woman living in an imaginary country, who has been married for three years and desires contraception. She has had several prior abortions and she fears any further abortions will limit her ability to have a safe pregnancy when she is ready. Abortion in her country is legal, safe and cheap. Contraception in her country, conversely, is expensive and scarce. In fact, the state funded health insurance does not cover contraception, as the population is below replacement level and the state is encouraging larger families. How would a Feminist and Utilitarian address this dilemma? Would their arguments differ or not? Why?

2. Ruby is a 21-year-old woman who is very excited by her recent engagement and upcoming wedding. Ruby is an active member of a conservative evangelical Protestant community and she shares her community's values and cultural habits. One important value for Ruby and her fiancée is that couples refrain from sexual activity until marriage. However, Ruby did have unprotected intercourse with a former boyfriend. Ruby recently went to have her first annual well woman exam, and discovered that she has a high-risk strain of the Human Papilloma Virus (HPV). Her Pap test was normal. The HPV test was ordered in error (per 2018 ACOG guidelines, HPV screening not begin on women until age 30. Ruby now knows that she has a sexually transmitted infection (STI) that she could potentially pass to her future husband. It is unknown what, if any, ill effects this strain of HPV has on men. Should Ruby tell her fiancée that she has an STI, thus admitting she has engaged in sexual activity before marriage? What ethical issues are involved in this case?

7.5. WEBSITES OF INTEREST TO ETHICS AND/OR WOMEN'S HEALTH

- **International Women's Health coalition:**
  https://iwhc.org/
- **World Health Organization – Women's Health:**
  https://www.who.int/topics/womens_health/en/
- **HHS Office of Women's Health:**
  https://www.womenshealth.gov/
- **American Society for Reproductive Medicine:**
  https://www.asrm.org
- **Health Professionals Advancing LGBTQ Equality:**
  https://glma.org
- **NIH Office of Research on Women's Health:**
  https://orwh.od.nih.gov
- **Our Bodies, Our Selves Organization:**
  https://ourbodiesourselves.org
- **Planned Parenthood:**
  https://planedparenthood.org
- **CDC WISEWOMEN Program:**
  https://cdc.gov/wisewomen/
- **Bioethics.com:**
  http://www.bioethics.com/womens-health
- **The Center for Bioethics and Human Dignity:**
  https://cbhd.org/category/issues/womens-health

- **Johns Hopkins Berman Institute of Bioethics:**
  http://www.bioethicsinstitute.org/research/public-health-research/womens-health
- **World Health Organization – Sexual and Reproductive Health:**
  https://www.who.int/reproductivehealth/topics/ethics/gender_guide_serg/en/
- **United Nations Doha Declaration – Module 9 Gender Dimensions of Ethics**
  https://www.unodc.org/e4j/en/integrity-ethics/module-9/key-issues/forms-of-gen der-discrimination.html

7.6. REFERENCES

ACOG (2016). Cervical cancer screening and prevention. Practice Bulletin # 168. *Obstetrics and Gynecology*, 128 (5).

Beauchamps, T.L. & Childress, J.F. (2009). *Principals of Biomedical Ethics*. New York: Oxford.

Chiang, J.W. & Berek, J.S. (2010). Gestational trophoblastic disease: Epidemiology, clinical manifestations and diagnosis. UpToDate. Retrieved from http://www.uptodate.com/contents/gestational-trophoblastic-disease-epidemiology-clinical-manifestations-and-diagnosis?source=search_resultandsearch=hydatiform+moleandsele ctedTitle=2%7E38#H19.

Cook, R.J. & Dickens, B.M. (2002). The injustice of unsafe motherhood. *Developing World Bioethics 2*: 64–81.

Cook, R., Dickens, B., & Fathalla, M. (2008). *Reproductive Health and Human Rights*. New York: Oxford.

Dodds, S. (2000). Choice and control in feminist bioethics. In: *Relational Autonomy* (pp. 213–235). C. Mackenzie and N. Stoljar (eds.). New York: Oxford.

Dickens, B.M. & Cook, R.J. (2007). Reproductive health and public health ethics. *International Journal of Gynecology and Obstetrics 99*: 75–79.

Feldman, S., Sirovich, B.E. & Goodman, A. (2012). Screening for cervical cancer: Rationale and recommendations. UpToDate. Retrieved from http://www.uptodate.com/contents/screening-for-cervical-cancer-rationale-and-recommendations?source=search_resultandsearch=pap+smearandselectedTitle=1 %7E137.

Gibson, S. (2004). The problem of abortion: Essentially contested concepts and moral autonomy. *Bioethics 18*: 221–233.

Grimes, D.A. & Wallach, M. (1997). *The Contraception Report*. New Jersey: Emron, Inc.

Lake, R. (1985). The metaethical framework of anti-abortion rhetoric. *Signs 11*: 478–499.

Mosciki, A.B., Shiboski, S., Hills, N.K., et al. (2004). Regression of low-grade squamous intra-epithelial lesions in young women. *Lancet 364*(9449): 1678–83.

Schlecht, N.F., Platt, R.W., Duarte-Franco, E., et al. (2003). Human papillomavirus infection and time to progression and regression of cervical intraepithelial neoplasia. *Journal of the National Cancer Institute 95*(17): 1336–43.

Shafer, M.A. (1998). Annual pelvic examination in the sexually active adolescent female: what are we doing and why are we doing it? *Journal of Adolescent Health 23*(2): 68–73.

Sherwin, S. (1992). *No Longer Patient: Feminist Ethics and Health Care*. Philadelphia: Temple.

Szarewski, A. & Sasieni, P. (2004). Cervical screening in adolescents—at least do no harm. *Lancet 364*(9446): 1642–4.

Townsend, J.W. (2007). Learning through conflict: Ethical debates in sexual and reproductive health. *Studies in Family Planning 38*: 225–228.

UN, Department of Public Information. (1995). *Platform for Action and Beijing Declaration, Fourth World Conference on Women*, Beijing, China, 4–15 September 1995. New York: UN.

Workowski, K.A., and Berman, S.M. (2006). Sexually transmitted disease treatment guidelines. *MMWR Recommendation Report, 55*(RR-11): 1–94.

CHAPTER 8

Ethical Business Practices Overview

JENNIFER A. SMITH
ANNE G. PEIRCE

8.1. INTRODUCTION

"In the evolutionary shift toward managed care, practitioners have been asked to embrace business values of efficiency and cost effectiveness, sometimes at the expense of their professional judgment and personal values. While some of these changes have been inevitable as our society sought to rein in out-of-control costs, it is not unreasonable for practitioners to call on payers, regulators and other parties to the health care delivery system to raise their ethical bar."
—D. Marcinko, The Business of Medical Practice, 2005

While not every nurse will set up his or her own practice, all will work within the context of a healthcare system that uses common business models and many will interact with insurance/managed care companies. Most health care professionals do not enter the field because they are intrigued by business or finance; in fact, to some it is considered 'anti-professional' to be concerned with the 'money end' of patient care. Nevertheless, it is important for providers to have a basic understanding of the financial under-pinning of the practices in which they work and the ethical and legal framework on which this is based. This chapter is meant to provide such an overview. While some examples described in this chapter may be physician-based, the principles apply to advanced practice nurses as well. It is to be hoped in the future that professional guidelines will cover some if not all of these subjects. Because of the diverseness of particular subject matter, individual topics are presented in alphabetical order for ease of reference.

8.2. ACCOUNTING

Kidder (2015) writes that, "The microscope on an organization's ethical standards often highlights it's financial decisions, and these are a direct result of financial reporting and judgments of accounting professionals." Financial information about a business is transmitted to the public via many mechanisms, foremost of which is accountancy, defined by the American Institute of Certified Public Accountants (AIPCA.org, accessed 2019) as "the art of recording, classifying and summarizing in a significant manner and in terms of money, transactions and events which are, in part at least, of financial character, and interpreting the results thereof." The principles of accounting, the language of business, apply equally to healthcare institutions and practices, both for profit and non-profit.

The accounting profession is guided by its own code of ethics, and those that utilize the services of accounting firms should expect that these codes are enforced and followed. Just as in other fields, these codes are meant to provide users of these services with the confidence that the work provided is ethically sound. There are three major accounting associations, including the American Institute of Certified Public Accountants (AICPA), the Institute of Management Accountants (IMA), and the Institute of Internal Auditors (IIA); all have codes of ethics which apply to their members. These codes of professional conduct direct behavior and provide guidelines for ethical performance, often above and beyond required laws and regulations (Duska and Duska, 2003). Similar to medical/nursing codes of ethics, all three of these accounting associations' codes require that accounting professionals must maintain client/professional confidentiality, possess professional competence and act with integrity and objectivity. Obviously, conflicts of interest may arise if an accountant has a vested interest in the company he/she is auditing or if the results of an audit may not be beneficial to the company, but are important for the shareholders to know, as it affects their investment.

Generally Accepted Accounting Principles (GAAP) are rules which currently frame financial accounting in the United States and are the basis for determining how accounting procedures are carried out. These are rules-based, as opposed to standards developed by the International Accounting Standards Board's International Financial Reporting Standards (IFRS), which are based on principles requiring professional judgment. Because of this, there is some question as to whether this is the proper basis for deciding accounting decisions; i.e., there is no context in which to inform decisions (Somerville, 2003). Work has been underway for several years by the Securities and Exchange Commission (SEC) to integrate IFRS and GAAP but as of 2017, it remains ongoing (https://www.sec.gov/news/statement/white-2016-01-05.html).

Multiple large financial scandals in the 1980s and 90s (Enron, AIG, Arthur Anderson, etc.) (Alexander et al., 2002) resulted not only in companies going out of business, but also the large accounting firms who were responsible for faulty/unethical accounting practices. In response, Congress passed the Sarbanes-Oxley Act of 2002 (also known as the Public Company Accounting Reform and Investor Protection Act of 2002). Sarbanes-Oxley is "to protect investors by improving the accuracy and reliability of corporate disclosures made pursuant to the securities laws . . ." and covers "public company accounting oversight board, auditor independence, corporate responsibility, enhanced financial disclosures, analyst conflicts of interest, commission resources and authority, studies and reports, corporate and criminal fraud accountability, white collar crime penalty enhancements, corporate tax returns, and corporate fraud and accountability." (SEC, 2002).

According to a survey of members of the International Federation of Accountants, some of the main factors which contribute to ethical failures for accountants are: "self-interest, failure to maintain objectivity and independence, inappropriate professional judgment, lack of ethical sensitivity, improper leadership and ill-culture, and failure to withstand advocacy threats." (Jackling et al., 2007)

Business schools across the country also began to include business ethics in their accounting and other curricula as a result of these scandals. https://www.topmba.com/mba-programs/importance-teaching-ethics-business-schools). As with all professions ethical goals are tied to standards of practice. For example:

- Relate accounting education to moral issues
- Recognize issues in accounting that have ethical implications
- Develop a sense of moral obligation or responsibility
- Develop the abilities needed to deal with ethical conflicts or dilemmas
- Learn to deal with the uncertainties of the accounting profession
- Set the stage for a change in ethical behavior
- Appreciate and understand the history and composition of all aspects of accounting ethics and their relationship to the general field of ethics (Loeb and Stephen, 1988; Dellaportas, 2006; Loeb, 1994).

Certified Public Accountants (CPAs) are regulated by individual states, which issue licenses to practice through the state board of accountancy. Because the state board may also include ethics language in its statutes, a breach of ethics may result in loss of license to practice. CPAs who audit financial statements of public corporations are also subject to regulation by the Securities and Exchange Commission (SEC). The SEC requires that all public firms' financial statements be audited by an independent CPA or accounting firm, thus promoting independence and avoiding potential conflicts of interest.

All APRNs should be aware of the importance of good accounting practices. It behooves nurses who work in freestanding or small group practices to make sure that CPAs are current in practice and aware of changing rules and regulations. If there are questions or concerns an independent auditor should always be brought in to make sure there is no criminal activity.

8.3. CONFLICTS OF INTEREST

In healthcare, conflicts of interest (COI) may arise when the best interests of a patient are put at risk because of a financial incentive or personal gain offered to their health care provider (perhaps by a pharmaceutical firm or medical device manufacturer) which goes against best evidence and standards of care (Conflict of Interest, 2017) Serra (2017) writes that harm occurs when the primary care giver is biased because of a secondary interest.

The ANA Code of Ethics Provision 2 states that "The Patient as Nursing's Foundational Commitment." While its provision 2.2 speaks directly about conflict of interest:

> *"An ethic of care recognizes that care, even good care, involves conflict in a number of ways, not the least of which is that "often care-givers will find that their needs to care for themselves come in conflict with the care that they must give to others. An actual conflict of interest refers to situations that place the nurse in a position where a choice must be made between the nurse's own self-interest and the patient's interests."*

> *"In situations of conflict of interest, the 2015 Code directs nurses to "address such conflicts in ways that ensure patient safety and that promote the patient's best interests while preserving the professional integrity of the nurse and supporting inter-professional collaboration." (Fowler, 2015, pp.31-32)*

An actual conflict of interest refers to situations that place the nurse in a position where a choice must be made between the nurse's own self-interest and the patient's interests. The moral presumption of the nurse–patient relationship in principle-based ethics is that the best interests of the patient will be served. In an ethic of care, conflict of interest strains the larger moral notions of attentiveness and responsibility and the overall framework of care. The existence of a conflict of interest does not, however, presume that the nurse will make a morally inappropriate choice, but only that the circumstances of the situation raise the risk of such decisions.

Several important relational elements come into play in a conflict of interest (Fowler, 2015):

1. A relationship must exist, whether personal or professional.
2. If it is a professional relationship, then there are common role-related expectations and responsibilities.
3. A professional relationship is one of trust with an expectation of loyalty.
4. The nurse's attentiveness has led to the identification of the patient's need(s) for care.
5. Some aspect of the nurse's own self-interest comes into play.
6. The nurse can choose to exercise self-interest over the care need of the patient.
7. Both the nurse's self-interest and the patient's care need(s) conflict.

There is a subtle but important difference between the ANA and the AMA that should be explored and discussed. The American Medical Association (1994) guideline is:

"Under no circumstances may physicians place their own financial interests above the welfare of their patients. The primary objective of the medical profession is to render service to humanity; reward or financial gain is a subordinate consideration. For a physician to unnecessarily hospitalize a patient, prescribe a drug, or conduct diagnostic tests for the physician's financial benefit is unethical. If a conflict develops between the physician's financial interest and the physician's responsibilities to the patient, the conflict must be resolved to the patient's benefit."

Conflict of interest also comes into play in publishing and research. Nurse scientists and authors are generally required to sign conflict of interest statements. The International Committee of Medical Journal Editors (www.icmje.org, accessed 2019) lists major disclosures that must be made prior to article publication including financial ties as well as any relationships that could be perceived to influence the work.

Similarities exist in research as well, where conflicts can have life and death repercussions. Lo and Grady (2017) note that even with the strict regulations of funded research there is still personal judgement and influence that may bias results. The NIH standard is:

"The NIH is committed to preserving the public's trust that the research supported by us is conducted without bias and with the highest scientific and ethical standards. We believe that strengthening the existing regulations on managing financial conflicts of interest is key to assuring the public that NIH and the institutions we support are taking a rigorous approach to managing the essential relationships between the government, federally-funded research institutions, and the private sector." (NIH, accessed, 2019)

The Institute of Medicine (IOM/NAM) Committee on Conflict of Interest in Medical Research, Education and Practice recommends that physicians should not:

- *accept items of material value from pharmaceutical, medical device, and biotechnology companies, except when a transaction involves payment at fair market value for a legitimate service;*
- *make educational presentations or publish scientific articles that are controlled by industry or that contain substantial portions written by someone who is not identified as an author;*
- *enter into consulting arrangements unless they are based on written contracts for expert services to be paid for at fair market value;*
- *meet with pharmaceutical and medical device sales representatives except by documented appointment and at the physician's express invitation; and*
- *accept drug samples, except in specified situations for patients who lack financial access to medications.*

(IOM/NAM, 2009, http://www.nationalacademies.org/hmd/Activities/Workforce/ConflictOfInterest.aspx)

The IOM/NAM also recommends that:

"Pharmaceutical, medical device, and biotechnology companies and their company foundations should have policies and practices against providing physicians with gifts, meals, drug samples (except for use by patients who lack financial access to medications), or other similar items of material value, and recommends against asking physicians to be authors of ghostwritten materials. Consulting arrangements should be for necessary services, documented in written contracts, and paid for at fair market value. Companies should not involve physicians and

patients in marketing projects that are presented as clinical research."
(IOM/NAM, 2009)

Many academic health centers and hospitals now require that all staff sign a yearly conflict of interest disclosure form that relates to research and patient care, if applicable, to prevent such issues. Columbia University's Conflict of Interest Policy states in part that:

"A financial conflict of interest (FCOI) is a situation in which an individual's private financial interest might interfere or appear to interfere with his or her professional obligations to Columbia or the conduct of the research. Such situations do not necessarily imply wrongdoing or inappropriate activities. However, in a research university setting, they can compromise, or be perceived as compromising, important academic values, research integrity, or the university mission.

Financial conflicts of interest in research have the potential to increase bias in research or create the appearance that research has been biased, regardless of whether or not that is the case. They also can present risk to human subjects participating in research." (Columbia University, accessed 2019).

While much of the policy applies to the legal ramifications of non-compliance, the bases of the policy are the moral under-pinnings of honesty and the performance of duty for the common good.

The American Nurses Association (2018) conflict of interest statement is directed towards the ANA corporate enterprise but speaks to the concerns nurses hold:

"Conflicts of Interest - The integrity of ANA and the activities it undertakes depends on the avoidance of conflicts of interest, or the even the appearance of conflicts. Conflicts of interest may arise when an individual's position or responsibilities with ANA present an opportunity for personal gain or profit separate and apart from that individual's earnings from ANA or where the individual's interests are otherwise inconsistent with the interests of ANA. A conflict of interest may arise in any number of situations and it is impossible to describe each and every instance. As a general matter, if an employee thinks that any situation may be a potential conflict of interest, he or she should consult with the Corporate Compliance Officer. (p5).

There are additional sections in many COI policies, including support for educational activities, gifts, consultation, continuing nursing education (CNE), non-CNE presentations and publications, travel, industry sponsored presentations, ghost authorship and ghost writing, inventions, drug and device representatives, and drug and device samples. Of course, not every contingency can be addressed, but these specifics do provide general guidance on conflict Conflicts of interest strike at the heart of trust between providers and patients (Fineberg, 2017). For this and many other reasons including bias and influence on judgement APRNs should be familiar with professional standards, specific institutional COIs standards as well as the concept in general. It is apparent that not all circumstances can be listed in any given COI document so APRNs must remain vigilant.

8.4. FRAUD

Fraud constitutes unlawful activities undertaken to enrich the person committing the fraud. Fraud includes theft, embezzlement, incorrect financial reporting or expense reports, conflict of interest, software piracy, falsified insurance submissions, counterfeit prescriptions, deceptive advertising, DRG falsities, duplicate billing, split billing, and other deceitful practices. Every business enterprise, including healthcare, must have safeguards in place to detect and prevent fraudulent behavior and systems to deal with any breaches in any such behavior. To state that such behavior is not only illegal, but unethical, is obvious.

Under the federal False Claims Act of 1863, an employee with knowledge of fraud against the government may file a lawsuit on behalf of the government. This law was created during the Civil War and was used against wartime defense contractors who billed the government for weapons that were not delivered as promised. It is now used by the Department of Justice in attacking healthcare fraud and abuse. Under its criminal statute, false claims are punishable by fine or imprisonment of up to five years, or both, for knowingly submitting a false statement for reimbursement. Innocent mistakes and mere negligence are not actionable under the False Claims Act, but acts such as bills for care not given, upcoding, providing substandard service but billing for standard care, or using someone else's Medicare/Medicaid number, are.

A key provision in the Act is entitled "qui tam", which allows an employee with knowledge of fraud against the government to file a lawsuit on behalf of the government (the employee is referred to as the *qui tam* plaintiff). Such plaintiffs are entitled to a percentage of any recovery as well as protection from being "discharged, demoted, suspended, threatened, harassed or in any other manner discriminated against" (CMS False Claims Act). This provision is commonly known as the Whistleblower Act. Employees are the most common whistleblowers, as knowledge of 'inside' information is usually required to prove alleged fraud (https://www.whistleblowers.org/faq/false-claims-act-qui-tam/).

The Civil Monetary Penalties Law (CMP) provides guidance for a variety of health care fraud violations. Different amounts of penalties and assessments may be authorized based on the type of violation. CMPs also may include an assessment of up to three times the amount claimed for each item or service, or up to three times the amount of remuneration offered, paid, solicited, or received. Each year, the Federal Government adjusts all CMPs for inflation. The adjusted amounts apply to civil penalties assessed after August 1, 2016, and violations after November 2, 2015. Refer to 45 CFR 102.3 for the yearly adjustments for inflation (CMS False Claims Act (2017), accessed January 2019).

Under the Deficit Reduction Act of 2005, Section 6032 requires that "any entity that receives or makes payments to the State Medicaid Program of at least $5 million annually, to provide Federal False Claims Act education to their employees." This was required because fraud costs the taxpayers huge amounts that could be otherwise spent on healthcare, as well as to alert all parties involved in the business side of health care to cut down on mistakes and negligence (CMS Deficit Reduction Act).

8.4.1. Stark Laws

The Stark laws are part of the Social Security Act and overseen by the Centers for Medicare and Medicaid Services. It is also known as the Physician Self-Referral Law and is intended to prohibit physicians from profiting from their own referrals. It states that a physician cannot refer a patient covered by Medicare/Medicaid to a clinical laboratory where the physician or an immediate family member of the physician has a financial relationship. The Acts were initially enacted in 1989 to only cover clinical lab services, but in 1993 they were expanded to cover the rest of the designated health services (DHS). Thus a physician may not refer a patient to certain DHS such as physical therapy, occupational therapy, radiation therapy, radiation services, durable medical equipment and supplies, parenteral and enteral nutrients, prosthetics, home health services, outpatient prescription drugs and other outpatient or inpatient services (CMS). In August of 2007, this was expanded to other business interests. The final revisions were in response to public comments and offered some flexibility when, for example organizations recruit physicians to rural areas, or when hospitals wish to show appreciation to their staffs in annual events. CMS published the Medicare Self-Referral Disclosure Protocol (SRDP) in September 2010 as part of the Patient Protection and Affordable Care Act (PPAC). This protocol enables providers and suppliers to "self-disclose actual or potential violations of the physician self-referral statute" and allows leeway in reducing amounts due for violations (CMS Physician Self Referral). In 2018 under the Bipartisan Budget Act policy changes were enacted including to the Stark Act (see 42 CFR 411.357). The changes include regulations about signatories and exceptions. In addition the CMS is calling for public recommendations about further changes needed.

CMS does allow some standard exceptions, including permitting the referral of a patient from one physician to another in the same group practice. In 2010, the in-office ancillary services exceptions were adopted that allow a physician within a group practice to refer a patient for MRI, CT or PET scans within the group practice, but at the time of referral must provide the patient with written notice that the patient may obtain these imaging services from a supplier other than the group practice and provide a list of alternatives. All this legislation is currently only applicable to physicians. (CMS Physician Self-Referral, 2015).

Additionally, CMS issued a rule in 2008 which requires physicians to disclose to their patients, at the time of referral, if they have ownership or an investment in the hospital as well as for physician-owned hospitals to disclose to their patients the names of any physicians (and immediate family members) who have an ownership or investment in the hospital (CMS Changes to Disclosure of Physician Ownership in Hospitals and Physician Self-Referral Rules, 2008). Exceptions are allowed if proof can be established of qualifications as a sole rural provider or hospital. The Patient Protection and Affordable Care Act (ACA) of 2010 added other requirements for hospitals in order to qualify for the rural provider and hospital exceptions to the ownership or investment prohibition. Section 6001 of the ACA limits expansion to hospitals that have physician ownership or investment and mandates certain disclosure obligations for physician-owned hospitals and referring physicians that have an ownership or investment interest in a hospital (CMS, 2015).

8.4.2. Anti-Kickback Statute

The Anti-Kickback Statute deals with "Anyone who knowingly or willfully solicits or receives, either directly or indirectly, any remuneration (including any kickback, bribe, or rebate) in exchange for referring an individual for services under any federal healthcare program or in return for purchasing, leasing, or ordering any good, facility, service, or item paid for under a federal health care program shall be guilty of a felony" (CMS Anti-Kickback Rule, see https://www.cms.gov/ Outreach-and-Education/Medicare-Learning-Network-MLN/MLN-

Products/downloads/fraud_and_abuse.pdf). Each offense is subject to a fine of up to $25,000 or imprisonment for up to 5 years or both. Often kickbacks involve payments from one party to another (physician to physician or hospital to physician) with the intent to induce or reward referrals. "The 'one purpose' test is used by the federal government to determine if a hospital has unlawfully compensated a physician. If one purpose of the physician compensation is to induce referrals, then the statute (Anti-Kickback Rule) has been violated even though the compensation was for a professional service" (Mustard, 2009).

In addition to the False Claims Act and the Federal Anti-Kickback Statute, the Department of Health and Human Services also employs the Civil Monetary Penalties Law (CMPL) as means to regulate some aspects of the physician/provider-industry interaction. The Office of the Attorney General may use the CMPL to enforce the Anti-Kickback Statute and "provides for monetary penalties of up to $50,000 for each illegal act, assessments of up to three times the amount of the kickback, and the exclusion from participation in federal health care programs" (Birkhahn et al., 2009). See also the Office of the Inspector General on fraud at https://oig.hhs.gov/fraud/enforcement/cmp/background.asp.

Even when heavy fines are levied, collecting them is not always easy. For example since 2005, the SEC and the Commodity Futures Trading Commission have imposed over $12.5 billion in fines (also including return of ill-gotten profits and repayment of restitution to investors for fraudulent activities). As of July 2011, only $8 billion has been recovered (WSJ, 2011).

8.4.3. HIPAA Viloations

Fraud involving HIPAA violations are now liable for criminal penalties enforced by the Department of Justice.

"An individual who knowingly obtains or discloses individually identifiable health information in violation of HIPAA faces a fine of $50,000 and up to one year imprisonment. The criminal penalties increase to $100,000 and up to five years imprisonment if the wrongful conduct involves false pretenses, and up to ten years imprisonment if the wrongful conduct involves the intent to sell, transfer, or use individually identifiable health information for commercial advantage, personal gain or malicious harm" (CMS Medicare HIPAA Eligibility).

The Criminal Health Care Fraud Statute (18 U.S.C. Section 1347) specifically forbids the defrauding of any health care benefit program (i.e., Medicare or Medicaid) or to obtain "by means of false or fraudulent pretenses, representations, or promises any of the money or property owned by, or under the custody or control of, any health care benefit program in connection with the delivery of or payment for health care benefits, items, or services" (CMS Criminal Health Care Fraud). Penalties for violating the statute may include fines, imprisonment, or both. For a current list of HIPAA violations and fines see the HHS Breach Portal at https://ocrportal.hhs.gov/ocr/breach/breach_report.jsf.

As is obvious, the government utilizes multiple entities to coordinate and monitor fraud, including CMS, the Center for Program Integrity, the Office of the Inspector General, the Health Care Fraud Prevention and Enforcement Action Team and the General Services Administration.

8.5. GIFTS

Gifts given for the 'joy of giving' and with no expectation of return or reward are usually received with willingness and enthusiasm by the recipient. However, gifts given to healthcare professionals with a *quid pro quo* expectancy constitute major concerns of legality and ethics.

There is a long history of companies, particularly pharmaceutical and medical device manufacturers, marketing their products to physicians through:

"gifts, even of relatively small items, including meals; payment for attendance at lectures and conferences, including on-line activities; CME for which physicians pay no fee; payment for time while attending meetings; payment for travel to meetings or scholarships to attend meetings; payment for participation in speakers bureaus; the provision of ghostwriting services; provision of pharmaceutical samples; grants for research projects; and payment for consulting relationships" *(Brennan et al., 2006).*

These gifts may compromise the professionalism and patient care given by physicians, and the guidelines suggested by such professional groups as the American Medical Association, the Accreditation Council for Continuing Medical Education and the American College of Physicians do not go far enough in protecting the welfare of patients or the integrity of research. Brennan *et al.* (2006) also dispute the commonly held belief that small gifts (pens, coffee mugs, etc.) do not influence physician behavior.

PhRMA, the Pharmaceutical Manufacturers Association, represents member companies and first issued guidelines regarding gifts to physicians in 2002. Their voluntary guidelines suggest that gifts valued at less than $100 were allowed if the physician could prove a value to patients and that modest meals were acceptable if in the context of an educational setting. These PhRMA guidelines were endorsed by the Office of the Inspector General, which also issued its own guidelines in 2003. A revision by PhRMA in 2009 was stricter, disallowing all gifts (even pens and mugs for example) other than meals that "are modest as judged by local standards; are not part of an entertainment or recreational event; and are provided in a manner conducive to informational communication", sample medications and educational gifts (PHRMA Code, 2009). But self-regulation by the industry did not change either public perception or practice and in 2010, as part of the Affordable Care Act national health reform law, the Physicians Payments Sunshine Act was passed. This Act now requires all pharmaceutical companies to report all payments to physicians above $10 and pay penalties if they fail to do so ($150,000 for failure to report and $1 million for knowingly doing so). (Mizik, 2010). CMS has updated its guidance (see https://www.cms.gov/Medicare/Health-Plans/ManagedCareMarketing/Downloads/CY-2018-Medicare-Marketing-Guidelines_Final072017.pdf) stating only gifts of minimal value are allowed. Interestingly states, including California and New Jersey, are considering banning gifts altogether.

The International Federation of Pharmaceutical Manufacturers (IFPMA) updated their code of conduct in 2019, In order to prevent undue influence they recommend the prohibition of all gifts except pens and paper used at meetings (https://www.ifpma.org/wp-content/uploads/2018/09/IFPMA_Code_of_Practice_2019.pdf)

The American Medical Association issued a number of guidelines to assist physicians regarding gifts. They state:

"Relationships among physicians and professional medical organizations and pharmaceutical, biotechnology, and medical device companies help drive innovation in patient care and contribute to the economic well-being of the community to the ultimate benefit of patients and the public. However, an increasingly urgent challenge for both medicine and industry is to devise ways to preserve strong, productive collaborations at the same time that they take clear effective action to prevent relationships that damage public trust and tarnish the reputation of both parties.

Gifts to physicians from industry create conditions that carry the risk of subtly biasing—or being perceived to bias—professional judgment in the care of patients.

To preserve the trust that is fundamental to the patient-physician relationship and public confidence in the profession, physicians should:

(a) Decline cash gifts in any amount from an entity that has a direct interest in physicians' treatment recommendations.

(b) Decline any gifts for which reciprocity is expected or implied.

(c) Accept an in-kind gift for the physician's practice only when the gift:

1. Will directly benefit patients, including patient education
2. Is of minimal value

(d) Academic institutions and residency and fellowship pro grams may accept special funding on behalf of trainees to support medical students', residents', and fellows' participa tion in professional meetings, including educational meetings, provided:

1. The program identifies recipients based on independent institutional criteria
2. Funds are distributed to recipients without specific attribution to sponsors"

(AMA Medical Code of Ethics, Opinion 9.6.2 https://www.ama-assn.org/delivering-care/ethics/gifts-physicians-industry).

Gifts from patients may present different challenges. According to the AMA Medical Code of Ethics opinion:

"Gifts that patients offer to physicians are often an expression of appreciation and gratitude or a reflection of cultural traditions, and can enhance the patient-physician relationship. . . . Physicians should make clear that gifts given to secure preferential treatment compromise their obligation to provide services in a fair manner. There are no definitive rules to determine when a physician should or should not accept a gift. No fixed value determines the appropriateness or inappropriateness of a gift from a patient; however, the gift's value relative to the patient's or the physician's means should not be disproportionately or inappropriately large" (AMA Code of Ethics—Gifts from Patients, 2003).

The ANA provides no official guidance to its members. Instead most regulation comes from the individual institutions. Given the increasingly independent practice by APRNs consideration should be given to developing gift policies. In the interim the AMA policies provide insight into the issue.

8.6. HUMAN RESOURCE MANAGEMENT

The workplace in healthcare consists of more than just patients and colleagues and requires specific and often complex knowledge of human resource issues, both legal and professional. The Society of Human Resource Management (SHRM) (2014) has published a Code of Ethics and also provides guidance to institutions who seek to develop their own. See https://www.shrm.org/about-shrm/pages/code-of-ethics.aspx.

Human resource management (HRM) related issues in the workplace today can be overwhelming: recruitment, performance appraisals, training, compensation, benefits (pay equity), labor relations (unions, strikes), discrimination (ageism, gender, race, religion, disabilities, and sexual harassment), termination, occupational health and safety, and privacy (workplace surveillance, drug testing, and whistleblowing). In other words, any aspect of the work force concerned with employees and employers. While many of these issues are regulated by government agencies and legal compliance, many rely on the culture of the institution and how attuned it is to the welfare of its employees. Decisions made in business about any of these issues affect people's livelihoods and chances for future employment. The 'bottom line' is that employees and employers should be treated fairly and equitably and human resources management plays an important role in making sure that all parties know and understand the culture and values of the institution (Rose, 2007).

Winstanley and Woodall (1996) note ethical concerns arising from HRM practices including:

- *"Increased job insecurity arising from flexible work practices, short-term and temporary employment, fear of job loss due to outsourcing, increased stress and a widening imbalance of power between management and workforce;*
- *Increase in surveillance and control ranging from the use of psychometric tests to electronic surveillance to random drug screening/testing;*
- *Deregulation of the market place which may be seen as pushing HR into compromising 'good' practice for business needs—i.e., 'doing well vs. doing good';*
- *A decline in management integrity which contrasts an emphasis on managing organizational culture with a highly formulaic approach in employment contracts."*

Margolis, Grant and Molinsky (2007) propose three standards for ethical management of human resources which take into consideration the organization itself, the target of any harmful action and the HR managers. They provide a thoughtful, yet simple framework, to consider:

- *"Advance the organization's objective. Execute the task in question so that progress is made towards the objective that calls for it to be done in the first place—in other words, hiring and firing decisions, performance appraisals, etc., should serve a central organizational objective that has been decided in advance and is available to all staff and managers.*
- *Enhance the dignity of those who may be harmed by the action. When managers distribute opportunities and benefits, there may be some who do not receive those opportunities and benefits—or receive fewer than others. When companies go through cycles of destruction—restructuring, downsizing—individuals get harmed. In both instances, those who lose out are due treatment that respects their standing, fosters their resilience, and enables them to continue to function effectively.*
- *Sustain the moral sensibility of those executing morally ambiguous tasks. Someone must deliver the poor performance appraisal, announce the lay-off, or close the manufacturing facility or office. The difficulty and ambivalence which may occur when performing these tasks reflects an underlying uneasiness about fair treatment and fair outcomes, and managers ought to remain attuned to that uneasiness."*

In the United States, the Sarbanes-Oxley Act of 2002, which covers all publicly traded companies, requires, among other things, that these companies have a code of ethics in place that includes detriments to financial wrong-doing and promotes integrity, specifically to senior financial officers and bans personal loans to executive officers or board of director members. A company must affirm that they are committed to honest and ethical conduct and avoidance of conflicts of interest. Under the Act, companies must prove to the Securities and Exchange Commission that its financial statements are accurate, complete, timely and understandable. They must also comply with any applicable laws and regulations.

The Act also requires companies to develop a complaint system and non-retaliation policy that is clearly explained to employees. This protects whistleblowers and applies not just to the employees of a publicly traded company, but to anyone who works for such a company including contractors, agents, etc. Because of the anti-retribution and whistleblower provisions in the Act:

"a company, officer, employee, contractor, subcontractor or agent is prohibited from discharging, demoting, suspending, threatening, harassing or otherwise discriminating in the terms and conditions of employment against an employee who...provides information or assists in an

investigation regarding conduct that the employee reasonably believes is fraudulent or a violation of a rule or regulation of the SEC when such information or assistance is provided to or the investigation is conducted by (1) a federal regulatory agency or law enforcement, (2) a member of Congress or a committee, (3) a person with supervisory authority over the person or (4) a person who has authority to investigate, discover or terminate misconduct" (Sarbanes-Oxley Act of 2002).

Being an ethically and socially responsible company can be an attraction for potential and current employees. Programs that encourage environmental responsibility, volunteerism and philanthropy, diversity, community and employee interactions, while ethically positive, are also good for business. Corporate social responsibility (CSR) is "a self-regulating business model that helps a company be socially accountable — to itself, its stakeholders, and the public" (https://www.investopedia.com/terms/c/corp-social-responsibility.asp, accessed February 2019). Non-publicly traded companies are also mirroring Sarbanes-Oxley requirements as the benefits of doing so are becoming more widely known. All impact HRM professionals. If employees know the rules, objectives and ethical expectations of the organization, and managers are expected to treat all employees fairly and are supported in their enforcement of rules and objectives, an ethical workplace will result.

8.7. INFORMATION TECHNOLOGY

According to Finn (accessed, January 2019):

"Healthcare is undergoing fundamental changes in reimbursement, care delivery models and the technology required to make these changes. Technology and information is no longer an adjunct to the business of healthcare — it is a strategic imperative. This information, however, is among the most regulated and protected information under the law. The data must be shared more widely with more people and organizations, all the while with stricter security and privacy controls." (https:// electronichealthreporter.com/top-health-it-issues-faced-by-hospitals/)

While Finn and others in the IT world tout the benefits of IT, of which there are many, there are also many problems. Kim, Coiera, & Magrabi (2017) note that IT can disrupt care, create new and often unpredictable errors and take unreasonable amounts of clinical care time.

Today information technology (IT) plays a major a major role in both business and personal lives. Employers are deciding whether or not to monitor emails and internet site visits and censorship, what security safeguards should be instituted to prevent hackers and spyware, should spam be utilized as a form of low cost marketing and what can and cannot be copyrighted when shared via IT (Reynolds, 2009).

The business side of health care is no different; from electronic health records (EHR) to computerized physician order entry (CPOE), to billing and claims systems to health information web sites to patient/practitioner emails, employers must develop policies and strategies for these and other contingencies. It is important that workplaces provide ethics instruction concerning IT issues to new employees and on a continuing basis in order to prevent unintentional violations and to provide information about consequences for unethical behaviors (Calluzzo and Cante, 2004).

Chief among the ethical issues involved with IT in healthcare is that of patient privacy/confidentiality. The Health Insurance Portability and Accountability Act of 1996 (HIPAA) was developed by the United States Department of Health and Human Services (HHS) in order to protect the privacy and security of certain health information. A Privacy Rule (the Standards of Privacy of Individually Identifiable Health Information, finalized in 2002) and a Security Rule (the Security Standards for the Protection of Electronic Protected Health Information, finalized in 2003) were established in order to implement HIPAA:

"The Privacy Rule standards address the use and disclosure of individuals' health information—called 'protected health information' by organizations subject to the Privacy Rule—called 'covered entities', as well as standards for individuals' privacy rights to understand and control how their health information is used. Within HHS, the Office for Civil Rights (OCR) has responsibility for implementing and enforcing the Privacy Rule with respect to voluntary compliance activities and civil money penalties. A major goal of the Privacy Rule is to assure that individuals' health information is properly protected while allowing the flow of health information needed to provide and promote high quality health care and to protect the public's health and well-being. The Rule balances necessary uses of information with protection of the privacy of people who seek health care. Because the health care marketplace has so many different participants, the Rule is designed to be flexible and comprehensive to cover the variety of uses and disclosures that must be addressed. HHS may impose penalties of $100 per failure to comply with a Privacy Rule requirement, not to exceed $25,000 per year for multiple violations. The Security Rule operationalizes the protections contained in the Privacy Rule by addressing the technical and non-technical safeguards that organizations called 'covered entities' must put in place to secure individuals' electronic protected health information (e-PHI)" (Health and Human Services Department, 2011).

Both of these rules have revolutionized the way healthcare is delivered for providers, patients, payers and for a myriad of firms whose sole businesses are consulting, developing and selling solutions to these requirements.

The Health Information Technology for Economic and Clinical Health Act (the HITECH Act) of 2009 (as part of the American Recovery and Reinvestment Act of 2009) allocated $27 billion over ten years to support adoption of electronic medical records (EMR) and provides payments to doctors and hospitals when they adopt EMRs and demonstrate that their use of EMRs improves the quality, safety and effectiveness of patient care. Included in the program are provisions to improve security and privacy of the records (CMS, 2009).

The U.S. government now mandates that all health care providers use a unique identifier, the National Provider Identifier (NPI). This includes all covered entities such as health plans and health care clearinghouses and the number must be used for all administrative and financial transactions adopted under HIPAA (CMS, 2011). This is another system designed to protect both providers and patients from unauthorized sharing of confidential information. Unfortunately algorithms and artificial intelligence, coupled with supercomputing are allowing breaches to this protective system (See chapters 1 and 2 for specific examples).

Individual hospitals, healthcare systems, and practices also have developed safeguards and methods of communicating with their patients. For example, Kansas State University now has an employee code of ethics that all must agree to sign, with the understanding that violation of the agreement may result in disciplinary action which could include dismissal and legal action. Some salient points include: "I will take reasonable precautions to prevent unauthorized access to passwords, user identifications, or other information; I will limit access to information contained in the systems to only authorized people . . . I will not share, record, copy, transmit, delete or in any way alter information in these systems except when required to perform my duties . . ." (Kansas State Information Technology Employee Code of Ethics).

The American College of Healthcare Executives has adopted a policy position that "in addition to following all applicable state laws and HIPAA, healthcare executives have a moral and professional obligation to respect confidentiality and protect the security of patients' medical records. As patient advocates, executives must ensure their organization obtains proper patient authorization to release information or follow carefully defined policies and applicable laws in those cases for which the release of information without consent is indicated" (Board of Governors of the American College of Healthcare Executives, 2016,

https://www.ache.org/about-ache/our-story/our-commitments/ethics/
ache-code-of-ethics/health-information-confidentiality).

The AMA's Code of Ethics clearly outlines systems that should be
in place to protect the confidentiality of patient records and the use
of computers and medical data stored in these computers and EMRs.
(AMA Opinion 5.07 Confidentiality: Computers). It also has clearly
defined standards for the use of email.

The AMA code also states that:

- *"Dedication to upholding trust in the patient-physician relationship, to
  preventing harms to patients, and to respecting patients' privacy and
  autonomy create responsibilities for individual physicians, medical
  practices and health care institutions when patient information is
  inappropriately disclosed. When there is reason to believe that patients'
  confidentiality has been compromised by a breach of the electronic
  medical record, physicians should:*
- *Ensure that patients are promptly informed about the breach and
  potential for harm, either by disclosing directly (when the physician has
  administrative responsibility for the EMR), participating in efforts by the
  practice or health care institution to disclose . . .*
- *Follow ethically appropriate procedures for disclosure . . . including
  describing what information was breached; how the breach happened;
  what the consequences may be; what corrective actions have been
  taken...and what steps patients themselves might take to minimize
  adverse consequences . . ." (AMA Opinion 5.10).*

The potential for breach of confidentiality, fraud and misuse of private information is growing exponentially along with the ease of use
and acceptance of IT in everyday life. According to the HIPAA Journal in "2017, there have been nine financial penalties issued to resolve
HIPAA violation cases. In 2016, a record year for enforcement of
HIPAA Rules, there were 12 settlements and one civil monetary penalty issued to resolve HIPAA violation cases" (https://www.hipaajournal.
com/hipaa-violation-cases/).

The use of IT is a world-wide phenomenon and Hongladarom and
Ess (2007) believe that there are global implications for rules of intellectual property and that this perspective must be considered, especially
in inter-cultural areas. The European Union recently implemented rules
regarding privacy which have global implications. Corporate IT ethics policies should be communicated clearly to all global partners and
corporate IT departments must remain current with worldwide laws and

regulations. See chapters 1 and 2 for how technology is challenging the ethical boundaries of health care.

8.8. LIMITED RESOURCES

Both the ANA and the AMA have provided guidance on the allocation of limited resources. The ANA (Fowler, 2015) focuses on the environment of care for nurses as follows:

Provision 6: The nurse, through individual and collective effort, establishes, maintains, and improves the ethical environment of the work setting and conditions of employment that are conducive to safe, quality health care.

6.3 Responsibility for the Healthcare Environment The ANA Nurse's Bill of Rights addresses environmental concerns of the workplace. It states:

To maximize the contributions nurses make to society, it is necessary to protect the dignity and autonomy of nurses in the workplace. To that end, the following rights must be afforded:

1. Nurses have the right to practice in a manner that fulfills their obligations to society and to those who receive nursing care.
2. Nurses have the right to practice in environments that allow them to act in accordance with professional standards and legally authorized scopes of practice.
3. Nurses have the right to a work environment that supports and facilitates ethical practice, in accordance with the Code of Ethics for Nurses with Interpretive Statements.

The AMA Code of Medical Ethics (2016) Opinion 11.1.3 states that the "Physicians' primary ethical obligation is to promote the well-being of their patients." Specifically:

Individually and collectively through the profession, physicians should advocate for policies and procedures that allocate scarce health care resources fairly among patients, in keeping with the following criteria:

(a) Base allocation policies on criteria relating to medical need, including urgency of need, likelihood and anticipated duration of benefit, and change in quality of life. In limited circumstances, it may be appropriate to take into consideration the amount of resources required for successful treatment. It is not appropriate to base allocation policies on social worth, perceived obstacles to treatment, patient contribution to illness, past use of resources, or other non-medical characteristics.

(b) Give first priority to those patients for whom treatment will
     avoid premature death or extremely poor outcomes, then to
     patients who will experience the greatest change in quality of
     life, when there are very substantial differences among patients
     who need access to the scarce resource(s).
(c) Use an objective, flexible, transparent mechanism to determine
     which patients will receive the resource(s) when there are not
     substantial differences among patients who need access to the
     scarce resource(s).
(d) Explain the applicable allocation policies or procedures to
     patients who are denied access to the scarce resource(s) and to
     the public.

Not having enough products or services to supply expectant
customers can have a disastrous effect on a company's business. In
health care shortages can result in loss of life. Unfortunately in many
health care settings, rather than health markers, profit (even for non-
profits), is used as a marker of excellence. Sometimes scarce resources
reflect an attempt to increase the bottom line and not actual scarcity.

As healthcare costs continue to rise, government officials, politicians
and most Americans have concerns about the system's ability to maintain support for funding programs already in existence, let alone future
expansions. Limiting access and services may be fiscally responsible
when attempting to balance budgets and woo voters, but presents equally compelling concerns such as rationing, quality of care and patients'
right to care. If healthcare providers determine what tests, procedures,
medications and treatments are necessary for the benefit of the patient,
and all of these choices have attending costs associated with them; how
then does this balance the conflicting rights of a provider to provide the
best possible (and obviously most appropriately evidence-based) care
against the various payers.

Most health care providers readily understand and agree with the
concept of triage, meant to ensure that the sickest patients, who need
immediate care, are taken care of first. This prioritizing of needs works
well in the emergency room and on the battle field and helped to develop a national system to allocate organs for transplants. But as evidenced by the absence of agreement about every health care reform
plan that has been proposed over the last several decades, the broader
concept of triage, which is conflated with rationing, is not without controversy. The public may say it wants fairness and economic frugality
for others in the system, but not when it applies to them as individuals.
While there is no guaranteed 'right to health care' in the Constitution,
allocation of limited and expensive health resources is now an integral

part of health policy decisions. For example, in 1998, Oregon began a plan to rank Medicaid patients' medical procedures according to cost/ benefit ratios—and reimburse accordingly. This was part of a cost savings strategy to enroll more Oregonians in the state health plan but was ultimately abandoned as too subjective (Jonsen, 1998; Fruits, 2010).

Some newer models evaluate allocation principles and suggest they be classified into four categories:

> *"treating people equally, favoring the worst-off, maximizing total benefits, and promoting and regarding social usefulness. No single principle is sufficient to incorporate all morally relevant considerations and therefore individual principles must be combined . . . recommend an alternative system which prioritizes younger people who have not yet lived a complete life, and also incorporates prognosis, saves the most lives, lottery and instrumental value principles" (Persad et al., 2009, p. 423).*

While intellectually satisfying, this model brings up many ethical concerns, including but not limited to fairness, justice and autonomy.

The American Medical Association's Code of Medical Ethics addresses financial barriers to health access in the following statements:

> *Health care is a fundamental human good because it affects our opportunity to pursue life goals, reduces our pain and suffering, helps prevent premature loss of life, and provides information needed to plan for our lives. As professionals, physicians individually and collectively have an ethical responsibility to ensure that all persons have access to needed care regardless of their economic means.*

In view of this obligation,
> *(a) Individual physicians should:*

> 1. *Take steps to promote access to care for individual patients, such as providing pro bono care in their office or through freestanding facilities or government programs that provide health care for the poor, or, when permissible, waiving insurance copayments in individual cases of hardship. Physicians in the poorest communities should be able to turn for assistance to colleagues in more prosperous communities.*
> 2. *Help patients obtain needed care through public or charitable programs when patients cannot do so themselves.*
>   *(b) Physicians, individually and collectively through their professional organizations and institutions, should participate in the political process as advocates for patients (or support those who do) so as to diminish financial obstacles to access health care.*
>   *(c) The medical profession must work to ensure that societal*

*decisions about the distribution of health resources safeguard
the interests of all patients and promote access to health
services.*

*(d) All stakeholders in health care, including physicians, health
facilities, health insurers, professional medical societies, and
public policymakers must work together to ensure sufficient
access to appropriate health care for all people.
(AMA Medical Code of Ethics Opinion 11.1.4).*

Critical care professionals were asked by survey in 1994 about
their attitudes about rationing, as noted by Bloomfield, "The results of
the study showed that quality of life of the patient, the probability of
surviving, whether the acute illness could be reversed or not and the
nature of a chronic disease all played a role in the provider's mind as
to whether resources could be distributed fairly. Economic background
of the patient did not play a role in this decision" (Bloomfield, 2009).

8.9. MANAGED CARE/THIRD PARTY PAYERS/BILLING AND COLLECTIONS

As is well known health care costs in the US are vastly higher than
the rest of the world, yet our utilization rate is not. Payment is a requirement of services provided in all businesses and is no less critical to
health care. However, the complicated relationship between patients,
providers and third party payers/insurance companies is more difficult
than 'regular' businesses where there is a product produced. The product of health care is care but it is difficult to measure and as a result
difficult to figure real and reasonable costs.

If a health care professional's primary obligation is to his or her patients, then interactions with insurance companies and managed care
organizations (MCO) may present ethical dilemmas related to issues
such as denial of care, postponement of care, choice of medications/
treatment and even provider choice. Terminology determined by business, which substitutes customer/client for patient and provider for
health care professional, further blur the distinction between a financial
transaction and appropriate patient care and stress competing interests.
Decisions regarding reimbursement may be made by non-healthcare
professionals, widening the gap between those who deliver the care and
those who say how it should be delivered (at least what will be paid
for). Professional organizations may not help, "although physicians
have an obligation to consider the needs of broader patient populations

within the context of the patient-physician relationship, their first duty must be to the individual patient.

The disruption of the patient-provider relationship may now be determined by reimbursement issues, rather than patient choice. Because managed care companies usually only pay for care provided by providers within their systems, patients may be forced to change providers if they wish their care to be covered by their insurance. Preferred provider groups will only reimburse fully to providers within their network, necessitating patients to 'pay extra' to continue to use an out-of network provider. Employers may change health plans offered to employees, employees may change jobs, and many MCOs require gatekeepers to specialists, all which can mean the loss of provider access.

Hospitals typically bill insured patients at a discounted or negotiated rate, but those who are uninsured or out of network are usually charged a much higher multiple of that rate (Hall and Schneider, 2008). In Darragh and McCarrick's "Managed Health Care: New Ethical Issues for All" article (*Kennedy Institute of Ethics Journal*, 1996), they present a literature review compiled during the early years of the Clinton administration's attempt at health care reform and provide a basis for understanding why these concerns are still with us in the United States in 2011. "These cost-containment features now play an intimate role in clinical practice. When a managed care plan contracts with a physician, the doctor becomes a 'double agent' with contractual obligations to the plan to provide a preset amount of services and professional responsibilities to each patient to authorize necessary treatment" (Darragh and McCarrick, 1996).

The American Medical Association's statement concerning managed care states that:

> "*The expansion of managed care has brought a variety of changes to medicine including new and different reimbursement systems for physicians with complex referral restrictions and benefits packages for patients. Some of these changes have raised concerns that a physician's ability to practice ethical medicine will be adversely affected by the modifications in the system . . . the following points were developed . . .*

> - "*The duty of patient advocacy is a fundamental element of the patient-physician relationship that should not be altered by the system of health care delivery. Physicians must continue to place the interests of their patients first.*
> - *When health care plans place restrictions on the care that physicians in the plan may provide to their patients . . . physicians must advocate for any care they believe will materially benefit their patients . . .*

- *When physicians are employed or reimbursed by health care plans that offer financial incentives to limit care, serious potential conflicts are created between the physicians' personal financial interests and the needs of their patients. Efforts to contain health care costs should not place patient welfare at risk . . .*
- *Physicians should encourage both that patients be aware of the benefits and limitations of their health care coverage and that they exercise their autonomy by public participation in the formulation of benefits packages and by prudent selection of health care coverage that best suits their needs" (AMA Medical Code of Ethics Opinion 8.054).*

For those who have no insurance, either by choice or not, the situation is often grim, yet affects even those who are covered. Rising insurance premiums, onerous labor contracts, and the exponentially rising costs associated with healthcare are some of the results of a system that must account for these millions of Americans. One example of the results of these escalating costs is described in a 2011 Wall Street Journal article (Anand, 2008) about Mennonites and Amish who believe that it is the religious duty of their community to provide care for each other when they are ill and consequently have never purchased any form of health insurance. However, as many of the children in these communities now suffer from genetic diseases (because of low rates of marriage to those outside these small communities), families are turning to the secular world's high-tech hospitals to provide care now available for hereditary diseases. While many healthcare systems offer some sort of charity care, which they must provide in order to receive tax subsidies from the government, the resulting bills can be astronomical and are a burden not only the patients, but the hospitals who must try to recover their costs. One of the hospitals in the article, Hershey Medical Center, said in a statement that "If a party chooses not to apply for medical assistance after we have counseled them and made the recommendation that they apply, they cannot be considered for charity care." (Anand, 2008).

The responsibility and understanding of what is covered/reimbursed (and what isn't) is not easily resolved, either for the patient or the providers who need to maximize their practices' profits. Authors Hall and Schneider suggest that physicians must decide between two different models of professionalism: "the transactional model which compares medical care to any other business transaction where payment is expected for services rendered, and the relational model which emphasizes the physician-patient relationship and discourages maximizing profit from this association" (Hall and Schneider, 2008).

Financial incentives for physicians are addressed by the AMA under their Code of Ethics. This opinion offers the following guidance:

- *"Although physicians have an obligation to consider the needs of broader patient populations within the context of the patient-physician relationship, their first duty must be to the individual patient. This obligation must override consideration of the reimbursement mechanism or specific financial incentives applied to a physician's clinical practice.*
- *Physicians, individually or through their representatives, should evaluate the financial incentives associated with participation in a health plan before contracting with that plan. The purpose of the evaluation is to ensure that the quality of patient care is not compromised by unrealistic expectations for utilization or by placing that physician's payments for care at excessive risk . . .*
- *Physicians also should advocate for incentives that promote efficient practice, but are not designed to realize cost savings beyond those attainable through efficiency . . .*
- *Patients must be informed of financial incentives that could impact the level or type of care they receive. Although this responsibility should be assumed by the health plan, physicians, individually or through their representatives, must be prepared to discuss with patients any financial arrangements that could impact patient care. Physicians should avoid reimbursement systems that, if disclosed to patients, could negatively affect the patient-physician relationship" (AMA Medical Code of Ethics Opinion 8.054).*

Similarly, the American College of Physicians' Center for Ethics and Professionalism, along with the Harvard Pilgrim Health Care Ethics Program and a sixteen member group of stakeholders, developed a statement of ethical principles; some of the points are:

- *Health plans, purchasers, clinicians and patients should be open and truthful in their dealings with each other;*
- *Health plans, purchasers, clinicians and patients should recognize and support the intimacy and importance of patient-clinician relationships and the ethical obligations of clinicians to patients;*
- *Resource allocation policy should be made through an open and participatory process;*
- *Clinicians have a responsibility to practice effective and efficient health care and to use health care resources responsibly;*
- *Health plans should engage purchasers in a discussion about what health care needs can reasonably be met, given a particular level of premium, and should explain the reasoning behind their coverage, exclusion, and cost determinations;*
- *Patients should have a basic understanding of the rules of their insurance;*
- *Health plans and health care organizations should not ask clinicians to participate in arrangements that jeopardize professional ethical standards. (Povar, 2004).*

8.10. MARKETING

Marketing is more than advertising—it is the entire spectrum of tools used to influence 'customers' to buy something, either a product or a service. Often considered pejoratively, it can be viewed as merely a basic communication tool necessary to provide essential information.

In the not so distant past, marketing of medical services was relegated to specialty journals rarely seen by the public. In *Goldfarb vs. Virginia State Bar*, the Supreme Court ruled that antitrust laws applied to professions and that restrictions on advertising by groups such as the American Medical Association were considered to unfairly restrict competition (Nisselson, 2008) Now, however, it is rare to not be bombarded by marketing campaigns known as direct-to-consumer advertising (DTCA) for hospitals, individual physicians, medications and insurance plans on television, billboards, Facebook and lay magazines.

There are a multitude of government agencies which are charged with protecting the public from unethical and/or false marketing claims. The Federal Trade Commission (FTC) and individual state agencies have responsibility for oversight of general marketing practices and for determining whether an advertisement is false, deceptive or misleading and for taking action against the advertiser. "Companies must support health advertising claims with solid proof. This is especially true for businesses that market food, over-the-counter drugs, dietary supplements, contact lenses, and other health-related products" (Federal Trade Commission, 2011).

The Food and Drug Administration (FDA) has responsibility for the safety of food and drug products and requires that "product claim ads give a fair balance of information about drug risks as compared with information about drug benefits" (FDA, 2011) Direct to consumer advertising began in the 1980s when drug companies began to provide consumers more information about their products instead of only to doctors and pharmacists. The FDA, under the Federal Food, Drug and Cosmetic Act, requires that advertisements for prescription drugs be accurate and not misleading. (FDA, 2011)

The Federal Communications Commission (FCC) regulates broadcast advertisements and "unless a broadcast advertisement is found to be in violation of a specific law or rule, the government cannot take action against it" (FCC, 2011). Consumers are advised, "depending on the nature of the advertisement, the appropriate agency should be contacted regarding advertisements that one believes may be false or misleading."

Misstating claims about the benefits of a product may not only be unethical, but may also be illegal. Weight loss products often overstate their success rates, or hide them in small print disclaimers or by using ambiguous language. Using sexual content and/or advertising products that could be seen as leading to promiscuous behavior such as condoms, birth control methods or sexual dysfunction medications, may be considered unethical to some consumers.

Because of the increasing scope of new unregulated media venues, many professional groups have developed their own ethical standards. The American Marketing Association's Statement of Ethics asks its members to remember that:

Values also serve as the criteria for evaluating our own personal actions and the actions of others. As marketers, we recognize that we not only serve our organizations but also act as stewards of society in creating, facilitating and executing the transactions that are part of the greater economy. In this role, marketers are expected to embrace the highest professional ethical norms and the ethical values implied by our responsibility toward multiple stakeholders (e.g., customers, employees, investors, peers, channel members, regulators and the host community). (American Marketing Association Statement of Ethics, 2017, accessed at www.ama.org/AboutAMA/Pages/Statement-of-Ethics.aspx)).

The American Medical Association's (2016) policy on advertising and publicity offers several key insights into healthcare marketing:

There are no restrictions on advertising by physicians except those that can be specifically justified to protect the public from deceptive practices. A physician may publicize him or herself as a physician through any commercial publicity or other form of public communication (including any newspaper, magazine, telephone directory, radio, television, direct mail, or other advertising) provided that the communication shall not be misleading because of the omission of necessary material information, shall not contain any false or misleading statement, or shall not otherwise operate to deceive. AMA Medical Code of Ethics Opinion 9.6.1—Advertising and Publicity).

All marketing codes of ethics reflect the basic principles of respect for patient autonomy and nonmaleficence, as any attempts to recruit patients must not misrepresent the value of a service offered and must always consider how the average person/patient might interpret the information. Any offensive material, whether by using stereotypes or that is demeaning to a specific demographic or that targets vulnerable populations such as children, the elderly, and developing countries' consumers, is clearly in conflict with the ethical mores and should be avoided.

In the United States, one of the most controversial and continuing ethical issues is regarding marketing of the legally available known carcinogen—cigarettes. All cigarette and tobacco advertising was banned on television and radio in the early 1970s as a public health initiative by the FCC (The Public Health Cigarette Smoking Act). Warnings from the Surgeon General must be included now on any advertisements and on all packaging. The Family Smoking Prevention and Tobacco Control Act of 2010 prohibit cigarette companies from sponsoring any athletic or cultural events or using their logos on items of clothing. In 2011, new graphic images depicting the effects of smoking were required to be placed on all packaging (FCC, 2011).

8.11. RISK MANAGEMENT

Risk entails a potential loss as a result of an action and applies to all aspects of life. Managing that risk is important to the financial health of a business, just as it is important to the physical health of patients and their care providers.

Risk management in corporations may involve 'managing' ethics in the workplace through policies and procedures designed to educate, reinforce, and regulate acceptable and non-acceptable behaviors. "The very exercise of developing a code is in itself worthwhile; it forces a large number of people to think through, in a fresh way, their mission and the important obligations they, as a group and as individuals, have with respect to society as a whole." (DeGeorge, 1994). All risk management programs are undertaken because corporations wish to minimize any negative effects on their bottom line, either by purposeful or accidental losses of their products, reputation, market share or income. In the light of several well-known scandals such as Enron, Tyco, AIG and Arthur Anderson, the public (specifically customers and stakeholders) is now very much aware that corporations must integrate and enforce codes of ethics as they determine what levels of risk are acceptable.

The Caux Round Table (CRT), an international consortium of business leaders whose goal is to promote ethical business practices in global society, suggests that there are ethical risk principles relating to customers, employees, stakeholders, owners, suppliers, competitors and the public that should be considered in a risk management strategy (see http://www.cauxroundtable.org/principles/). By answering questions and outlining possible scenarios in each of these categories, a framework for ethical corporate responsibility can be developed and used as a standard for all communities of interest.

Internal and external audits for financial reporting (Institute of Internal Auditors (IIA) Code of Ethics, (2013) are two of the main resources used in a risk management program, yet alone they do not address the underlying reasons such audits are necessary and legally required. A company must analyze all types of risks involving individual employees, management, board directors, investors, customers, and competitors—everything that concerns corporate legal compliance https://na.theiia.org/special-promotion/PublicDocuments/Code%20of%20 Ethics.pdf. The U.S. Sentencing Commission in 2005 and updated in 2018, amended its guidelines to require companies to expand their programs to include "compliance and ethics as a means to prevent and detect criminal conduct and foster an organizational culture that encourages ethical conduct and a commitment to legal compliance" (Federal Sentencing Guidelines Manual and Appendices, United States Sentencing Commission, effective2018 https://www.ussc.gov/guidelines/2018-guidelines-manual). This emphasis on organizational culture and corporate responsibility implies that compliance and ethics must be pervasive in a company, from top management on down.

Risks associated with compliance violations and ethics may include:

- *"accounting breakdowns including fraud, inaccurate record keeping, inappropriate record retention or destruction and noncompliance with the requirements of Sarbanes-Oxley;*
- *Business ethics failures, such as the exposure of confidential client information, conflicts of interest and giving and receiving inappropriate gifts;*
- *Employment related risks such as equal opportunity violations, workplace harassment and immigration offenses;*
- *Fair trading laws, which cover price fixing, abuse of dominance and collusion;*
- *Customer and workplace violations; for example, aiding and abetting illegal customer acts and creating unsafe workplace conditions and;*
- *Product issues such as product safety failures and intellectual property violations" (LRN/Ethics and compliance risk management, 2007, p.3).*

Public perception of a company's reputation is also a risk which may affect a company's performance and is now influenced by an ever growing world of twenty-four hour live communication channels. Public relations professionals who are specialists in handling the fallout of bad publicity are now plentiful and are frequently employed by firms wishing to minimize the risk of financial damage resulting from a change in public opinion.

Risk management that is solely focused on legal compliance and requirements will not be effective unless there is an underlying culture that encourages ethical behavior through continuing education and support systems, while clearly and consistently enforcing code violations.

8.12. STAKEHOLDER ISSUES

In the broadest sense, a stakeholder is a constituent who can be affected by an organization's actions, while shareholders are those who own stock in a company. There are many different stakeholders and stakeholder groups in business and all are important, even those without a financial impact on the organization. Healthcare stakeholders range from patients to the largest healthcare systems/hospitals and everything in between. For an example of the many stakeholders in health care see https://www.stakeholdermap.com/examples-stakeholders-healthcare. html#health, accessed January, 2019.

Stakeholders differ from shareholders because, in theory, a corporation's responsibility to its shareholders is purely fiduciary, while the responsibility to stakeholders goes beyond financial responsibility. Stakeholders may include investors, employees, suppliers, customers, and also prospective employees and customers, trade associations, government bodies, competitors, the environment and the public. As explained by Grunig and Repper, the public differs from stakeholders because problems arise around issues and stakeholders are 'connected to the organization by consequences" (Grunig, 1992, pp. 171-57). As noted by Collins, ". . . the actions of individuals within the health care industry impact more than just the stockholders of the organization. In health care organizations, errors in management strategies and poor leadership decisions can impact all stakeholders and shareholders alike. This is mainly due to the fact that unlike most other industries, those in the health care industry understand that their actions could potentially create life-threatening consequences" (Collins, 2010, p. 343).

Research by Bowen demonstrates that many organizations showed "a preference for legalistic codes of ethics and governance documents seemed to pervade all but the most exemplary organizations in this sample." (Bowen, 2010). R. Edward Freeman (1984) suggests an idea of 'stakeholder theory' which states that a corporation/business firm should be managed in a way that achieves balance among the interests of everyone who bears a substantial relationship to the firm, i.e., its stakeholders. In one of his many lectures for the Darden School of Business's Business Roundtable Institute for Corporate Ethics, Freeman said, "Stakeholder theory says if you just focus on financiers, you miss what makes capitalism tick. What makes capitalism tick is that shareholders and financiers, customers, suppliers, employees, communities can together create something that no one of them can create alone" (Freeman, 2009).

Section 406 of the Sarbanes-Oxley Act of 2002 mandates that top officers in an organization have a code of ethics and defines a code of ethics as "standards as are reasonably necessary to promote honest and ethical conduct, including the ethical handling of actual or apparent conflict of interest between personal and professional relationships; full, fair, accurate, timely, and understandable disclosure in the periodic reports required to be filed by the issuer; and compliance with applicable governmental rules and regulations" (http://www.gpo.gov/fdsys/pkg/PLAW-107publ204/html/PLAW-107publ204.htm). Enactment of Sarbanes-Oxley has also motivated companies to put in place (and make public) policies and procedures that address ethical issues, not only for their employees, but for all stakeholders. Similarly, professional organizations are incorporating ethical behavior guidelines regarding stakeholders/shareholders into their codes of conduct (Association of Chartered Certified Accounts, 2007).

The 2010 Dodd-Frank act, put in place after the 2008 financial crisis, requires publicly held companies to give shareholders a 'say on pay' about executive compensation. In 2011, of 2,532 companies reporting, "shareholders at 39 of them rejected executive pay plans" (WSJ, July 8, 2011, B1), perhaps suggesting that excessive executive compensation may not meet the ethical standards of fair pay to company shareholders.

This emphasis on shareholder value being affected by ethics is not just occurring in the United States. Globalization and corporate social responsibility is now the norm in multi-national corporations. Archie Carroll has developed a pyramid framework for global institutions that states:

- *"Make a profit consistent expectations for international businesses (economic responsibility);*
- *Obey the law of host countries as well as international law (legal responsibility);*
- *Be ethical in its practices, taking host country and global standards into consideration (ethical responsibility); and*
- *Be a good corporate citizen, especially as defined by the host country's expectations (philanthropic responsibility)." (Carroll, 2004, p. 118)*

Corporate social responsibility may be initiated by stakeholders/shareholders rather than the 'conscience' of management, who may urge companies to 'do the right thing', but studies and surveys have shown that customers' purchasing decisions are increasingly influenced by the ethical conduct of the company and companies are listening (Kanovich, 2007).

8.13. TRANSPARENCY

Information is critical to patients, providers and systems yet the necessary information in health care is far from transparent. Transparency in healthcare and business may take various forms, from publishing results of specific studies in the lay press, to detailing specific political background of supporters, to making financial reporting more readily accessible. According to Rio and McAvey (2018) transparency is necessary to competition.

The All Payer Claims Databases (APCDs) are growing phenomenon. Many states are developing these information repositories aimed at increasing transparency (see https://www.apcdcouncil.org/state/map, accessed January 2018). New Hampshire provides an example of one site, see https://nhhealthcost.nh.gov/. However, there are still unresolved issues about transparency as evidenced by the 2016 Supreme Court of the United States 6-2 ruling that ERISA preempts Vermont law regarding some aspects of transparency in Gobeille v. Liberty Mutual Insurance Company.

Beyond legal and financial requirements, many companies now realize the benefits of providing the public clear transparent statements of their ethical values and social responsibility (Bernard and Lacrosse, 2005; Jacobs, Cerfolio and Sade, 2009). Ernst and Young, the accounting firm, has a general section on their website about its corporate Code of Conduct and transparency which says:

"We promote a culture of integrity among our professionals. The EY Global Code of Conduct provides a clear set of principles that guide our actions and our business conduct, and are to be followed by all EY personnel. The Code of Conduct is divided into five categories:

- *Working with one another*
- *Working with clients and others*
- *Acting with professional integrity*
- *Maintaining our objectivity and independence*
- *Respecting intellectual capital*

Through our procedures to monitor compliance with the EY Global Code of Conduct, and through frequent communications, we strive to create an environment that encourages all personnel to act responsibly, including *reporting misconduct without fear of retaliation (https://www.ey.com/ Publication/vwLUAssets/ey-us-transparency-report-2017/$FILE/ey-us-transparency-report-2017.pdf)"*

The Commonwealth Foundation published a report in 2006 that said, "Transparency and better public information on cost and quality are essential for three reasons: (1) to help providers improve by benchmarking their performance against others; (2) to encourage private insurers and public programs to reward quality and efficiency; and (3) to help patients make informed choices about their care." The authors believe that to achieve transparency in our health system, the following steps should be taken:

- *"Medicare can assume a leadership role in making cost and quality information by provider and by patient condition publicly available...*
- *Create a National Quality Coordination Board within the U.S. Department of Health and Human Services, as the Institute of Medicine has recommended. The board will set priorities, oversee the development of appropriate quality and efficiency measures, ensure the collection of timely and accurate information on these measures at the individual provider level, and encourage their incorporation in pay-for-performance payment systems operated by Medicare, Medicaid, and private insurers.*
- *Invest in health information technology . . .*
- *Make fundamental changes in current payment methods . . .*
- *Modify HSA legislation to reduce its potentially harmful effects on vulnerable populations . . ." (Commonwealth Fund, 2006).*

In 2010, Health and Human Services in 2010 began an initiative, the Community Health Data Initiative (CHDI), which will provide free government health data directly to the public. Their mission is to "(1) raise awareness of community health performance, (2) increase pressure on decision makers to improve performance, and (3) help facilitate and inform action to improve performance." The U.S. Department of Health and Human Services (HHS) faces increasingly complex challenges One initiative to be more transparent to the public addresses access to public data as follows:

"From across the U.S. Department of Health and Human Services (HHS), its many agencies collect a vast array of data to better understand the health of the nation. The Office of the CTO has been a leader in the federal government in enabling the public release of more than 1,500 data sets collected by HHS for use by researchers and entrepreneurs. The Open Data movement continues to be a focus of the Department

and the Office of the CTO is committed to making data available for the public to do research, develop applications, and create new products to improve health.

HHS is also examining how it is currently using its own data assets to make more evidence-based policy decisions. Sharing data internally at HHS and across its many different agencies is a priority. The Data Initiative is exploring HHS' data assets across all agencies and the ways in which data can be shared and connected in responsible ways to improve how HHS delivers on its mission. The Office is interested in identifying models of effective sharing and looking for opportunities to address inefficiencies."

(https://www.hhs.gov/cto/initiatives/data-initiative/index.html, accessed January 2019).

Perhaps nothing could be less 'transparent' in the healthcare professions than admitting to medical errors. Ethically sound, but fraught with concerns about malpractice, any admission of guilt has long been considered an unwise decision. However, in a study published in the Annals of Internal Medicine in 2010, a study was conducted of the University of Michigan Health System (UMHS), which began to fully disclose and offer compensation to patients for medical errors in 2001. The purpose of the study was to compare liability claims and costs before and after the new program—in other words, whether or not it cost more to 'do the right thing.' Brin (2018), states "While the open approach may feel counterintuitive to administrators, physicians, and malpractice attorneys, studies and anecdotal accounts suggest transparency and accountability policies can save hospitals, patients, and families years of grueling litigation that typically ends in settlement." (https://news.aamc.org/patient-care/article/best-response-medical-errors-transparency)

Different strategies in error reduction have been proposed, most of which include transparency as one element. Lambert et al (2016) report on the results of implementing the "Seven Pillars"of safety. The pillars (McDonald et al, 2010) include:

1. Incident reporting
2. Investigation
3. Early communication with patient and family
4. Full disclosure, apology and remedy
5. System improvement
6. Data tracking and evaluation
7. Education and training.

The Lambert et.al (2016) study used hospital information to look at the effectiveness of the "Seven Pillars". They found that the system increased incidence reports, but reduced claims, legal fees, claims and insurance costs. When it may be that only 41% of the medical profession actually reported medical errors, there is an obvious need for education about the need for transparency (Anwer & Abu-Zaid, 2014).

8.14. CASE STUDIES

1. One of your patients with difficult to control hypertension has responded well to some drug samples for a new beta blocker that you gave him. You write him a prescription for the medication and are told by your office staff later that week, that the patient has called and told them that his insurance plan only covers the generic version of the drug. How should you handle the patient's request for the brand name drug? What if you believe there is no difference in efficacy? What if you believe there is reason to prescribe the brand name but it is far more expensive? What effects do requests such as these have on the health care system? Should you have used drug samples in the first place? Is it your responsibility, the managed care company's, the pharmaceutical firm's or the government's to determine what is in a patient's best interest, regardless of cost?

2. An undocumented, uninsured migrant worker is brought into the emergency room of a local community hospital with shortness of breath and chest pain. He was admitted to the hospital for evaluation and testing. Further exams showed congestive heart disease and severe atrial regurgitation. It is determined that the patient requires a valve replacement. Without being eligible for Medicaid because of his immigration status, and no way to pay for this expensive operation, what is your responsibility as a health care provider? What is the hospital's responsibility? How involved should the patient be in the decision making process? Do the principles of justice and beneficence hold here? Are there justifiable limits to the amount of care provided? What about allocation of scarce resources?

3. Mrs. X was at her annual gynecological exam with her nurse practitioner, Dr. Jones. Mrs. X is a healthy 45 year old who doesn't smoke, exercises regularly, and maintains her weight through good nutrition. All age appropriate and recommended screening tests have been negative in the past. Today she states

that a new imaging center has opened up in her neighborhood and they are advertising a whole body CT scan. She asks Dr. Jones to prescribe this for her, 'just in case' there's a problem that could only be seen by the scan. What is Dr. Jones responsibility to the patient? To the patient's insurance company? What ethical principles are at stake here or in any case when a patient requests a test or procedure that is not medically indicated? Is the imaging center utilizing ethical marketing practices by going directly to the consumer and implying there is a need for their product? Are patients entitled to expensive diagnostic procedures?

4. You have been invited by a pharmaceutical company to lead an informal discussion about high blood pressure, particularly in post-menopausal women. The discussion will be held in a restaurant and will be hosted by the company. There will be as many as twenty nurse practitioners attending, all with prescriptive privileges in your state. The pharmaceutical company sells a new and very expensive prescription product for reducing blood pressure. You are offered $500 to help recruit attendees and to lead the discussion. What ethical issues are involved? Are there any legal or professional concerns? Would you be more likely to prescribe this company's medication rather than another's or over lifestyle changes? If you sign a contract with a drug company to help recruit participants and lead an informal discussion, are you required to disclose this to your current employer's conflict of interest policy?

5. A patient of yours is experiencing premature ejaculation and has asked for your help. The anti-depressant medication sertraline (Zoloft) is commonly prescribed to treat this condition. The patient's insurance plan will pay for Zoloft only for treatment of depression. You wonder whether it is 'insurance fraud' to help the patient have the cost of his medication covered by his insurance company, by prescribing Zoloft for depression instead of for premature ejaculation treatment. What other issues might be involved? If you proceed with ordering the Zoloft, how would you chart/justify the reasons for doing so? Is this a legal issue? Would/should you involve the patient in the decision?

6. Your practice sees a mix of Medicare, Medicaid and privately insured patients. Over the past year, reimbursements from all these sources have been steadily declining and you are now forced with a choice: lay off two of your long-time front office/billers who are the main source of income for their families or stop taking insurance altogether. You know that if you do stop

taking insurance, you will lose many of your patients because they will not be able to afford your new charges. What are the main ethical dilemmas presented by this case?

8.15. SELECTED WEBSITES

- **American Association of Colleges of Nursing**
  https:// www.aacn.org
- **American Medical Association:**
  https://www. https://www.ama-assn.org
- **American Association of Colleges of Medicine:**
  https://aacm.org
- **American Nurses Association:**
  https://www.nursingworld.org
- **Office of the Inspector General:**
  https://www.OIG.hhs.gov
- **Centers for Medicare and Medicaid Services:**
  https://www.cms.gov
- **National Organization of Nurse Practitioner Faculties:**
  https://www.nonpf.org
- **National Council for State Boards of Nursing:**
  https://www.ncsbn.org
- **Agency for Healthcare Quality and Research:**
  https://www.ahrq.gov
- **National Committee for Quality Assurance:**
  https://www.ncqa.org
- **Center for Affordable Quality Healthcare:**
  https://www.caqh.org
- **The Joint Commission:**
  https://www.jointcommission
- **Center for Affordable Quality Healthcare:**
  https://www.caqh.org

8.16. REFERENCES

Introduction
Marcinko, D. (Ed.) (2005) The Business of Medical Practice: Advanced Profit Maximization Techniques for Savvy Doctors, 2nd Edition. Springer Publishing Company.

Accounting
AICPA Code of Professional Conduct. (1988) Jersey City, NJ: American Institute of Certified Public Accountants.

AICPA Committee on Terminology. (1953) Accounting Terminology Bulletin No. 1, Review and Resume.

Alexander, D., Burns, G., Manor, R., McRoberts, F., and Torriero, E.A. (2002) The fall of Anderson. Hartford Courant. http://www.courant.com/news/nationworld/chi-0209010315sep01,0,2343149.story.

Dellaportas, S. (2006) Making a difference with a discrete course on accounting ethics. Journal of Business Ethics, 65: 391-404. DOI 10.1007/s10551-006-0020-7.

Duska, R. and Duska, B. (2003) Accounting Ethics. Wiley-Blackwell, p. 28. ISBN 0-631-21651-0. http://books.google.com/?id=Y4LgynCsC&printsec=frontcover&dq=Understanding+Accounting+Ethics.

Institute of Internal Auditors. (1988) IIA Code of Ethics. Altamonte Springs, FL: Institute of Internal Auditors.

Institute of Management Accounts. (1997) Statements on Management Accounting: Objectives of Management Accounting, Statement No. 1B. New York, NY: Institute of Management Accounts.

Jackling, B., Cooper, B., Leung, P., and Dellaportas, S. (2007) Professional accounting bodies: perceptions of ethical issues, causes of ethical failure and ethics education. Managerial Auditing Journal 22(9): 928-944. Doi:10.1108/02686900710829426. http://proquest.umi.com.libproxy.sdsu.edu/pqdweb: did=1347117971&sid=1&Fmt=3&clientId-17862&RQT=309&VName+PQD.

Kidder, R. (2015). Ethics in accounting. http://cuidadosrespiratorios.com/ethics-in-accounting.html.

Loeb, S. (1988) Teaching students accounting ethics: some crucial issues. Issues in Accounting Education 3: 316–329. http://proquest.umi.com.libproxy.sdsu.edu/pqdweb?did=7569002&sid=1&2Fmt=7&clientId=17862&RQT=309&VName=PQD. Retrieved April 7, 2011.

Loeb, S. (1994) "Ethics and accounting doctoral education." Journal of Business Ethics, 13: 817–828.

Sarbanes-Oxley Act of 2002. www.sec.gov/about/laws/soa2002.pdf.

Smith, K. and Smith, L. Business and Accounting Ethics, http://acct.tamu.edu/smith/ethics/ethics.htm. Retrieved April 7, 2011.

Somerville, L. (Feb. 28, 2003). Accounting changes boil down to principles vs. rules. The Business Journal. http://www.bizjournals.com/triad/stories/2003/03/03/focus2.html. Retrieved April 7, 2011.

Conflict of Interest

AMA Code of Medical Ethics – Opinion 8.03 – Conflicts of Interest: Guidelines http://www.ama-assn.org/ama/pub/physician-resources/medical-ethics/code-medical-ethics/opinion803.page?

AMA Code of Medical Ethics—Opinion 10.018—Physician Participation in Soliciting Contributions from Patients. http://www.ama-assn.org/ama/pub/physician-resources/medical-ethics/code-medical-ethics/opinion10018.

ANA Enterprise: Code of ethical conduct and compliance program (2018). https://www.nursingworld.org/~49a7fc/globalassets/docs/ancc/anaenterprisecodeofethicalconductandcomplianceprogram.pdf.

Bernard, R. and Lacrosse, C. (2005) Corporate transparency: code of ethics disclosures. The CPA Journal.

Brennan, T.J., Rothman, D.J., et al. (2006) Health industry practices that create conflicts of interest: a policy proposal for academic medical centers. JAMA 295: 429–33.

Campbell, E.G., Weissman J.S., et.al. (2007) Institutional academic industry relationahips. JAMA 298: 1779–86.

Carreyrou, J. (2011) Senators look into Medtronic, doctors. Wall Street Journal, June 29, 2011, B1.

Columbia University (accessed, January 2019) Conflict of Interest FAQs. Retrieved from https://research.columbia.edu/content/conflict-interest-faqs.

Conflict of Interest Theme Issue (2017). JAMA 317 (17), 1705-1812.

Fineberg, H.V. (2017). Conflict of interest: Does it matter? JAMA 317 (17), 1717-1718.

International Committee of Medical Journal Editors: Author responsibilities- Conflicts of Interest (accessed 2019). http://www.icmje.org/recommendations.

IOM/NAM (2009). Conflict of Interest in Medical Research, Education, and Practice. http://www.nationalacademies.org/hmd/Activities/Workforce/ConflictOfInterest.aspx.

Lo, B. and Field, M.J. (Eds.). (2009) Conflict of Interest and Medical Research, Education and Practice. Washington (DC): National Academies Press, 2009.

Lo, B & Grady, D. (2017). Payments to physicians: does the amount of money make a difference? JAMA 317 (17), 1723-4.

NIH (accessed 2019). Financial conflicts of interest. https://grants.nih.gov/grants/policy/coi/index.htm.

Jacobs, J., Cerfolio, R., and Sade, R. (2009) The ethics of transparency: publication of cardiothoracic surgical outcomes in the lay press. The Annals of Thoracic Surgery. 87: 679–686.

Pinzur, MS. (2017). Conflict of interest. Foot and Ankle International 38 (7), 820.

Serra, M.E. (2017). Conflict of interest: Nuances between principles and the aim. Arch Argent Pediatr 115 (5), 501-504.

Technology Transfer: Administration of the Bayh Dole Act by Research Universities. US General Accounting Office report to congressional committees. GAO/RCED-98–126, 1998. www.gao.gov/archive/1998/rc98126.pdf.

Fraud

Birkhahn, R., et al. (2009) A review of federal guidelines that inform and influence relationships between physicians and industry. Academic Emergency Medicine 2009: 16: 776–781.

Buppert, C. (2012) Nurse Practitioner's Business Practice and Legal Guide. Sudbury, MA: Jones and Barlett Learning, LLC.

CMS Anti-Kickback https://www.cms.gov/compliance/safe-harbor-regulations.

CMS Changes to Disclosure of Physician Ownership in Hospitals and Physician Self-Referral Rules, Federal Register, October 3, 2008 https://www.cms.gov/acuteinpatientpps/ipps/itemdetail.asp?itemid=CMS1227598.

CMS Deficit Reduction Act https://www.cms.gov/DeficitReductionAct/Downloads/Checklist1.pdf.

CMS False Claims Act (2017) Medicare Fraud & Abuse: Prevention, Detection, and Reporting. Retrieved from https://www.cms.gov/Outreach-and-Education/Medicare-Learning-Network-MLN/MLNProducts/downloads/fraud_and_abuse.pdf. Accessed January 2019.

CMS Health Care Fraud Statute https://www.cms.gov/MLNProducts/downloads/Fraud_and_Abuse.pdf.

CMS Medicare HIPAA Eligibility https://www.cms.gov/Medicare HIPAA/Eligibility-TransactionSystemInquiriesRulesofBehavior.pdf.

CMS Physician Self Referral (2015) https://www.cms.gov/Medicare/Fraud-and-Abuse/ PhysicianSelfReferral/. Accessed January 2019).

Mustard, L. (2009) Questionable hospital financial relationships with physicians. Medical Practice Management, July/August 2009, pp. 41–43.

Patient Protection and Affordable Care Act, 2010, Public Law 111–148 http://www. gpo.gov/fdsys/pkg/PLAW-111publ148/content-detail.html.

Gifts

AMA Medical Code of Ethics Opinion 8.061—Gifts to Physicians from Industry http:// www.ama-assn.org/ama/put/physiican-resources/medical-ethics/code-medical-ethics/opinion8061.page?

AMA Medical Code of Ethics Opinion 10.017—Gift from Patients http://www. ama-assn.org/ama/put/physiican-resources/medical-ethics/code-medical-ethics/ opinion10017.page?

Brennan, T.J., Rothman, D.J., et al. (2006) Health industry practices that create conflicts of interest: a policy proposal for academic medical centers. JAMA 295: 429–33, 2006.

Columbia University School of Nursing. (2009) Accepting Gifts from Students Policy. CUSON Faculty Handbook, CUSON Intranet.

Mizik, N. (2010) The pharmaceutical industry interactions with physicians: the cost, the ethics, and the patient welfare. Columbia CaseWorks, Columbia Business School, pp. 1–7).

Pharmaceutical Research and Manufacturers of America. (2010) Code on Interactions with Healthcare Professionals. Washington, DC: Pharmaceutical Research and Manufacturers of America; c2010 [Revised 2008 Jun]. http://www.phrma.org/ code_on_interactions_with_healthcare_professionals.

Yukhananvov, A. (2011) Drugmakers get more time to record gifts to doctors. Reuters, Dec. 14, 2011. http://www.reuters.com/article/2011/12/15/us-cms-sunshine-idUSTRE7BE04N20111215.

Human Resources

Kim, M..I; Coiera, E.; & Magrabi, F. (2017). Problems with health information technology and their effects on care delivery and patient outcomes: a systematic review, Journal of the American Medical Informatics Association, 24, (1) pp.246–250, https://doi.org/10.1093/jamia/ocw154.

Lehigh University Code of Ethics. http://www.lehigh.edu/~inhro/code_of_ethics.html.

Margolis, J., Grant, A., and Molinsky, A. (2007) Expanding ethical standards of hrm: necessary evils and the multiple dimensions of impact. In: Human Resource Management Ethics and Employment, pp. 237–251. A. Pinninton, R. Macklin and T. Campbell (Eds.). New York: Oxford University Press.

Rose, A. (2007) Ethics and Human Resource Management. McGraw Hill Publishers. http://highered.mcgrawhill.com/sites/dl/free/0077111028/536508/EHR_CO2.pdf)).

Society for Human Resource Management (2014). Ethics. Accessed at https://www. shrm.org/about-shrm/pages/code-of-ethics.aspx, January 2018.

Sarbanes-Oxley Act of 2002 www.sec.gov/about/laws/soa2002.pdf.

Winstanley, D. and Woodall, J. (1996) Business ethics and human resource management. Personnel Review, 25(6): 5–12.

Information Technology

AMA Code of Medical Ethics—Opinion 5.07—Confidentiality: Computers http://

www.ama-assn.org/ama/put/physician-resources/medical-ethics/code-medical-ethics/opinion507.page?

AMA Code of Medical Ethics—Opinion 5.10—A Physician's Role Following a Breach of Electronic Health Information Mail http://www.ama-assn.org/ama/put/physician-resources/medical-ethics/code-medical-ethics/opinion510.page?

American College of Healthcare Executives http://www.ache.org/policy/hiconf.cfm.

Calluzzo, V. and Cante, C. (2004) Ethics in information technology and software use. Journal of Business Ethics, 51: 301–302.

CMS https://www.cms.gov/EHRIncentivePrograms/.

HIPAA http://www.cms.gov/NationalProvidentStand/.

Hongladarom, S. and Ess, C. (Eds.) (2007) Information Technology Ethics: Cultural Perspectives. Hershey, PA: Idea Group Reference, 2007. (ISBN 1-59904-310-6).

Kansas State University. Information Technology Employee Code of Ethics. https://www.ksu.edu/infotech/ethics/.

LA Times. (2007) http://latimesblogs.latimes.com/lanow/2011/07/ucla-pays-865500-to-settle-celebrity-medical-record-snooping-case.html.

Reynolds, G., 2009. Ethics in Information Technology. Cengage Learning, Boston, MA.

Limited Resources

AMA Medical Code of Ethics Opinion 9.051 http://www.ama-assn.org/ama/pub/physician-resources/medical-ethics/code-medical-ethics/opinion90651.page?

Bloomfield, E. (2009) The ethics of rationing of critical care services: Should technology assessment play a role? Anesthesiology Research and Practice, Article ID 915197, 8 pages.

Fruits, E. (2010) The Oregon Health Plan, A Bold Experiment that Failed. Portland, Oregon: Cascade Policy Institute.

Jonsen, A. (1998) Resource Allocation: Ethical Topic in Medicine. University of Washington School of Medicine. http://depts.washington.edu/bioethx/topics/resall.html.

Persad, G., Wertheimer, A., and Emanuel, E. (2009) Principles for allocation of scarce medical interventions. The Lancet January 31, 2009; 373: 423–31.

Managed Care/Third Party Payers/Billing and Collections

AMA Medical Code of Ethics Opinion 8.054—Financial Incentives and the Practice of Medicine, http://www.ama-assn.org/ama/pub/physician-resources/medical-ethics/code-medical-ethics/opinion8054.page?

AMA Medical Code of Ethics Opinion 8.13 – Managed Care, http://www.ama-assn.org/ama/pub/physician-resources/medical-ethics/code-medical-ethics/opinion813.page?

American College of Physicians. The Changing Practice Environment. In: ACOP Ethics Manual Sixth Edition, http://www.acponline.org/running_practice/ethics/manual/manual6th.htm#finance.

Anand, G. (2008) Opting out. Wall Street Journal June 28, 2008, A1.

Darragh, M. and McCarrick, P. (1996) Managed health care: new ethical issues for all. National Reference Center for Bioethics Literature, Scope Note 31, Kennedy Institute of Ethics Journal, 1996.

Hall, M.A. and Schneider, C.E. (2008) Patients as consumers; courts, contracts and the new medical marketplace. Michigan Law Review 106(4): 643–649.

Hall, M.A. and Schneider, C.E. The professional ethics of billing and collections. JAMA 300(15): 1806–1808.

Povar, G. et al. (2004) Ethics in Practice: Managed Care and the Changing Health Care Environment, Medicine as a Profession Managed Care Ethics Working Group Statement. Annals of Internal Medicine, July 20, 2004, 141(2): 131–136.

University of Washington School of Medicine. Managed Care, Ethics in Medicine. http://depts.washington.edu/bioethx/topics/manag.html.

Marketing

American Dental Association. Principles of Ethics and Code of Professional Conduct, With Official Advisory Opinions Revised to January 2005. Chicago: ADA.

American Marketing Association. Statement of Ethics. http://www.marketingpower.com/AboutAMA/Pages/Statement%20of%20Ethics.aspx.

American Medical Association. Medical Code of Ethics http://www.ama-assn.org/ama/put/physisicn-resources/medical-ethics/code-medical-ethics/opinion502.page?

American Psychological Association. (2002) Ethical principles of psychologists and code of conduct. American Psychologist, 57: 1060–1073.

Ethical Moment—What ethical considerations are involved in offering introductory discounts to attract new patients?, Journal of the American Dental Association, 139(6): 769–771.

Ethics and Plastic Surgery: ASAPS position. July 20, 2000. http://www.surgery.org/media/news-releases/ethics-and-plastic-surgery-asaps-position

Federal Communications Commission. http://www.fcc.gov/cgb/consumerfacts/advertising.html.

Federal Communications Commission. http://transition.fcc.gov/mb/audio/decdoc/public_and_broadcasting.html#_Toc202587565.

Federal Communications Commission. http://transition.fcc.gov/mb/audio/decdoc/public_and_broadcasting.html#_Toc202587565.

Federal Drug Administration. http://www.fda.gov/Drugs/ResourcesForYou/Consumers/PrescriptionDrugAdvertising/ucm072025.htm.

Federal Trade Commission http://business.ftc.gov/advertising-and-marketing/health-claims.

Taylor, M, (2011). The impact of the "business" of pain medicine on patient care. Pain Medicine 12: 763–772.

Wong, W., Camp, M., Camp, J., and Gupta, S. (2010). The quality of internet advertising in aesthetic surgery: an in-depth analysis. Aesthetic Surgery Journal, 30(5): 735–743.

Risk Management

2005 Federal Sentencing Guidelines 8B2.1(a)(2). 2005 Federal Sentencing Guidelines Manual and Appendices, United States Sentencing Commission, effective 1 November 2005, http://www.ussc.gov/guidelin.htm.

DeGeorge, R. (1994) In:, Military Ethics: Reflections on Principles – The Profession of Arms, Military Leadership, Ethical Practices, War and Morality, Education the Citizen-Soldier, p. 28. M. Wakin (Ed.). Diane Publishing.

Dienhart, J. (2010) Enterprise Risk Management: Why Ethics and Compliance Function Adds Value. Seattle, WA: The Ethics Resource and the ERC Fellows Risk Assessment Group, Seattle University.

Grunig, J.E. and Repper, F.C. (1992). Strategic management, publics and issues. In: Excellence in Public Relations and Communication Management, pp. 171–57. J.E. Grunig (Ed.). Hillsdale, NJ: Lawrence Erlbaum Associates.

Head, G. (2005) Why Link Risk Management and Ethics. International Risk Management Institute, February 2005. http://www.irmi.com/expert/articles/2005/head02.aspx.

Institute of Internal Auditors (IIA) (1988) Code of Ethics. Altamonte Springs, FL: Institute of Internal Auditors.

LRN (2007) Ethics and compliance risk management, pp. 3,12.

Young, P. (2004) Ethics and risk management: building a framework. Risk Management: An International Journal, 6(3): 23–34.

Stakeholders

Association of Chartered Certified Accounts. (2007) Business Ethics Contribute Towards Shareholder Value. http://www.acca.co.uk/page/3011288.

Bowen, S. (2010) An examination of applied ethics and stakeholder management on top corporate websites. Public Relations Journal 4(1).

Carroll, A. (2004) Managing ethically with global stakeholders: a present and future challenge. Academy of Management Executives 18(2): 114–119.

Collins, S. (2010)."Corporate social responsibility and the future health care manager. The Health Care Manager 29: 4: 339–345.

Corporate Disclosures Act. http://www.gpo.gov/fdsys/pkg/PLAW-107publ204/html/PLAW-107publ204.htm.

Freeman, R.E. (1984) Strategic Management: A Stakeholder Approach. Boston: Pitman.

Freeman, R.E. (2009) What is Stakeholder Theory? Business Roundtable Institute for Corporate Ethics, www.youtube.com/watch?v=bIRUalLcvPe8.

Grunig, J. (1992) Strategic management, publics and issues. In: Excellence in public relations and communication management, pp. 171–57. J.E. Grunig (Ed.).

Kanovich, E. (2007) Stakeholder Theory, Ethics and the Return on Customer. http://www.slideshare.net/ekanovich/stakeholder-theory-ethics-and-the-return-on-customer.

Transparency

Anwar, L.A. & Abu-Zaid, A. (2014) Transparency in medical error disclosure: The need for ormal teaching in undergraduate medical education curriculum, Med Educ Online. 19: 10.3402/meo.v19.23542.Published online 2014 Jan 31. doi: 10.3402/meo.v19.23542.

Bernard, R. and Lacrosse, C. (2005) Corporate transparency: code of ethics disclosures. The CPA Journal.

Brin, D.W. (2018, January 16). The best response to medical errors? Transparency. AANC news. Retrieved from: https://news.aamc.org/patient-care/article/best-response-medical-errors-transparency/.

Caux Round Table. Retrieved from http://www.cauxroundtable.org/principles/, accessed January 2019.

Collins, S. and Davis, K. (2006) Transparency in Health Care: The Time Has Come. The Commonwealth Fund, March 15, 2006.

Ernst and Young. (2011) Corporate Values.www.ey.com/US/en?About-us/Our-values

Jacobs, J., Cerfolio, R., and Sade, R. (2009) The ethics of transparency: publication of cardiothoracic surgical outcomes in the lay press. The Annals of Thoracic Surgery 87: 679-686.

Kachalia, A., et al. Liability claims and costs before and after implementation of a medical error disclosure program. Annals of Internal Medicine 153(4): 213–221.

McDonald,T.B.; Helmchen, L.A.; Smith, K.M.; Centomani, N.; Gunderson, A.; Mayer, D. & Chamberlin, W.H. (2010). Responding to patient safety incidents: "The Seven Pillars", Quality and Sifter in Health Care, 19 (6), e11.

Merck Ethics Policy http://www.merck.com/responsibility/ethics-and-transparency/home.html.

US Government Department of Health and Human Services. (2010) Community Health Data Initiative, 2010. http://www.hhs.gov/open/plan/opengovrnmentplan/initiatives/initiative.html.

US Government Department of Health and Human Services. (2010) Community Health Data Initiative, 2010. http://www.hhs.gov/open/plan/opengovrnmentplan/initiatives/initiative.html.

CHAPTER 9

Legal Issues for Advanced Practice Nurses

KIM A. O'HARA

9.1. INTRODUCTION

Health care delivery in the United States (US) is at an important crossroads with health care reform and system change (Institute of Medicine (IOM/NAM), 2010). A confluence of events, including the repeal, replacement and substantial modification of health care laws have created new challenges to operationalizing population health strategies, managing cost and improving the efficiency and effectiveness of care delivery. Further complicating matters are the many inconsistencies that exist from jurisdiction to jurisdiction in regard to regulation of practice. For the Advanced Practice Registered Nurse (APRN) practitioner, an understanding as to how these laws function is essential, as reconceptualization of the APRN role may be necessary in order to fulfill new obligations as they pertain to licensing, regulation, practice settings, scopes of practice and education. This chapter is designed to acquaint the reader with fundamental legal and regulatory principles that underpin professional practice. Contemporary issues of liability, ethical and regulatory practice constraints will be explored. Online resources are provided to encourage further prospect and understanding. APRNs are cautioned to use this information only as a resource and to seek legal counsel when necessary.

9.2. APRN PRACTICE GOVERNANCE

Regulatory mechanisms underpin APRN practice, yet it is well acknowledged that there is a lack of uniformity among the 50 states with respect to role recognition, titling, educational standards and competencies, legal scopes of practice, prescriptive authority and expectation of collaboration (Kleinpell, et al., 2014). Because the actions of healthcare

321

professionals can pose a potential risk to the public, the state has the obligation to enact laws to regulate practice and maintain the health, safety and welfare of its citizens (Russell, 2012). Jurisdictional differences created by state-level regulatory policies have created conflict between what the APRN can and may do, perpetuating discordance in hiring practices, misunderstanding by consumers and increasing potential for liability (Poghosyan, Liu & Norful, 2017).

9.3. NURSE PRACTICE ACT

APRN practice is governed by some integration of statute and regulation, each state with its own unique combination. These statutes or codified statements of law are passed by the state legislature and declare, proscribe or command something, often conditions and scopes of practice and more (Legal Information Institute) (LII), 2018). Commonly entitled "The Nurse Practice Act" (NPA), it is essentially the "who, what, where, when, why and how" of professional APRN practice within the geographic boundaries of that jurisdiction (American Nurses Association (ANA), 2018). Although the language and mandates vary among states, most NPAs typically include:

- Requirements for licensure and certification;
  –Types of nursing titles and licenses
  –Title protection
- Educational program accreditation standards;
  –Standards and scope of practice
- Authority, power, and composition of a Board of Nursing (BON);
- Grounds for disciplinary action and remedies for those noncompliant (Russell, 2018).

To date, only Michigan is without a stand-alone nurse practice act. In Michigan, all professional health care provider practice (dental hygienists, dental therapists, nurse practitioners, physician assistants and 21 others) is regulated by a consolidated practice act imbedded in their public health code.

9.4. BOARD OF NURSING

It is within the NPA mandate that state legislatures' delegate authority to a state governmental agency like a BON, to oversee nursing practice. While some BON's are independent agencies within a state government, others independent agencies outside state government or are an individual boards within an umbrella state agency (National Council of State Boards of Nursing (NCSBN) 2017), each are usually given responsibility and regulatory power by the NPA to:

- Set nursing education standards;
- Develop nursing standards of practice;
- License qualified applicants;
- Ensure continuing competency;
- Monitor nursing compliance with the rules and regulations of the NPA;
- Take action (discipline) for noncompliance (Russell, 2018).

Although from a legal perspective statutes and regulations have equal weight, a regulation dictated by a BON can never contradict a statute's directive. It is solely within the purview of the state legislature to adopt or modify practice acts to which the BON must adhere, legally obligating the APRN to comply or suffer consequences. Variance in the law and unpredictability of the health care system demands that APRN's do not act in the absence of explicit authority (statute or regulation).

Complaints reported to a board of nursing can come from a variety of sources including but not limited to patients, employers, co-workers, and members of the general public (Brous, 2012). How the complaints are processed and how the investigatory process unfolds varies from state to state. In all states, the nurse has the right to due process which includes fair treatment, full disclosure and the opportunity to respond and contest (appeal) accusations and judgments against them. It is only after a thorough investigation and sufficient basis to conclude the APRN violated the act, a BON may take action. Once a complaint is filed with a board of nursing, the boards have a complaint process that they follow from review to resolution. This process is summarized in the NCSBN video Board of Nursing Complaint Process: Investigation to Resolution (NCSBN, accessed January, 2019). Many APRN's mistakenly believe a BON will only act on practice deviations while on the job or in relation to a nurse-patient relationship. It is well within the BON's authority to discipline an APRN for activities that take place in their private life. Disciplinary actions are often grouped into the following categories. Practice related, drug-related, boundary violations, sexual misconduct, abuse, fraud and positive criminal background checks (NCSBN, 2009) and can encompass unprofessional or unethical conduct, unsafe, incompetent practice, scope of practice issues, willful misconduct (diverting narcotics, fraud and deceit, writing illegal prescriptions, presenting illegal prescriptions), alcohol and substance abuse allegations and criminal convictions to name a few (Brous, 2012). Although the terminology used to describe the types of discipline and remedies available to a BON is dictated by the NPA and varies among states, typical board action may include:

- Fine or civil penalty;
- Public reprimand or censure for minor violation of nurse practice act often with no restrictions on license;
- Limitation or restriction of one or more aspects of practice (e.g., probation with certain restrictions, limiting role, setting, activities, hours worked);
- Separation from practice for a period of time (suspension) or loss of license (revocation or voluntary surrender);
- Imposition of requirements for monitoring, remediation, education or other provisions tailored to the particular situation;
- Referral to an alternative discipline program for practice monitoring and recovery support (drug or alcohol dependent nurses, or in some other mental or physical conditions) (NCSBN, 2018)

9.5. NURSYS® AND THE NATIONAL PRACTITIONER DATA BANK (NPDB)

Professional disciplinary actions, nursing licensure verification, education and practice privileges are considered public information. While each state has a unique process for verifying a nurse's license and obtaining disciplinary information, most post information on Nursys®, a national database maintained by NCSBN, that provides centralized access to information supplied by participating state boards of nursing and all states in the Enhanced Nurse Licensure Compact (eNLC) nurse. org, 2019).

9.5.1. The Nursing Licensure Compact States & Nurse Licensure

As of July 2019, there are 29 states, with others pending, that are part of the eNLC:

- Alabama (Starting Date: TBD)
- Arizona
- Arkansas
- Colorado

- Delaware
- Florida
- Georgia
- Idaho
- Indiana (Starting: 1/1/2020)
- Iowa
- Kansas
- Kentucky
- Louisiana (Registered Nurse and Practical Nurse)
- Maine
- Maryland
- Mississippi
- Missouri
- Montana
- Nebraska
- New Hampshire
- New Mexico
- North Carolina
- North Dakota
- Oklahoma
- South Carolina
- South Dakota
- Tennessee
- Texas
- Utah
- Virginia
- West Virginia (Registered Nurse and Practical Nurse)
- Wisconsin
- Wyoming

For those states who do not post or who are not part of the compact, ProPublica (U.S.), an independent, nonprofit organization provides state by state guidelines to assist with an inquiry. The information can be accessed by placing the following link in your browser: https://projects.propublica.org/graphics/investigating-nurses.

It is important to understand that an APRN can be disciplined on the basis of their own state or another state's disciplinary action that implicates the individual's ongoing ability and likelihood to practice professionally and safely. The purpose of this retained jurisdictional authority is to prevent the nurse from evading disciplinary action merely by fleeing the state where the incident occurred.

In addition to state disciplinary licensure mandates, federal law also requires that adverse actions (disciplinary actions) taken against a health care professional's license also be reported. The National Practitioner Data Bank (NPDB) a confidential information clearinghouse estab-lished by Congress in 1986, compiles comprehensive data on the credentials of health care practitioners, entities, providers, and suppliers (NPDB, 2015). Reports in its public use file include details regarding medical malpractice payments, adverse clinical privileges actions, federal and state licensure and certification actions, professional society membership actions, peer review organization actions, private accreditation actions, exclusions from federal or state health care programs, and other adjudicated actions or decisions (NPDB, 2015). Unlike the Nursys® database, reportable state licensure actions (as determined by the law) are accessible from the NPDB only by authorized "eligible entities" such as hospitals, health centers, health plans, state licensing and certification authorities, and medical malpractice payers, as well as the subjects of the reports (NPDB, 2015). Adverse actions taken by a BON and reported to the NPDB remain in the NPDB indefinitely, visible to future employers and other eligible entities. Data bank listings may have dire consequences as they can compromise clinical privileges, professional society membership, participation in Medicare and Medicaid, collaborative practice agreements, and employability (Brous, 2012). In its most current research brief published by NCSBN in 2009, an analysis of Nursys® disciplinary data from 1996-2006, there were over 50,000 nurses reported by the 44 BONs for a disciplinary and over 114,000 violations. Of those, only a small percentage, 1% (n=1,052) were against APRN's (NCSBN, 2017). Despite the small percentage of disciplinary actions against APRN's, prudence dictates that the APRN should become an active member of an APRN collective or organization to obtain current information regarding education and practice obligations. Given that each state regulates APRN practice with statutes that differ and boards of nursing empowered with different responsibilities, it is imperative that all APRNs read their practice act regularly, become familiar with their respective BONs depth and breath of power and keep abreast of all legislative initiatives that affect practice.

9.6. CODE OF ETHICS FOR NURSES WITH INTERPRETIVE STATEMENTS "THE CODE"

In 2015, the Code of Ethics for Nurses with Interpretive Statements ("The Code") was revised by the ANA to provide a more succinct, prescriptive statement of the "ethical values, obligations, duties and professional ideals of nurses individually and collectively" that adequatly reflects "the contemporary context of nursing and anticipative advances in healthcare" (ANA, 2015b). As the system and practice changes, one can anticipate changes in the Code, therefore, it is critical

---

Box 9.1 - Resource links

- **NCSBN summarizes a general Board of Nursing Complaint Process in their video Board of Nursing Complaint Process: Investigation to Resolution:**
  https://youtu.be/fzEwtCxaTmI.
- **A list of APRN organizations:**
  https://onlinenursepractitionerprograms.com/professional-organizations/
- **Up to date contact information for each states BON:**
  https://www.ncsbn.org/contact-bon.htm:
- **General information pertaining to a BON's complaint process:**
  https://www.ncsbn.org/673.htm
- **Streamlined approach to ascertaining all APRN scope of practice laws by state, Barton Associates has compiled an interactive scope of practice law guide:**
  https://www.bartonassociates.com/locum-tenens-resources/
  nurse-practitioner-scope-of-practice-laws
- **The most recent APRN state by state legislative updates:**
  https://ruralprep.org/wp-content/uploads/2018/02/30th-APRN-Legislative-Update.pdf.

---

that the APRN read the Code often and become familiar with its tenets. The use of logic and self-awareness can often thwart unintended lapses.

Within complex systems arise complex problems. Everyday APRN's are faced with ethical dilemmas that require both decision and action. As professionals these decisions must be made utilizing specific knowledge and skills and the application of professional ethical tenets. These tenets are the foundation of values, morals and ideals of a profession that is "an expression of its own understanding of its commitment to society" (ANA, 2015b). Often deriving from the law, institutional policies/practices, policies of professional organizations, professional standards of care or fiduciary obligations (Brock and Mastroianni, 2014), its principles and standards are non-negotiable and may be referenced by a BON, court or other public body (APA, 2016). Whether or not an APRN has violated the Code does not solely determine legal liability, however, compliance with or violation of the Code may be admissible as evidence in some legal proceedings (Peterson, 2018). Until recently, courts have viewed ethical codes as something to which professionals merely aspire. Some have accepted ethical rules as a standard of practice and use the rules to determine professional responsibility, while others dismiss them as merely suggestions (Peterson, 2018). Recently, however, more state courts have determined that "ethical rules have legal significance and that failing to adhere to ethical standards can result in court-imposed civil liability" (Peterson, 2018). It is important to remember that actions that violate ethical codes may lead to the imposition of sanctions by professional associations and groups, BON's and health care service payer's, providers and the courts (Epstein and Turner, 2016). Some common Code violations include but are not limited to:

• Privacy violations;
• Withholding information;
• Allowing personal beliefs to interfere with patient care;
• Failure to pay spousal or child support or student loans;
• Failure to wear an identification badge with one's name and status prominently displayed;
• Bullying;
• Failure to respect professional boundaries with patient (Brous, 2012).

9.7. LEGAL

As health care delivery continues to evolve, APRNs will continue to play a critical role in meeting the needs of an increasing and diversifying population. This growth in demand along with practice scope expansion, will subject the APRN to increased responsibility, accountability and exposure to legal risk. APRNs can be named as a defendant and/or be asked to testify on behalf of another. The differences in the rules that govern a case differ based on whether the act is to be adjudicated under civil or criminal procedure.

9.7.1. Civil Actions

Civil actions deal with disputes between individuals or entities. A civil action is punished under the tort system, "which seeks to deter negligence by monetarily punishing negligent providers and compensating the injured parties with those monies" (Sohn, 2013). An APRN can become involved in a civil action such as professional negligence or medical malpractice, personal injury lawsuits, workers compensation or employment disputes against themselves or others. While dis-

---

Box 9.2 - Resource links

• **The ANA (2015b), provides recommendations as they pertain to The Code, that can be helpful at any level of practice:**
https://www.nursingworld.org/practice-policy/nursing-excellence/ethics/code-of-ethics-for-nurses/

ciplinary actions for ethical and regulatory breaches are difficult and often life-changing it is the prospect of being accused of professional negligence or medical malpractice that causes the most angst. Medical malpractice law is based on common law, whose general rules and governing principles have been established through judicial precedent or judge-made law, or case law.

Medical malpractice is considered to be "a type of professional negligence that results when the practitioner fails by act or omission to exercise the degree of skill and learning expected of a reasonably prudent, reputable member of their respective profession" (Black, 1979). It is legal theory that describes a failure to exercise the standard of care that a reasonably prudent practitioner (APRN with similar education, experience, years of practice) would exercise in like circumstances (practice area, patient condition). In order to obtain a favorable judicial outcome the individual bringing the claim (often the patient or their estate), must prove that the practitioner had a duty of care to them, breached that duty and as a result suffered injury or harm. The APRN duty typically arises within the context of a patient-provider relationship that commonly takes place during office hours or over the phone. However, advice given outside of the workplace with a patient or even a neighbor, may also be construed as a relationship depending on individual state case precedent. APRNs should note that the definition of relationship is not fixed but ever changing.

A breach occurs when the APRN's conduct (act or omission) falls below the standard of care in same or similar circumstances. Causation, although somewhat complex, is established when it is determined that the conduct of the APRN caused an injury or harm. This can be established if the harm or injury would not have occurred "but for" the conduct of the defendant (Black, 1979). If it would have occurred otherwise there is no causation and no negligence. Creating this link is often challenging. The jury must be convinced that the harm suffered was caused solely by the negligence; not other factors such as genetics, lifestyle choices, or an intervening event to name a few. The harm or injury can be either physical or emotional and can include but is not limited to pain, mental anguish. disfigurement, loss of enjoyment of life or aggravation of a pre-existing condition. If there is no harm there is no case.

9.7.2. Criminal Actions

Criminal law is a system of laws concerned with punishment of individuals who commit crimes. Both the states and the federal government have codified conduct that rises to the level of a crime justifying criminal sanction (punishment). These laws vary among states but are essentially designed to punish conduct that has harmed not only a victim but society as a whole. Unlike the purpose of a civil ligation (to resolve disputes and provide compensation), the purpose of criminal litigation is to punish and deter. APRN's can be charged with intentional crimes such as murder and fraud or criminally prosecuted for negligent behavior. In order to be culpable for criminal negligence, the APRN needs to have failed to perceive a "substantial and unjustifiable risk of such nature a degree that failure to perceive it constitutes a gross deviation from the standard of care that a reasonably prudent APRN would have observed in same or similar circumstances". The distinction between how grossly deviant from the standard of care the APRN was is often not clear or consistently applied varying state by state. In A *Review of Criminal Convictions Among Nurses, 2012-2013*, Zhong, McCarthy and Alexander (2016), found that nurses with criminal convictions accounted for approximately 10% of the disciplinary actions taken by BONs between 2003 and 2013, the majority of which were not patient related. Following are a series of case studies that illuminate the hurdles involved in establishing all of the elements of professional malpractice (negligence).

It is important to remember that not all harms are a result of negligence but rather result from the inherent risks present in the care or treatment, adverse events or system errors (Sohn, 2013), and while one can never predict what compels a patient to sue, the literature supports that a positive relationship between patient and provider with open, honest communication may be one way in which to protect practice (Joel, 2013).

Nevertheless a lawsuit can be harmful and costly regardless of ultimate outcome. According to the NPDB (2016), from 2012 to 2016, 11,095 claims were paid out by malpractice insurance companies on behalf of all practitioners, including physicians and advanced practice providers. For APRN's malpractice rates remain low with only 1.9% having been named as a primary defendant during that time (NPDB, 2016), (less than physicians (31.9%) and physician assistants (52.8%) respectively), (Brock, Nicholson and Hooker, 2016). The most frequent claims against them took place primarily in adult medical/primary care (41.2%) and behavioral health (15.3%) typically in physician practice settings (36%). The majority of allegations developed from a failure to diagnose properly (32.8%) improper prescription and management of medications (29.4%) and overall treatment and care management (22.3%). Only (4.2%) were related to scope of practice (NSO, 2017).

9.7.3. Case Studies

9.7.3.1. Case One: Established Duty

The APRN takes the day off to go to his son's little league game. Sitting in the stands he strikes up a conversation with his neighbor who asks what he suggests he should use to remedy his son's cough. The APRN asks appropriate questions regarding the youngster's state of health and ultimately suggests that the parent administer an over the counter cough suppressant. Although the drug prescribed was appropriate given the child's symptoms, the following day the APRN is informed that the child died after developing an allergic reaction. The father purports that the APRN did not ask if his son had any allergies. The APRN is ultimately sued for professional malpractice.

1. Have all the elements of professional negligence (malpractice) been met?
2. Does the APRN's actions rise to the level of a crime?
3. What defense if any can be raised on behalf of the APRN?
4. What responsibility does the parent have, if any?

9.7.3.2. Case Two: Criminal Negligence

The APRN in a collaborative office practice arrangement cares for a patient she has never seen before. The patient is returning to obtain results from a series of diagnostic tests done the previous week. Following a review of the tests, the APRN mistakenly tells the patient that she is cancer free when she is not. Continuing to have symptoms the patient seeks advice from another practitioner only to find out that the cancer has spread. Several weeks later, the patient dies and the APRN is charged with criminally negligent homicide.

1. Is the APRN criminally negligent?
2. What arguments can be made on her behalf?
3. What is it about the cancer diagnosis that makes this case unique?
4. Could the first provider who saw the patient the previous week be liable?

9.8. PROFESSIONAL LIABILITY INSURANCE (PLI)

Although there is a lack of consensus regarding whether an APRN should hold their own professional malpractice (liability) insurance policy, (whether employed, self-employed in independent practice, or in training), it is imperative that the practitioner take a pragmatic approach when reviewing the literature on the pros and cons. Most professional liability insurance policies cover the costs of a defense attorney and any settlement or judgment against the nurse, up to the policy limits. Depending on the policy, disciplinary, licensing and termination proceedings may also be covered. In certain instances malpractice coverage may be denied. Should the APRN decide to forgo a policy and rely solely on the employers insurance, it is important to remember that should a settlement or judgment against the nurse occur, the employer could seek to recover monies spent in defending the nurse (sue the nurse). Additionally, if the judgment exceeds that of the policy limits of the employer, the nurse may be legally obligated to pay the rest. This payment may be recovered from the APRN's personal savings, belongings or future earnings. Typically the employer will also be named as a defendant by mere virtue of the employer/employee relationship. Under the legal theory known as "vicarious liability", employers are customarily liable for the negligence of their employees if the employee

---

Box 9.3 - What to do if you are sued

1. **RESPOND IMMEDIATELY.** In most jurisdictions failure to do so within 20-30 days could result in a judgment against you (you lose right at the starting gate);
2. If have you have insurance from your workplace contact the risk management-legal department. They will initiate the response and advise you accordingly.
3. If you have your own insurance, **READ THE POLICY.** It will provide you with specific instructions on what to do, usually asked to forward the complaint. Do so certified mail. The insurance company will notify you after reviewing the complaint.
4. If you are uninsured, contact your state nurses association, the American Association of Nurse Attorney's (TAANA), or a local bar association to furnish you with an attorney that could help. Make sure the attorney has experience in these matters.
5. **DO NOT** under any circumstances, unless directed by your attorney, disclose any information about the case to anyone.
6. Some nurses choose to hire their own attorney regardless of whether they have insurance or otherwise. It is up to you.

Box 9.4 - Resource links

There is a plethora of published up to date information on how to evaluate risk exposure in practice and how to's on how to avoid them.

- **NSO, 2018 provides a Risk Control Self-assessment Checklist which can be accessed by placing the link in your browser:**
  https://docplayer.net/4872421-Cna-and-nso-risk-control-self-assessment-checklist-for-nurse-practitioners-1-self-assessment-topic-yes-no-actions-needed-to-reduce-risks.html:

Carolyn Buppert a nurse attorney and former nurse practitioner provides a nice overview regarding malpractice insurance in a YouTube video entitled

- **"Malpractice insurance for nurse practitioners: Claims made or occurrence"**, which can be accessed by placing the link in your browser and clicking on the following link:
  https://youtu.be/jL1FLrq2SGY.:

---

was acting within the scope of their employment when the negligent act or omission occurred. While an array of elements must be met, the court will examine the nature of the employer/employee relationship and how much control the employer had over the employees practice and performance. Should there be a failure on the part of the employee to follow procedures as dictated by policies of the facility, the facility may choose to sue the employee directly.

9.8.1. Case Three: Vicarious Liability

The APRN is an employee of a hospital working for the pain team. He visits a patient with end-stage metastatic pancreatic cancer in excruciating pain, who despite all efforts to date has had no relief. He decides to place an epidural catheter with the appropriate concentrations of fentanyl and bupivacaine. The hospital policy requires he be supervised, yet, despite the lack of supervision at this time, he decides to proceed. Fifteen minutes following a skillful insertion of the catheter, and careful post procedure monitoring by the nursing staff, the patient respiratory arrests and dies.

1. Is the APRN liable for professional negligence (malpractice)?
2. Does his actions rise to the level of a crime?
3. What defense can be raised in support of his actions?
4. Is the hospital liable?
5. What defense can be raised on their behalf?

9.9. CONTEMPORARY PRACTICE ISSUES

9.9.1. Practice Barriers

There is a growing shortage of medical providers often resulting in the inability of seniors and people in rural and underserved communities to access care. Ample research suggests that care delivered by APRNs, compared to care delivered by doctors, generates similar or better health outcomes for a broad range of patient conditions (Laurant, et al., 2018). Despite the shortage and evidence of high quality care, APRN's continue to be barred from practicing to full extent of their education and skill set (NCSBN, 2018). These barriers result in part from state practice acts, institutional rules, federal statutes and regulations from the Centers for Medicare and Medicaid Services (CMS) and political lobbies (American Medical Association (AMA), placing restrictions on how APRN's practice and how they will be paid for their services (Fauteux, Brand, Fink, Frelick & Werrlein, 2017).

Across the country these barriers include but are not limited to:

- State collaborative agreement and supervision mandates;
- Refusal of some hospitals to grant privileges;
- Restrictions on APRNs' authority to prescribe medications (DEA obstacles) and medical equipment;
- Reduced reimbursement from some private payers;
- Lack of access to affordable professional malpractice or liability insurance;
- Centers for Medicare & Medicaid Services (CMS) rules limiting services APRNs may provide in skilled nursing facilities;
- CMS billing eligibility and reimbursement requirements;
- Failure to recognize the CNS as an APRN ((Fauteux, Brand, Fink, Frelick & Werrlein, 2017);
- Inability to move fluidly across state boundaries (Holding one multi-state license and privileges to practice in other compact state (APRN Compact) (NCSBN, 2015).

In 2008, a collaborative effort between the APRN Consensus Work Group and the National Council of State Boards of Nursing (NCSBN) APRN Advisory Committee began work to break down these barriers by establishing national standards for uniform regulation of APRNs in all states (NCSBN, 2008). From their efforts and input from participating APRN certifiers, accreditors, public regulators, educators and employers, The *APRN Joint Dialogue Group Report* was published from which the The APRN Consensus Model emerged. This model and its 5 foundational recommendations for uniform regulation of APRN licensure, accreditation, certification, and education (collectively known as LACE), set forth as follows.

All nurses wishing to practice as an APRN must:

• Have a graduate education (Masters or doctoral level) from an institution nationally accredited by an organization recognized by the U.S. Department of Education (USDE) and/or the Council for Higher Education Accreditation (CHEA);
• Be licensed and regulated by a state board of nursing;
• Be certified by a national nursing certification body such as the American Nurses Credentialing Center (ANCC) or the American Academy of Nurse Practitioners Certification Board (AANPCB);
• Use the APRN title followed by the specific population foci role the APRN is authorized to practice (CNP, CNS, CRNA, or CNM).

Despite all efforts to date, a uniform model of regulation of APRNs across states has not been actualized. Clearly, the adoption of the APRN Consensus Model recommendations will provide numerous benefits for consumers, employers, current and future practitioners, boards of nursing and legislators (NCSBN, 2018). However, it will require APRN persistence. The Amer ican Association of Nurse Practitioners (AANP) in its 2016 strategic plan identified the following as "high priority" objectives for future APRN practice:

• Removal of practice barriers;
• Eliminate payment disparities;
• Increase the number of states with full practice authority;
• Decrease physician-specific language in statutes, regulation and the healthcare industry;
• Increase general knowledge and public awareness about APRN's;
• Increase political presence and influence on state and federal legislation pertaining to practice (AANP, 2016).

All APRNs have a legal and ethical mandate to stay abreast of current legal and regulatory changes affecting practice and anticipate incorporating continued legal, ethical and regulatory education into their continuing education practice. Becoming active in nursing organizations working to eliminate barriers is essential.

Box 9.6 - Resource links

- **A more comprehensive understanding of the model is available on the NCSBN website:**
  https://www.ncsbn.org/aprn-consensus.htm
- **Consensus model implementation status:**
  https://www.ncsbn.org/5397.htm: NCSBN
- **Published up to date information on the implementa-tion status of the model in each state along with grassroots action initiatives are published by both the NCSBN and the NursingAmerica organization:**
  https://nursingamerica.org/ NursingAmerica: NursingAmerica Campaign for Ac-tion (grassroots initiatives)
- **NCSBN publishes up to date contact information on the state to state status of this legislation:**
  https://www.ncsbn.org/aprn-compact.htm

9.10. THE EMPLOYMENT CONTRACT

The employment contract, is a legally binding agreement between an employer and employee that states the terms of the working relationship and details of employment obligations. In many states, unless there is a written contract, (and sometimes even with a contract depending on the state) employment is considered to be at will, meaning that the employee or the employer can terminate employment without cause at any point in time. Most state laws provide some protection for employees who face termination without contract protection, but accessing this protection may be a lengthy process requiring legal action (Jansen and Blair, 2015). Most employment contracts provide details as to salary, benefits, liability insurance coverage, productivity expectations, job functions, and hours of work (Jansen and Blair, 2015). Some will contain restrictive covenants, (non-compete clause), a clause in the contract that typically restrict the employee from practicing in a certain specialty within a certain number of miles from the employer for a certain period of time. They are designed to protect the employers legitimate business interest and are often legal and enforceable. In addition to the restrictive covenant, most contracts contain a termination clause that describes events that are the basis for termination of the employee "with cause." These events may include but are not limited to, loss of license or certification, professional negligence or criminal behavior.

In some states, the APRN is required to maintain a written practice agreement with a physician. Those that do will ask that the APRN sign a formal agreement which may contain APRN practice details, (what the APRN is permitted and not permitted to do), protocols, standing orders, liability insurance details and grounds for dissolution of the contract. Before signing an employment contract, the APRN should carefully review the contract, negotiate areas of confusion, review their individual state directive and see an attorney. The APRN at signing must make sure the agreement is in adherence to all state laws, allows for optimal practice and is based upon interdisciplinary collaboration.

9.11. SUMMARY

There is no doubt that 270,000 APRN's represent a powerful segment of the health care workforce. Providing primary, acute and specialty care across the lifespan, they are well-suited to continue to play a decisive role in the care of patients and communities. With the inevitability of independence, now is the time to take greater command of all aspects of their practice and continued design of its future.

9.12. REFERENCES

American Association of Nurse Practitioners (AANP) (2016). Strategic Plan. Retrieved from: https://www.aanp.org/

American Nurses Association (ANA) (2018). Definition of The Nurse Practice Act. Retrieved from: https://www.nursingworld.org/practice-policy/scope-of-practice/.

American Nurses Association (ANA) (2015b). Code of Ethics for Nurses: with Interpretive Statements (The Code). Retrieved from: https://www.nursingworld.org/practice-policy/nursing-excellence/ethics/code-of-ethics-for-nurses/.

American Psychological Association (APA) (2016). Ethical Principles of Psychologists and Code of Conduct. Retrieved from: https://www.apa.org/ethics/code/.

Black, I.E. (1979). Negligence. *Legal Med. Q, 3(123).*

Brock, L.V. & Mastroianni, A. (2014). Clinical ethics and law. *Ethics in Medicine Online*. Retrieved from: https://ssrn.com/abstract=2475191.

Brous, E. (2012). Common misconceptions about nursing licensure. *American Journal of Nursing (AJN), 112*(10), 55-59.

Epstein, B. & Turner, M. (2015). The Nursing Code of Ethics: Its value, its history. *The Online Journal of Issues in Nursing, 20*(2).

Fauteux, N., Brand, R., Fink, J.L.W., Frelick, M. & Werrlein, D. (2017). Charting nursing's future. Robert Wood Johnson Foundation. Retrieved from: https://www.rwjf.org/en/library/research/2017/03/the-case-for-removing-barriers-to-aprn-practice.html.

Institute of Medicine (IOM) (2010). The Future of Nursing: Leading Change, Advancing Health. Retrieved from: https://www.nursingworld.org/practice-policy/iom-future-of-nursing-report/.

Institute of Medicine (IOM) (2015). Assessing Progress on the IOM Report The Future of Nursing Retrieved from: http://iom.nationalacademies.org/Reports/2015/Assessing-Progress-on-the-IOM-Report-The-Future-of-Nursing.aspx.

Jansen, M. & Blair, K.A. (2015). Advanced Practice Nursing, Fifth Edition: Core Concepts for Professional Role Development. New York: Springer Publishing Company, LLC.

Joel, L. (2013). *Advanced practice nursing: Essentials for role development.* (3rd edition). Philadelphia, PA.: F.A. Davis Company.

Kleinpell, R., Scanlon, A., Hibbert, D., Ganz, F., East, L., Fraser, D., Wong, F., Beauchesne, M. (2014). Addressing issues impacting advanced nursing practice worldwide. *The Online Journal of Issues in Nursing, 19*(2).

Laurant, M., van der Biezen, M., Wijers, N. Watananirun, K., Kontopantelis, E. & van Vught, A.JAH. (2018). Nurses as substitutes for doctors in primary care. *Cochrane Database of Systematic Reviews, 7*(3), 1-121.

Legal Information Institute (LII) (2018). Definition of statute. Retrieved from: https://www.law.cornell.edu/.

National Council of State Boards of Nursing (NCSBN) (2018). APRN Joint Dialogue Group Report. Retrieved from: https://www.ncsbn.org/Consensus_Model_for_APRN_Regulation_July_2008.pdf.

National Council of State Boards of Nursing (NCSBN) (2018). APRN campaign for consensus: Moving toward uniformity in state laws. Retrieved from: https://www.ncsbn.org/campaign-for-consensus.htm.

National Council of State Boards of Nursing (NCSBN) (2017). About U.S. Boards of Nursing. Retrieved from: https://www.ncsbn.org/about-boards-of-nursing.htm.

National Council of State Boards of Nursing (NCSBN) (2015). APRN Compact. Retrieved from: https://www.ncsbn.org/aprn-compact.htm

National Council of State Boards of Nursing (NCSBN) (2009). Changes in healthcare professions' scope of practice:Legislative considerations. Retrieved from: https://www.ncsbn.org/ScopeofPractice_09.pdf.

National practitioner databank (NPDB) (2016). NPDB research statistics. Retrieved from: https://www.npdb.hrsa.gov/resources/npdbstats/npdbStatistics.jsp#contentTop.

Nursing America (2018). Campaign for Action. Retrieved from: https://nursingamerica.org/

Nurses Service Organization (NSO) (2017). Nurse Practitioner Claim Report: 4th Edition Executive Summary. Retrieved from: https://www.nso.com/.

Nursing Service Association (NSO), (2018). Risk Control Self-assessment Checklist. Retrieved from:https://docplayer.net/4872421-Cna-and-nso-risk-control-self-assessment-checklist-for-nurse-practitioners-1-self-assessment-topic-yes-no-actions-needed-to-reduce-risks.html.

Ornstein, C. & Waldman, A. (2015). How to investigate nurses. ProPublica. Retrieved from: https://projects.propublica.org/graphics/investigating-nurses.

Peterson, F.J. (2018). Legal consequences of unethical behavior. Retrieved from: https://www.mcrazlaw.com/legal-consequences-of-unethical-behavior/.

Phillips, S.J. (2018). Improving access to healthcare one state at a time: 30th annual legislative update. Retrieved from: https://ruralprep.org/wp-content/uploads/2018/02/30th-APRN-Legislative-Update.pdf.

Poghosyan, L., Liu, J. & Norful, A.A. (2017). Nurse practitioners as primary care providers with their own patient panels and organizational structures: A cross-sectional study. *International Journal of Nursing Studies 74*, 1–7.

Registered nursing.org (2019). How Nurses Can Avoid the Most Common Ethics Violations. Retrieved from: https://www.registerednursing.org/how-avoid-common-ethics-violations/.

Russell, K.A. (2012). Nurse practice acts guide and govern nursing practice. *Journal of Nursing Regulation, 3*(3), 36-42.

Scala, E. (2018). Top Professional Organizations for Nurse Practitioners. BLOG Retrieved from: https://onlinenursepractitionerprograms.com/professional-organizations/.

Sohn, D. (2013). Negligence, genuine error, and litigation. *Int J Gen Med,* (6), 49–56.

Starr, K.T. (2018). You've been served: Responding to a malpractice summons. *Nursing 2018, 48*(8), 11-12

Stokes, F. (2016). Use of Code of Ethics and The Nurse Practice Act. Retrieved from: https://www.ncsbn.org/2016IRE_FStokes.pdf.

Zhong, E., McCarthy, H., Carey, A. (2016). A review of criminal convictions among nurses 2012-2013. *Journal of Nursing Regulation, 7*(1), 27-33.

9.13. APPENDIX: 2019 NURSE PRACTITIONER STATE PRACTICE ENVIRONMENT

The American Association of Nurse Practitioners (AANP) broadly defines three scope-of-practice statuses nationwide. Limits and restrictions on specific elements of practice may be lifted in certain states and circumstances while other states have no law. Additional practice requirements may include: continuing education, a specific number of practice hours, a collaborating physician practice protocol and/or specific patient population.

The three scope-of-practice statuses are as follows:

- **Full practice:** "State practice and licensure law fully provides for all nurse practitioners to evaluate patients, diagnose, order and interpret diagnostic tests, initiate and manage treatments and prescribe medication under the exclusive licensure authority of the state Board of Nursing".
  Alaska, Arizona, Connecticut, Colorado, District of Columbia, Hawaii, Idaho, Iowa, Maine, Maryland, Minnesota, Montana, Nebraska, Nevada, New Hampshire, New Mexico, North Dakota, Oregon, Rhode Island, South Dakota,Vermont, Washington and Wyoming.
- **Reduced practice:** "State practice and licensure law reduces the ability of nurse practitioners to engage in at least one element of NP practice. State law requires a regulated collaborative agreement with an outside health discipline in order for the NP to provide patient care or limits the setting or scope of one or more elements of NP practice."
  Alabama, Arkansas, Delaware, Illinois, Indiana, Kansas, Kentucky, Louisiana, Mississippi, New Jersey, New York, Ohio, Pennsylvania, Utah, West Virginia, Wisconsin

- **Restricted practice:** "State practice and licensure law restricts the ability of a nurse practitioner to engage in at least one element of NP practice. State requires supervision, delegation, or team-management by an outside health discipline in order for the NP to provide patient care."
  California, Florida, Georgia, Massachusetts, Michigan, South Carolina, Texas, Tennessee, Missouri, North Carolina, Oklahoma, Virginia

Under the exclusive authority of a state's Board of Nursing or regulatory authority the following chart sets out the current state by state dictate of the APRN's practice independence. It is not meant to be all inclusive. Specific details regarding individual state practice latitude can be found by referencing the statute. (Table 9.1., pages 341-355)

TABLE 9.1.

State	Primary Care provider status	Write admitting orders	Assess, diagnose, develop and implement treatment plans	Make referrals	Prescribe Schedules II-V drugs	Sign polst, post, molst, most/colst forms	Sign death certificates	Statutory or legislative authority references
Alabama	Yes	Yes with collaborative agreement	Yes with collaborative agreement	Yes with collaborative agreement	Yes with a physician protocol and special permit	No law	No law	Ala. Code §A34-21 et.seq. and Ala. Admin. Code r. 610-X-6 et. seq.
Alaska	Yes	Yes	Yes	Yes	Yes	Yes	Yes	A.S. 08.68 seq. and 12 ACC 44 et. seq.
Arkansas	No law	No law	Yes with collaborative agreement	Yes with collaborative agreement	May not	May not	Yes	A.C.A. 17-87 et. seq.
Arizona	Yes	Yes	Yes	Yes	Yes	Yes	No law	A.R.S. § R4- 19 et seq.

(continued)

TABLE 9.1. *(continued)*

State	Primary Care provider status	Write admitting orders	Assess, diagnose, develop and implement treatment plans	Make referrals	Prescribe Schedules II-V drugs	Sign polst, post, molst, most/colst forms	Sign death certificates	Statutory or legislative authority references
California	Yes	Yes with collaborative agreement	Yes with collaborative agreement	Yes with collaborative agreement	Yes with physician oversight	Yes with collaborative agreement	May not	Cal. Com Code § Cal. Code Reg. tit. 16 § 1485; Cal. BPC. Code § 2834-2837 et. Seq.
Colorado	Yes	Yes	Yes	Yes	Yes, with "prescribing mentorship" by physician	Yes	May not	Colo. Rev. Stat. Ann. § 12-38 et Seq.
Connecticut	Yes	Yes	Yes	Yes	Yes with collaborative agreement	Yes	Yes	Conn. Gen. Stat. Ann. 378-20-87a to378-20-102a et. seq.

(continued)

TABLE 9.1. (continued)

State	Primary Care provider status	Write admitting orders	Assess, diagnose, develop and implement treatment plans	Make referrals	Prescribe Schedules II-V drugs	Sign polst, post, molst, most/colst forms	Sign death certificates	Statutory or legislative authority references
Delaware	Yes	Yes with collaborative agreement	Yes with collaborative agreement	Yes with collaborative agreement	Yes with collaborative agreement	Yes with collaborative agreement	Yes with collaborative agreement	Del. Cod. Ann. Tit. 24 1900 et. seq.
District of	Yes	Yes	Yes	Yes	Yes	No law	May not	D.C. Code § 3-12 et.seq.
Florida	Yes	Yes with collaborative agreement	Yes with collaborative agreement	Yes	May not	No law	May not	Fla. Stat. Tit. XXXII Ch. 464 et. seq.
Georgia	No law	Yes with collaborative agreement	Yes with collaborative agreement	No law	May not	Yes in some circumstances	Yes with collaborative agreement	GA. Code Ann § 43-26 et. Seq. GA Comp R & Regs. R. 410-12 et. seq.

(continued)

TABLE 9.1. (continued)

State	Primary Care provider status	Write admitting orders	Assess, diagnose, develop and implement treatment plans	Make referrals	Prescribe Schedules II-V drugs	Sign polst, post, molst, most/colst forms	Sign death certificates	Statutory or legislative authority references
Hawaii	Yes	Yes	Yes	Yes	Yes	Yes	May not	Haw. Rev. Stat. § 457 et. seq. Haw. Admin. Rules § 16-89 et. seq.
Idaho	Yes	Yes	Yes	Yes	Yes	Yes	Yes	Idaho Code Ann. § 54-14 et. seq., Idaho Admin. Code § 23.01.01:280
Illinois seq. Ill. Code	Yes	Yes with collaborative agreement	Yes with collaborative agreement	Yes	Yes with collaborative agreement	Yes	May not	225 Ill. Comp. Stat. § 65/15-5 et. Admin. tit. 68, pt. 1300, sub-pt. D et. seq.

(continued)

TABLE 9.1. (continued)

State	Primary Care provider status	Write admitting orders	Assess, diagnose, develop and implement treatment plans	Make referrals	Prescribe Schedules II-V drugs	Sign polst, post, molst, most/colst forms	Sign death certificates	Statutory or legislative authority references
Indiana	No law	Yes with collaborative agreement	Yes with collaborative agreement	Yes	Yes with collaborative agreement	May not	May not	Ind. Code § 25-23 et. seq.; Ind. Admin. Code. Tit. 848., r. 4-5 et. seq.
Iowa	Yes	Yes	Yes	Yes	Yes	Yes	Yes	IA. Admin. Code r. 655.7 et. seq.
Kansas	No law	Yes with collaborative agreement	Yes with collaborative agreement	Yes	Yes with written physician protocol agreement	No law	May not	Kan. Stat. Ann § 65.1130-1134 Kan. Admin. Regs. §60-11-101 – 60-11-121

(continued)

TABLE 9.1. (continued)

State	Primary Care provider status	Write admitting orders	Assess, diagnose, develop and implement treatment plans	Make referrals	Prescribe Schedules II-V drugs	Sign polst, post, molst, most/colst forms	Sign death certificates	Statutory or legislative authority references
Kentucky	Yes	Yes	Yes with collaborative agreement	No law	Yes with a written collaborative agreement w/ supervising physician or other healthcare provider	May not	Yes	KY. Rev. Stat. Ann. § 314 et.seq.; 201 Ky. Admin. Regs. § 20:057 et. seq.
Louisiana	No law	No law	Yes	Yes	Yes with collaborative agreement	No	No	LA. Rev. Stat. 37L911 et. seq.; La. Admin. Code. Tit. 46, § XLVII et. seq.

(continued)

TABLE 9.1. (continued)

State	Primary Care provider status	Write admitting orders	Assess, diagnose, develop and implement treatment plans	Make referrals	Prescribe Schedules II-V drugs	Sign polst, post, molst, most/colst forms	Sign death certificates	Statutory or legislative authority references
Maine	Yes	Yes	Yes	Yes	Yes	Yes	Yes	ME. Rev. Stat Ann tit. 32 § 2101 et. seq., Code Me. R. 8 02 380 § 8 et. seq.
Maryland	Yes	Yes	Yes	Yes	Yes	Yes	Yes	COMAR 10.27 et. seq.
Massachusetts	Yes	Yes	Yes	Yes	Yes with written collaborative agreement w/ physician	Yes	Yes	244 Code Mass. Rules § 4.00 et. seq.

(continued)

TABLE 9.1. (continued)

State	Primary Care provider status	Write admitting orders	Assess, diagnose, develop and implement treatment plans	Make referrals	Prescribe Schedules II-V drugs	Sign polst, post, molst, most/colst forms	Sign death certificates	Statutory or legislative authority references
Michigan	No law	Yes	Yes	Yes	Yes with physician oversight	Yes	No	There is no statutory or regulatory nurse practitioner scope of practice There is no nurse PracticeAct. All rules promulgated by Board of Nursing or embedded in Public Health Code Act 368, Part 172 et. seq. Doctors may delegate authority to practice (including to prescribe) at their discretion Mich. Comp. Laws §333.16215(1).

(continued)

TABLE 9.1. *(continued)*

State	Primary Care provider status	Write admitting orders	Assess, diagnose, develop and implement treatment plans	Make referrals	Prescribe Schedules II-V drugs	Sign polst, post, molst, most/colst forms	Sign death certificates	Statutory or legislative authority references
Minnesota	Yes	Yes	Yes	Yes	Yes	Yes	Yes	Minn. Stat. Ann. § 148.171 et. seq.
Mississippi	No law	No law	Yes	Yes	Yes	May not	May not	Miss. Code Ann. § 73-15-17-20; Miss. Admin. Code. Tit. 30 § 2840
Missouri	No law	No law	Yes	Yes	May not	No law	May not	Mo. Ann. Stat. § 335 et. seq.; Mo. Code. Regs. tit. 20 § 2200 et. seq.
Montana	Yes	Yes	Yes	Yes	Yes	Yes	Yes	Mont. Code Ann. § 2-15-1734 et. seq.; Mont. Ad min R. Mont. 24.159.1401 et. seq.

(continued)

TABLE 9.1. (continued)

State	Primary Care provider status	Write admitting orders	Assess, diagnose, develop and implement treatment plans	Make referrals	Prescribe Schedules II-V drugs	Sign polst, post, molst, most/colst forms	Sign death certificates	Statutory or legislative authority references
Nebraska	No law	Yes	Yes	Yes	Yes	No law	Yes	Neb. Rev. Stat. § 38-2301 et. seq.; 172 NAC 100 et. seq.
Nevada	No law	Yes	Yes	Yes	Yes	Yes	May not	Nev. Admin. Code § 632 et. seq.
New Hampshire	Yes	Yes	Yes	Yes	Yes	Yes	Yes	N.H. Rev. Stat. Ann. § 326-B:1 et seq.
New Jersey	Yes	Yes	Yes	Yes	Yes with written collaborative agreement	Yes	Yes	N.J. S.A. § 45:1 et seq.; N.J.A.C. 13:37.
New Mexico	Yes	Yes	Yes	Yes	Yes	Yes	Yes	N.M. Stat. Ann. § 61.3 et. seq.

(continued)

TABLE 9.1. (continued)

State	Primary Care provider status	Write admitting orders	Assess, diagnose, develop and implement treatment plans	Make referrals	Prescribe Schedules II-V drugs	Sign polst, post, molst, most/colst forms	Sign death certificates	Statutory or legislative authority references
New York	Yes	Yes	Yes	Yes	Yes written collaborative agreement	May not	Yes in certain situations	N.Y. Educ. Law, Art. 139 §6900 et. seq.
North Carolina	No law	Yes	Yes	Yes	Yes written collaborative agreement	Yes	Yes	21 N.C.G.S. § 90-171.19 et. seq.; N.C.A.C. 36.0101 et seq.
North Dakota	Yes	Yes	Yes	Yes	Yes	Yes	Yes	N.D. Cent. Code § 43-12-1-01et. seq.; N.D. Admin. Code § 54-05-03.1
Ohio	Yes	Yes	Yes	Yes	Yes with collaborative agreement	No law	May not	Ohio Re. Code Ann. § 4723.01 et seq.

(continued)

TABLE 9.1. (continued)

State	Primary Care provider status	Write admitting orders	Assess, diagnose, develop and implement treatment plans	Make referrals	Prescribe Schedules II-V drugs	Sign polst, post, molst, most/colst forms	Sign death certificates	Statutory or legislative authority references
Oklahoma	Yes	Yes	Yes	Yes	Yes with collaborative agreement	May not	May not	59 O.S. § 567.1 et. seq.; Okla. Admin. Code § 485: 10-15-1 et.seq.
Oregon	Yes	Yes	Yes	Yes	Yes	Yes	Yes	O.R.S. § 851-050-63 et seq
Pennsylvania	Yes	Yes	Yes	Yes	Yes with collaborative agreement	Yes	Yes	49 PA Code § 21.251 et. seq.; 49 PA Code 21.801 et. seq.
Rhode Island	Yes	Yes	Yes	Yes	Yes	Yes	Yes	R.I. Gen. Laws § 5-34, R.I.R. R5-34-Nur/Ed
South Carolina	No law	No law	Yes	No law	Yes written protocol/ collaborative agreement	May not	May not	S.C. Code Ann. § 40-33-5 et. seq.

(continued)

TABLE 9.1. (continued)

State	Primary Care provider status	Write admitting orders	Assess, diagnose, develop and implement treatment plans	Make referrals	Prescribe Schedules II-V drugs	Sign polst, post, molst, most/colst forms	Sign death certificates	Statutory or legislative authority references
South Dakota	Yes	Yes	Yes	Yes	Yes with collaborative agreement	No law	Yes	S.D. Codified Laws § 36-9A et. seq.
Tennessee	Yes	Yes	Yes	Yes	Yes physician supervision	Yes	May not	T.C.A. § 63-7 et. seq.
Texas	Yes	Yes	Yes	Yes	May not	Yes	May not	Texas Admin. Code § 221.1-17 et. seq.; TOC § 301 et. seq.
Utah	No law	Yes with collaborative agreement	Yes with collaborative agreement	Yes with collaborative agreement	Yes with collaborative agreement	Yes with collaborative agreement	Yes with collaborative agreement	Utah Code. Ann. § 58-31b-101 et seq, Utah Adm. Code r. 156 et. seq.

(continued)

TABLE 9.1. *(continued)*

State	Primary Care provider status	Write admitting orders	Assess, diagnose, develop and implement treatment plans	Make referrals	Prescribe Schedules II-V drugs	Sign polst, post, molst, most/colst forms	Sign death certificates	Statutory or legislative authority references
Vermont	No law	Yes	Yes	Yrs	Yes	Yers	Yes	Vt. Stat. Ann.Tit. 26 § 1572(4); Vt. Code R. Ch. 4 Subchapter 8, 111
Virginia	No law	Yes	Yes	Yes	Yes as part of a patient team (With physician members)	Yes	Yes	Code of Virginia Ch. 29 § 54. 1-2900-§ 54.1-2957.03.; 18 Va. Admin Code § 90-30-120A
Washington	Yes	Yes	Yes	Yes	Yes	Yes	Yes	Wash. Rev. Code§ 18.79.250, Wash Admin Code § 246.840-300.

(continued)

TABLE 9.1. (continued)

State	Primary Care provider status	Write admitting orders	Assess, diagnose, develop and implement treatment plans	Make referrals	Prescribe Schedules II-V drugs	Sign polst, post, molst, most/colst forms	Sign death certificates	Statutory or legislative authority references
West Virginia	Yes	Yes	Yes	Yes	May not	Yes	Yes	W. Va. Code § 30-7-15 et. seq.
Wisconsin	No law	Yes	Yes	Yes	Yes with collaborative agreement	No law	May not	Wis. Admin Code § N8
Wyoming	Yes	Yes	Yes	Yes	Yes	Yes	Yes	Wyo. Stat. Ann. § 33-21-120(a)(i).

Index

vulnerable populations, 52, 61, 143ff.,
178 (*see also* Belmont Report,
Common Rule)
and research, 58
care of, 143ff.
conceptual model, 108, 147
international, 84ff.
mentally ill, 185

whistleblowers, 282, 290–291
Willowbrook State School, 47, 85, 195
withholding and withdrawing care/treat-
ment, 31–32, 34, 131
Wilson, D.S., 3
women as research subjects, 62 (*see also*
pregnancy)
World Health Organization (WHO), 154,
263
World Medical Association Declaration
of Ethical Considerations Regarding
Health Databases and Biobanks, 79
whole-body scan, 312
whole exome sequencing, 238
whole-genome sequencing, 75, 238
and privacy, 77ff.
withdrawing life support,
infants and children, 245
principles of, 32